Strategies for Teaching At-Risk and Handicapped Infants and Toddlers: A Transdisciplinary Approach

SHARON A. RAVER

Old Dominion University

Merrill, an imprint of
Macmillan Publishing Company
New York

Collier Macmillan Canada, Inc.
Toronto

Maxwell Macmillan International Publishing Group
New York   Oxford   Singapore   Sydney

Cover photo: Victor Paul, Media Resource Center, Meyer Rehabilitation Institute. A University Affiliated Program, University of Nebraska Medical Center.

Editor: Ann Castel
Production Editor: Jonathan Lawrence
Art Coordinator: Ruth A. Kimpel
Photo Editor: Gail Meese
Cover Designer: Robert Vega
Production Buyer: Pamela D. Bennett

This book was set in Garamond.

Photo credits: pp. 14, 34, 91, 173, 285, 350, 374 by Jorge Chazo; p. 155 Courtesy Children's Hospital of the King's Daughters, Norfolk, Virginia; and pp. 66, 250 Courtesy Photographic Services of Auburn University.

Macmillan Publishing Company
866 Third Avenue, New York, NY 10022

Collier Macmillan Canada, Inc.

Library of Congress Cataloging-in-Publication Data
Raver, Sharon A.
    Strategies for teaching at-risk and handicapped infants and toddlers: a transdisciplinary approach / Sharon A. Raver.
        p.   cm.
    Includes bibliographical references and index.
    ISBN 0–675–21202–2
    1. Infants—Diseases—Treatment.   2. Children—Diseases—Treatment.   3. Infants—Development.   4. Handicapped children—Development.   5. Handicapped children—Family relationships.
    I. Title.
    RJ135.R38   1991
    362.1'9892—dc20
                                                                                    90–46743
                                                                                    CIP

Printing: 1   2   3   4   5   6   7   8   9   Year: 1   2   3   4

To Greg and Emily

Preface

Strategies for Teaching At-Risk and Handicapped Infants and Toddlers: A Transdisciplinary Approach has been written to assist interventionists and families in developing state-of-the-art practices for producing optimal developmental growth in children younger than age 3. The material is designed to comprehensively cover procedures that link theory and research to form best practices in serving infants, toddlers, and their families. Although each child and family is unique, some strategies have proven to be more effective than others. This book brings those practical strategies together under one cover.

The book is organized around the transdisciplinary approach to early intervention services. Consequently, the contributors were selected because of their discipline expertise as well as their direct experience with at-risk and handicapped infants, toddlers, and their families. A goal of this book is to translate discipline-specific techniques and jargon for interventionists so that integrated, comprehensive, and meaningful services are more accessible.

The family-centered approach to early intervention has shaped this book's organization. The child is seen as inextricably connected to the family. Consequently, efforts to assist the child's development must simultaneously address the characteristics and needs of the child's family. The book is divided into five parts. Part I presents historical and introductory information on infant intervention in the last 3 decades. Part II presents specific techniques for stimulating the development of children with different exceptionalities and needs. Part III offers procedures for medical-oriented settings. Intervention strategies for specific populations, and techniques for low-incidence and specialized disabilities such as sensory impairments, are found in Part IV. Part V addresses issues and skills pertinent to working with families, such as communication strategies and writing Individualized Family Service Plans (IFSPs).

Appreciation is extended to the families who allowed their stories to be told in the case studies. Although the information is theirs, names have been changed to protect their identities. Further appreciation is extended to the professionals who allowed their candid comments to be shared. As they requested, their identities are protected, also.

I would like to thank my colleagues in the Child Study/Special Education Department of Old Dominion University for their personal support. Sincere appreciation is extended to the reviewers who guided the completion of this text: David W. Anderson, Lock Haven University of Pennsylvania; Nancy K. Klein, Cleveland State University; Carol J. Sears, George Mason University; Ramona E. Patterson, McNeese State University; M. Diane Klein, California State University, Los Angeles; Helmi C. Owens, Pacific Lutheran University; David M. Finn, University of Alabama at Birmingham; and James S. McCrory, Mary Baldwin College. Thanks go to the copyeditor, Janet Brown McCracken, for her work on the manuscript. A final acknowledgment must be given to all the infants and their families who have enriched my life. This book is the product of what they have taught, and continue to teach, me.

S. A. R.

Contents in Brief

Contents

PART I

FOUNDATIONS OF INFANT AND TODDLER INTERVENTION

1

Trends Affecting Infant and Toddler Services

Sharon A. Raver

OVERVIEW

This chapter discusses the development of services for at-risk infants and toddlers and those with disabilities, including:

- □ the principal objectives of intervention
- □ trends in intervention
- □ results of intervention research with at-risk and handicapped infants and toddlers
- □ legislative cornerstones in the evolution of services for very young children and their families
- □ major competencies needed by infant and toddler interventionists

Most professionals involved with very early intervention enthusiastically report that their efforts offer opportunities to prevent, reduce, or avoid deficits in children at risk for developmental problems. They indicate that this intervention also permits opportunities to reduce stress in families and prevent or reduce family dysfunction. Despite such strong endorsements, services for children younger than 3 have been the exception, not the rule. After nearly 3 decades of effort, a portion of Public Law (P.L.) 99–457 (The Infant/Toddler Program, Part H), passed in 1986, calls for the establishment of statewide services beginning at birth for all handicapped children and their families. Because of this legislation, many now hope that services eventually will be available to every child and every family who desire them (Garwood & Sheehan, 1989).

The authors of P.L. 99–457, Part H, wrote the legislation so individual states could maintain control of the type of services they provide as well as define which children and families are eligible for services (Ballard, Ramirez, & Zantal-Wiener, 1987). These new responsibilities have prompted policymakers and professionals to closely examine the objectives of existing very early intervention services and objectives for new statewide service delivery systems.

OBJECTIVES OF INTERVENTION

Infant intervention is a term used to describe any service, or cluster of services, made available to at-risk and handicapped children and their families at any time from the child's birth to the time of the child's third birthday. The time from birth to 12 months tends to be described as the infancy period and 13 to 35 months is usually considered the toddler period. Typically, infant and toddler service delivery systems are managed differently than preschool service options. **Preschool intervention** is a term used to describe services provided for at-risk and handicapped children between 3 and 5 years of age. When infant and preschool services are discussed together the term **early intervention** is frequently used. Recent research in child development, adult-child relationships, and family dynamics is shaping the way professionals now view intervention efforts and services systems provided in the first 3 years of life.

At present, there is little uniformity in infant services among states. In fact, services within the same state may have different components as well as different objectives. Despite the broad range of service options for at-risk and special needs infants, most services are grounded in four major premises of infant development.

First, the initial years of life are viewed as critical to subsequent development and behavior (Bricker, 1986; Piaget, 1952). During the first 3 years, the foundations of all higher-functioning skills—communication, thinking, social relationships—are developed. The parent-child bond, one of the most significant and lasting attachments, is secured during this developmental period. Further, the complex, dynamic transaction between innate temperament and the environment begins to be played out.

Second, infants and toddlers are recognized as active learners, influencing their environment, as well as being influenced by their environment (Lamb, Garn, & Keating, 1981; Yarrow, Rubenstein, & Pedersen, 1975). The notion of the passive infant is no longer accepted. Early intervention services tend to increase the child's participation in all experiences.

Third, most of these services are anchored in the understanding that intervention is best when it is begun as soon as possible. Research confirms that initiating intervention during infancy with at-risk and disabled children can ameliorate some developmental problems (Guralnick & Bennett, 1987).

Finally, most services geared toward infants and toddlers accept that development during this period is influenced by family life, culture, and other external circumstances (Bendell, Culbertson, Shelton, & Carter, 1986; Clarke & Clarke, 1976; Field, Goldberg, Stern, & Sostek, 1980). Any of the conditions facing contemporary families, such as single-parent homes, decreased family size, working parents, and multiple caretakers, may dramatically affect a child's passage through infancy. Children who are at risk and those with special needs may contend with these circumstances in addition to other problems and stresses associated with their condition. Although other premises of child and family development are certainly acknowledged, these four premises tend to be most reliably reflected in best practices with very young children.

Drawing from these premises, most very early intervention services for at-risk and/or special needs children tend to have one or more of these principal objectives:

☐ to provide information, support, and assistance to families dealing with the needs associated with the infant or toddler who is at risk for delayed development, or the one who is identified as having developmental delays
☐ to build parental confidence as the primary facilitator of their child's development and principal advocate for their child
☐ to foster effective interactions between parent, family, and child that promote mutual feelings of competence and enjoyment

Infant and toddler services are founded on the assumption that they will, in some way, improve the developmental functioning of the child and the well-being and/or functioning of the child's family. The means to accomplish these objectives vary greatly among services and across states.

In addition to a general consensus on the principal objectives of infant intervention, there is agreement about the lack of services for children already identified as needing services. In fact, many policymakers and service providers are overwhelmed by the number of young children who may qualify for services under the Infant/Toddler Program (Part H) of P.L. 99–457.

NUMBER OF CHILDREN NEEDING SERVICES

The number of infants and toddlers who may qualify for services through Part H of P.L. 99–457 is staggering. Considering the many ways young children may be placed at risk in their development (e.g., drug exposure, poverty, inadequate maternal health, congenital conditions) some states are just coming to grips with the number of children they may need to serve. The number of children who may be eligible for services may be inferred from these national statistics:

1. Almost 250,000 babies are born each year weighing less than $5\frac{1}{2}$ pounds, and of these more than 43,000 weigh less than $3\frac{1}{2}$ pounds. Premature, low birth-weight infants are 10 times more likely to be mentally retarded than full-term infants (National Center for Clinical Infant Programs, 1986).
2. 100,000 to 150,000 infants (3 to 5%) are born each year with congenital anomalies that lead to mental retardation (National Center for Clinical Infant Programs, 1986).
3. 4.2% of all children between birth and 5 years of age have poor health (National Center for Clinical Infant Programs, 1986).
4. Adolescent mothers have a higher rate of still births, and mentally retarded, malformed and developmentally delayed infants. The incidence of adolescent mothers continues to increase (National Center for Clinical Infant Programs, 1986).

5. 15% of pregnant mothers report using illegal drugs or alcohol during pregnancy. Some experts fear that the real percentage may be far higher (Greer, 1990).

States are making efforts to identify more precise figures. However, it is evident that the number of children eligible for infant services will increase during the 1990s, especially because some risk categories such as drug exposure are projected to rise. Even before the passage of P.L. 99–457, a shortage of trained professionals to serve the small number of at-risk and handicapped infants and toddlers who received services had been reported (National Center for Clinical Infant Programs, 1985; 1986). In 1986, nearly 90% of the states responding to a national survey reported they lack personnel to adequately serve children with disabilities from birth through age 2 (Weiner & Koppelman, 1987). A similar personnel shortage has been documented in related services of physical, occupational, and speech therapy (Thorp & McCollum, 1988).

P.L. 99–457, Part H, presents policy issues that affect personnel shortages as well as the way in which very early interventionists are trained. The content and standards of training are influenced by certain prominent trends in very early intervention today.

TRENDS IN INFANT AND TODDLER INTERVENTION

The specialization of infant and toddler intervention is undergoing rapid change. Trends related to intervention teaming, prevention, and family-focused intervention and empowerment are shaping the development of intervention policy, service delivery systems, and personnel training.

Intervention Teaming

Historically, there has been much common ground shared by special education and child-related disciplines such as psychology, speech and physical therapy, nursing, child development, and early childhood education. Infant and toddler intervention has traditionally drawn personnel from different disciplines as a means of adjusting to personnel shortages, and as a means of best serving families.

Intervention teaming involves professionals, often from different discipline backgrounds, who work collaboratively to identify and implement services for children and families. Effective teamwork involves systematically teaching skills to team members while learning skills from team members. The degree to which skills are shared depends on the specific team approach adopted by the team. Team approaches to early intervention are discussed in Chapter 2. This type of skill sharing may be helpful for interventionists because many speech and language therapists, occupational therapists, and social workers do not receive specialized training about infants and toddlers when they are trained in their own discipline (Thorp & McCollum, 1988).

Even the field of medicine is beginning to acknowledge the value of learning across disciplines. Pediatric residents at the University of Washington in Seattle, for example, have a 2-month rotation at the University's Child Development and Mental Retardation Center under the direction of a developmental pediatrician. Following this experience, 85% of the pediatricians returning questionnaires indicated that the experience in the cross-disciplinary approach had been beneficial and that their understanding of and empathy for handicapped children increased (Bennett, 1982). The clearly stated multidisciplinary emphasis of P.L. 99–457, Part H, will probably further weaken rigid discipline boundaries.

Prevention

The Infant/Toddler Program of P.L. 99–457, Part H, has created opportunities for states not only to provide quality services to developmentally delayed and disabled children, but also to design and implement more comprehensive prevention efforts. Certain risk factors increase the probability of the need for very early services. For instance, low socioeconomic status (SES) and single parenthood are correlated with higher-than-expected incidences of developmental difficulties in children (Peterson, 1987). Drug use during pregnancy presents significant concern for the child and for the quality of the child's later home environment which may continue to be influenced by drug use (Greer, 1990).

Child development appears to be strongly influenced by the dynamics of family functioning. Intervention directed toward significant areas of family functioning may prevent or reduce developmental deficits (Kochanek, Friedman, Bagnall, & Fazzio, 1988). Services aimed at strengthening families' resources, families' social support networks, and the caregiving environment may reduce some of the deleterious effects observed in infants and toddlers who are at risk for disabilities (Kochanek et al., 1988). Chapter 8 addresses prevention issues in detail.

Family-focused Intervention and Empowerment

The unique dependence of infants and toddlers on their families necessitates a **family-focused approach** to intervention. The family-focused approach involves focusing intervention equally on the child and the child's family. Successful family-focused intervention may require rethinking on the part of interventionists working in the field. These interventionists may have been trained from a traditional model of working with the child, not the family (Karnes & Stayton, 1988).

The family-focused approach is a *process* designed to facilitate and nurture parental confidence and self-assurance by allowing families to make decisions about their lives. Infant and toddler intervention may be the beginning of many years of services for families. Consequently, by allowing families to decide in what way, and to what degree, they wish to participate, they are assisted in building self-advocacy skills, and feel reduced helplessness. A true family-focused approach means that families' expectations and limits are acknowledged and parents are encouraged to be involved as parents, not as professionals (Garland & Linder, 1988).

As a complement to the family-focused orientation to services, some professionals advocate using the term, **early facilitation**, instead of early intervention. Supporters of this terminology suggest that it may more appropriately describe the way

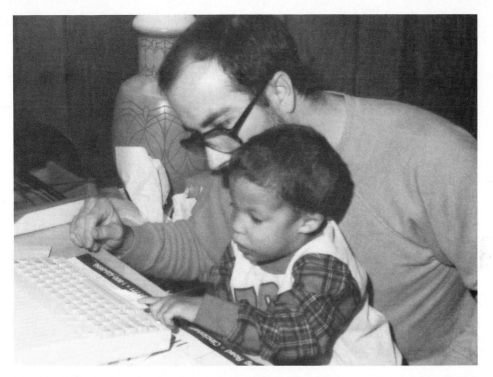

The family-focused approach attempts to facilitate and nurture parental confidence and self-assurance.

in which infant interventionists support the development of infants and their families. The manner in which a family-focused approach will be manifested depends on the unique characteristics of the child and the family, the family's cultural background, and ultimately, the family's wishes.

One father reported his attitudes about the family-focused approach this way: "As I look back on the first 2 years of my son's life, I see that I was a zombie. I did what I was told. I tried to be a good parent to handle the hopelessness I felt. But now, I can't, for the life of me, remember any details of those years. I know they happened. I have pictures from that time, but I was just in shock. I was insane. I wouldn't allow myself—or anyone in my family, either—to discuss how horrible our situation really was. I would have agreed to anything, anyone would have suggested. . . . But now since Rory is 6, I will not let anyone make a decision for me. I am sure I drive them (his teachers) crazy but I have to know why they are doing what they're doing!"

Helping families make decisions about their lives has encouraged the use of another term, family **empowerment**. Empowerment, in general, is the process of assisting families in recognizing and developing their own competence (Dunst, Trivette, & Deal, 1988). Family empowerment has been misunderstood because some professionals believe the term implies that professionals *give* power to parents which, of course, is not the case. To facilitate empowerment, interventionists must find a balance between promoting competence and independence in families, on one hand, and providing needed expertise and emotional support on the other.

These trends have evolved from best practices developed by model infant and toddler services, and form the foundation for recent legislation. As professionals and researchers continue efforts to identify the most effective characteristics of very early intervention services and service delivery options, these trends may change as understanding of these variables increases.

EFFICACY OF INFANT AND TODDLER INTERVENTION

A general frustration surrounds attempts to evaluate the utility, or efficacy, of infant and toddler intervention research. **Efficacy** refers to positive effects or impact of a program, strategy, approach, or procedure on a target population. The frustration with intervention research is related to methodological problems in this body of literature. Common methodological problems involve differences in populations of children, appropriate measures of change, research designs and analyses, and the relationship between dependent and independent variables (Bricker, Bailey, & Bruder, 1984). Because many intervention research analyses are flawed, a definitive statement about the effectiveness of early intervention research is difficult to make (Odom, Yoder, & Hill, 1988; Ottenbacher, 1989).

Nonetheless, despite acknowledged methodological weaknesses in the early intervention literature, the House Report 99–860 (U. S. House of Representatives, 1986) that accompanied P.L. 99–457 cited strong support for the effectiveness of infant and toddler intervention. This report stated that testimony from families and research indicated that very early intervention and preschool services achieve the following:

- help enhance intelligence in some children
- produce substantial gains in physical development, cognitive development, language and speech development, psychosocial development, and self-help skills
- help prevent secondary handicapping conditions
- reduce family stress
- reduce societal dependency and institutionalization
- reduce the need for special class placement in special education programs at school age for some children
- save substantial costs to society and the nation's schools. (pp. 4–5)

Although the prevailing attitude regarding the efficacy of early intervention of service providers and families is very positive, research support varies. This evidence may vary depending on whether the research was conducted primarily with at-risk or handicapped children, or focused on the family.

Research with At-risk Children

The results of research studies with at-risk infants and toddlers tend to be more encouraging than the results reported for those with biological impairments. This appears to be related to the fact that investigations with at-risk children tend to have control groups that provide valid comparisons. Results tend to be more interpretable because standardized measures are used in at least some developmental areas (Bricker et al., 1984). Very young children considered to be at risk in their development do not form a homogeneous group. Although there are a number of ways to categorize at-risk conditions during the first 3 years, most at-risk definitions include these four categories (Smith, 1988b):

Established risk or disability.   These are children with identified conditions or disabilities that can adversely affect development. Cerebral palsy, spina bifida, and Down Syndrome fall into this category. Chapters 8, 9, 10, and 11 discuss children with established risks and/or disabilities.

Developmental delay.   Children with or without an established diagnosis who have fallen significantly behind developmental norms are considered developmentally delayed.

Biological risk.   Children who do not have an identified disability or delay, but who, because of biological circumstances such as low birthweight or prematurity have a higher than normal chance of developmental problems, are viewed as biologically at risk. Chapters 6, 7, and 8 discuss issues pertinent to the biologically at-risk population.

Environmental risk.   Children without identifiable biological risk factors whose development is seen as vulnerable because of environmental conditions are referred to as environmentally at risk. Poverty, drug exposure, alcohol abuse, teenage parents, and mental illness in parents are just a few of the factors associated with a higher than average risk of developmental problems. Chapter 8 discusses issues relating to all at-risk categories.

Naturally, it is possible for children to fall into more than one risk category. For example, a child may have a biological risk such as congenital deafness and also experience environmental risks because the child's mother is drug dependent and unemployed.

The Syracuse University Family Development Research Program is an example of a successful intervention research program targeted toward infants who were primarily at risk due to environmental factors (Lally, Mangione, Honig, & Wittmer, 1988). Ten years after participation in this project, the program group of children from impoverished backgrounds had a 6% rate of juvenile delinquency compared to a 22% rate for children in the control group. Not only was the control group delinquency rate almost four times greater, but the offenses were more severe. The costs to the court and probation departments for handling the cases were estimated at only $12,000 for the children in the program group; the costs for those in the control group were $107,000.

In general, intervention research with at-risk populations seems to reveal positive benefits. Unfortunately, the results of very early intervention studies with children who have severe and/or identified handicaps tend to be more difficult to interpret.

Research with Handicapped Children

Bricker and her colleagues (1984) state that it is not possible to draw conclusions about the efficacy of intervention research with handicapped children due to definition difficulties and the lack of methodological commonalities. The wide range of disabilities and severity found in populations of children identified as handicapped or disabled in intervention research, and the range of interventions and evaluation procedures used in this research literature, make conclusive statements difficult (Ottenbacher, 1989). For example, Simeonsson (1985) analyzed the nature and quality of evidence from 10 early intervention studies. He reports that although causal inferences can be drawn from most studies, methodological problems limit the generalizability of the findings. After an analysis of more than 300 studies, White (1986) concludes that early intervention appears to have positive effects, but good and consistent research, particularly regarding the long-term effects of specific types of intervention, is needed.

Despite these confounding factors, sufficient individual research studies report positive impacts on children's development for the benefits of early intervention to be confidently accepted. As an example, Hanson (1985) reports that children with moderate and severe handicaps experienced positive behavioral changes, and that their parents experienced measured positive changes due to their involvement in infant intervention services. No relationship was found, however, between the amount of child developmental progress and parenting behavior. Similarly, Bagnato and Neisworth (1985) found that interdisciplinary assessment and treatment of infants and preschoolers with congenital and acquired brain injury produced significant gains for both groups.

The majority of policymakers, service providers, and families contend that early intervention is clearly worthwhile. With Part H of P.L. 99–457 in place, this may be the time for early intervention research to move beyond the traditional measurement of short-term effects and move toward the examination of long-term impacts. Toward this end, the efficacy of infant and toddler programs should be judged by positive changes in child development, as well as positive changes in the family's adaptation to life with a child with special needs (Healy, Keesee, & Smith, 1989).

Research with Families

Parent participation during infancy and toddlerhood may have a greater effect on child outcomes than participation during the preschool years, with children who are developmentally vulnerable (Shonkoff, Hauser-Cram, Krauss, & Upshur, 1988). Child skills tend to increase when parents participate in home programs with their developmentally delayed infants (Moxley-Haegert & Serbin, 1983; Safford, Gregg, Schneider, & Sewell, 1976).

Many programs have emphasized the importance of parent involvement in facilitating their child's developmental progress. For example, Allen (1980) reports positive results with the Family Consultation Project, a transdisciplinary, noncategorical early intervention program serving infants with known handicaps or infants at risk due to genetic disorders or severe **perinatal** (occurring during birth) medical complications. This project used arranged interventions that encouraged mutual pleasure in parent-infant interactions and increased parents' sense of competence in affecting their children's development. After 9 months of participation, program families scored higher than control families on measures of maternal responsiveness, comfort in interaction, verbal exchange, and pleasure in contact between parents and infants. Infants in the intervention program improved on developmental assessments; infants in the control group fell further behind.

Basically, intervention services that focus on increasing parent and family competence appear to produce positive effects on children and their families. Family-focused interventions may offer economic incentives for society as well.

Cost-Benefits of Early Intervention

When examining the results of early intervention research efforts, the cost-benefit potential of services must be considered. Infant and toddler services may reduce the need for costly residential or institutional care for some children. Considerable savings in educational costs may be gained when very early intervention increases the likelihood of regular educational placement. For children who need long-term special education services, long-term savings tend to be realized if intervention begins before school age (Bricker et al., 1984). Many consider the economic benefits of early intervention to outweigh, or at least justify, the expenditures for early intervention (Bricker et al., 1984).

The costs of early intervention programs vary significantly. The Early Intervention Research Institute at Utah State University (Smith, 1988b) reports that as of 1988 a one-time per month, home-based program that meets all of the guidelines of P.L. 99–457 can be delivered for as little as $1500 per child per year. A center-based program which provides half-day, 5 days per week of services for infants and toddlers with mild and moderate disabilities costs about $4500 per child per year. The same program for infants and toddlers with severe handicaps costs approximately $12,000 per child per year. Of course, these costs are approximations because the cost of staff, caseloads, facilities, and comprehensiveness of programs vary. However, it is hoped that cost will not be the only consideration used to select program models because it is still unknown which program model is most efficacious or cost-effective for different disabling conditions and different families.

Cost-benefit investigations indicate that for every $1 invested in early intervention services, there is a $3 reduction in long-term, public special education costs (Berrueter-Clement, Schweinhart, Barnett, Epstein, & Weikart, 1984). A follow-up study of 42 children, up to 14 years of age, who had participated in a home-based infant stimulation program indicates the variability of long-range benefits (Widerstrom & Goodwin, 1987). This study found that approximately 66% of the children were in full-time special education programs, 20% were mainstreamed, and 15% were in regular classrooms full time. These results were undoubtedly influenced by the fact that most of the children involved had serious developmental disabilities.

When the positive influences on the child and the child's family and the possibility for long-term cost savings are considered, the utility of infant and toddler services is difficult to deny. This growing understanding has spearheaded federal legislative efforts toward the development, and later the expansion, of services for the youngest exceptional children.

EVOLUTION OF FEDERAL POLICY ON EARLY INTERVENTION

Only 25 years ago, no early intervention policy existed for at-risk and special needs children in the United States. The federal government's commitment to provide quality early intervention services for young at-risk and handicapped children and their families has expanded dramatically since the 1960s. Now the majority of states have legal mandates for services for 3- to 5-year-old children and a number have mandates for children from birth to 3 years (U. S. Department of Education, 1987).

Early intervention services were initially developed for children considered at risk for school and health problems due to socioeconomic conditions. Poverty increases the chances of a number of environmental risk conditions. Some risk factors such as prematurity, for example, are higher in lower-SES environments. In fact, poverty is the statistical factor most predictive of problems in children, in health and in nearly any other aspect of development (Healy et al., 1989). The first early intervention projects were designed to assist in making the unequal circumstances of economically disadvantaged children more equal.

Later, services to prevent, ameliorate, or help compensate for disabilities were introduced in states. The goals of these programs were to assist children with disabilities to overcome or lessen the impact of their disability (Edgar, 1988). Federal policy has furnished strong leadership to states for providing programs for at-risk and handicapped children. Although the early federal initiatives may not have focused on children younger than 3, later federal legislative actions brought attention to this population and increased the chances of mandated services.

Model Programs

Project Head Start was the first national attempt to intervene directly with preschool children with the specific goal of improving their development through a variety of services—educational, medical, nutritional, and parent training. Begun in 1965 to help low-income preschool children realize their potential, Head Start attempts to remedy the damaging effects of poverty through early intervention (Smith, 1988a).

In the early 1970s, Public Laws 92–924 and 93–644 established that 10% of the enrollment in Head Start programs should be filled with handicapped children. These laws make Head Start the largest provider of **mainstreamed** services for preschool handicapped children in the country. More than 60,000 handicapped children were enrolled in Head Start programs in 1985 (U. S. Department of Health and Human Services, 1986).

A variety of other national efforts have stimulated the development of model programs to serve infants and toddlers. One example is P.L. 90–248, which established the Early and Periodic Screening, Diagnosis and Treatment (EPSDT) program in 1967. A component of Medicaid, EPSDT focuses on early identification and treatment as a method to prevent medical and developmental problems.

In 1968, P.L. 90–538, the Handicapped Children's Early Education Assistance Act, was passed. This legislation established the landmark Handicapped Children's Early Education Program (HCEEP), which provides federal support for the development of effective model programs and methods, and encourages state-wide planning and policies in early intervention for handicapped children. HCEEP, a seed money program, assists the development of exemplary services for handicapped children from birth to 8 years of age, and their families. Since 1968, more than 500 projects have developed model practices in curricula, assessment, and training nationwide (Smith, 1988a). HCEEP demonstration programs focusing on infants and toddlers have increased significantly in the last decade. Between 1982 and 1986, approximately 83% of the 131 HCEEP projects included services for infants (Suarez, Hurth, & Prestridge, 1987).

P.L. 94–142, the Education of the Handicapped Act passed in 1975, did not require services for children younger than school age, but encouraged states to serve handicapped preschoolers through the Preschool Incentive Grant program. This program was strictly voluntary. P.L. 94–142 was reauthorized by P.L. 99–457 in 1986 and services for preschool children were expanded at that time.

As federal initiatives expanded, state policies for early intervention also increased, so that by 1984 more than half of the states offered services to some portion of their population of 3- to 5-year-olds, and about 10 states offered services from birth to at least some exceptional children (Smith, 1988a). In 1984, to stimulate further state action, Congress passed P.L. 98–199, which established a new state planning component in HCEEP providing federal funds to states for planning, developing, and implementing comprehensive services for at-risk and handicapped children from birth to 5 years of age, as well as their families (Smith, 1988a).

Each legislation has provided additional incentives for states to serve younger handicapped children. The goal of comprehensive services for children from birth to school age nearly became a reality with the passage of P.L. 99–457.

Public Law 99–457

On October 8, 1986, President Ronald Reagan signed P.L. 99–457, the Education of the Handicapped Act Amendments of 1986. This landmark legislation was the culmination of 20 years of policy-making for the early education of the handicapped. P.L. 99–457 contains provisions for handicapped children of all ages. The significance of this legislation is that it comes close to a national policy of providing services for all handicapped and at-risk children, birth to 5 years of age, and their families (Garwood & Sheehan, 1989).

This law includes two initiatives that lead to expanded and improved services to at-risk and handicapped infants, toddlers, and preschool children. One provision extends P.L. 94–142 to include all handicapped children from 3 years of age and increases funding for this group. As of the 1991–1992 school year, all states applying

P.L. 99–457 offers the hope that all children and their families who desire infant and toddler services will receive them.

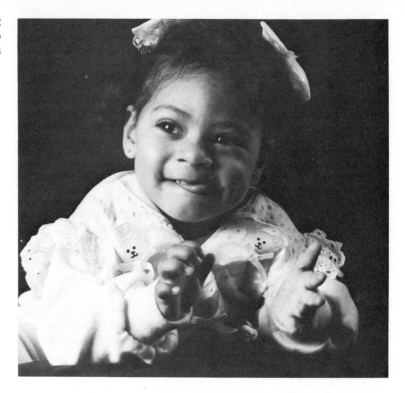

for P.L. 94–142 funds must assure they are providing a free, appropriate public education to handicapped children ages 3 to 5 (The Council for Exceptional Children, 1988).

The second provision is a discretionary program to assist states in serving all handicapped children from birth through age 2. This provision, The Infant/Toddler Program (Part H), provides financial assistance to states that elect to offer services. The financial incentive (Smith, 1988a) is for:

☐ developing and implementing statewide, comprehensive, coordinated, multidisciplinary, and interagency services

☐ facilitating the coordination of early intervention resources from federal, state, local, and private sources

☐ enhancing states' capabilities to provide high-quality infant intervention services

As of 1987, 14 states had mandated at least partial services to the birth to 2-year-old population (U. S. Department of Education, 1987). Participation in this program is strictly voluntary.

Eligibility for the Infant/Toddler Program.   Because this volume focuses on services to children from birth through age 2, discussion is limited to Part H of P.L. 99–457.

Part H acknowledges the needs of children from birth to their third birthday who need early education due to:

□ developmental delays in one or more of the following domains: cognitive, physical, language and speech, psychosocial, or self-help skills (each state determines criteria)

□ a physical or mental condition that has a high probability of resulting in delay (e.g., cerebral palsy, Down Syndrome)

□ being at risk medically or environmentally for substantial developmental delays if early education is not provided (determined at each state's discretion) (Fraas, 1986)

Further, families of at-risk and handicapped children may receive services that facilitate their ability to assist in their child's development.

State responsibilities for the Infant/Toddler Program.   When states apply for funding under Part H of P.L. 99–457, they must meet all requirements of the law. In the first 2 years (1987–1988), states had to

1. Establish an Interagency Coordinating Council made up of parents, state agency representatives, personnel trainers, state legislature representatives, and others.
2. Establish a lead agency.
3. Ensure that funds were used to plan, develop, and implement statewide services.

By the third and fourth years, states had to adopt a policy that ensures a statewide system, including:

1. A definition of the term *developmentally delayed*.
2. A timetable for ensuring services are available to all eligible children by the 5th year of participation.
3. A multidisciplinary evaluation system for eligible children and their families.
4. A provision for a written **Individualized Family Service Plan** (IFSP) for all eligible children.
5. A comprehensive **Child Find** system and a system for making referrals to service providers (primary service providers may include educational programs, hospitals, physicians, other health care professionals and agencies, and child care facilities).
6. A public awareness program focused on early identification.
7. A central directory of state resources, services, experts, and research and demonstration projects.
8. A comprehensive system of personnel development, including training public and private service providers and primary referral sources, as well as preservice training.
9. A **lead agency**, which is a single line of authority established by the governor to carry out the general administration, supervision, and monitoring of infant/toddler programs and activities (Chapter 13 discusses lead agencies).

10. A policy pertaining to the contracting or making of other arrangements with local service providers.
11. A procedure for securing timely reimbursement of funds between state and local agencies.
12. A procedural system for settling disagreements between families and providers, including:
    □ the right to appeal
    □ the right to confidentiality of information
    □ the opportunity to examine records
    □ the assignment of surrogate parents
    □ the right to prior written notice to parents in their native language
    □ the establishment of procedures to ensure the provision of services pending the resolution of complaints
13. A policy and procedures for the establishment and maintenance of personnel training, hiring, and certification/licensing standards.
14. A system for compiling data on the early intervention programs that can be accomplished through sampling techniques.

The statewide system had to be in effect no later than the beginning of the 4th year, except for the assurance of full services to all eligible children. By 1990 to 1991, the fifth and succeeding years, states must ensure that the system is in effect, and that full services are available to all eligible children. Infant services may range from least restrictive (prevention and monitoring) to most restrictive (residential programs) options, depending on the child's and the family's needs. Figure 1–1 shows the continuum of infant intervention services that may be offered.

All infant services must include a multidisciplinary assessment and a written IFSP developed by the team and the family (P.L. 99–457, 1986). Services designed to meet the developmental needs of the child and the family are specified in the IFSP. The multidisciplinary team may include professionals from special education, speech and language therapy, audiology, occupational therapy, physical therapy, psychology, counseling, and health professions. Family training and counseling, transition services, and medical services for diagnostic purposes may be provided as needed. To coordinate necessary services, case management is included for every child and

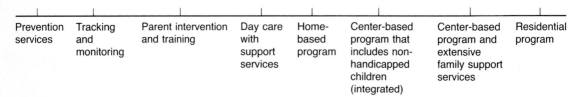

FIGURE 1–1
Early intervention continuum of services. (From "Early Childhood Special Education in the Next Decade: Implementing and Expanding P.L. 99–457" by B. Smith and P. Strain, 1988, *Topics in Early Childhood Special Education, 8,* p. 41. Copyright © 1988, PRO-ED, Inc. Reprinted by permission.)

family. These services must be provided free of cost, except where federal and state law provides for payment on a sliding fee basis.

States have offered preschool handicapped services through the special education divisions of local school systems. However, Part H of P.L. 99–457 designates that each state must select a lead agency to manage their infant services (U. S. Department of Education, 1987). Table 1–1 shows the frequency of agencies designated as lead agencies for early intervention programs funded under P.L. 99–457 as of 1988. As can be seen, the majority of states continued to place early intervention programs under the control of education departments.

Because of the broad parameters written into P.L. 99–457, Part H, there is variety among states' policies and services for at-risk and handicapped infants and toddlers. No intervention service component is mandated nationally, so variability in the type and quality of services also exists.

This law introduces many new challenges for professionals. The emphasis on family-focused services and the broad range of service options suggests the need for inservice and preservice training. The focus on interagency coordination to control redundancy in services presents a formidable challenge to programs accustomed to operating independently. Low funding levels, inconsistent eligibility criteria, and inconsistent state regulations have been recognized as obstacles to efficient interagency coordination (Meisels, Harbin, Modigliani, & Olson, 1987). Further, a shortage of trained infant professionals and a pressing need for teacher certification standards in infant and toddler intervention challenge the implementation of Part H of P.L. 99–457. Recently, universities, state agencies, and national education and advocacy organizations have identified some of the major competencies needed by professionals serving at-risk and special needs children and their families.

INTERVENTION COMPETENCIES

Certification requirements for early intervention can be a controversial issue (Gilkerson, Hilliard, Schrag, & Shonkoff, 1987). One concern is that states and local school systems faced with extreme personnel shortages that jeopardize the successful implementation of P.L. 99–457, Part H, may lower or waive certification requirements (Burke, McLaughlin, & Valdivieso, 1988). This practice would have serious deleterious effects on the quality of services rendered to families. Another concern is that states may resort to short-term, episodic forms of preservice and inservice training to handle personnel shortages. Short-term training, as a whole, has been found to be less effective in developing quality personnel than long-term, field-based training programs (Gilkerson et al., 1987). The shortage of trained pediatric speech, occupational, and physical/developmental therapists and interventionists is expected to last well into the 1990s. The establishment of linkages with local universities is considered by some to be the best choice for comprehensive personnel development (Campbell, Bellamy, & Bishop, 1988) for infant and toddler intervention.

Some of the skills necessary for professionals serving infants and toddlers differ from those needed for preschool-aged intervention (McCollum, 1987). Thorp and

TABLE 1–1

Lead agency for early intervention programs funded under P.L. 99–457 as of 1988.

Education	Health	Health and Social Services	Developmental Disabilities	Human Resources	Other Agency	Interagency Coordinating Council
Alabama	Hawaii	Alaska	Arizona	Arkansas	Indiana	Maine
Colorado	Kansas	Washington	California	Dist. of Columbia	Maryland	Rhode Island
Connecticut	Massachusetts	Wisconsin	Idaho	Georgia	Virginia	Texas
Delaware	Mississippi	Wyoming	Montana	Kentucky		
Florida	New Mexico		Oregon	Nevada		
Illinois	New York			N. Carolina		
Iowa	Ohio			N. Dakota		
Louisiana	S. Carolina			Pennsylvania		
Michigan	Utah					
Minnesota	W. Virginia					
Missouri						
Nebraska						
New Hampshire						
New Jersey						
Oklahoma						
S. Dakota						
Tennessee						
Vermont						

Source: Mapping the Future of Children with Special Needs (p. 128) by B. Smith (Ed.), 1988, Iowa City: University of Iowa Press. Copyright © 1988, University of Iowa Press. Reprinted by permission.

McCollum (1988) indicate that infant interventionists require competencies in a common infancy core, whatever their previous discipline training. They identify the common infancy core as having 4 broad categories of knowledge and skill: infant-related, family-related, teaming-related, and interagency/advocacy-related competencies.

Child-related Competencies

A strong foundation in typical and atypical infant development is necessary to work with very young handicapped children. A sensitivity to the rate of development and an understanding of the interdependence of **domains**, different developmental areas such as fine and gross motor, is important. Although it is possible to discuss domains separately, developmental skills are often interrelated and interdependent in infancy. Attachment, for example, is significantly interrelated with all modes of learning and social development (Healy et al., 1989). Although Part II of this book (Chapters 3, 4, and 5) is roughly organized by domains, it is counterproductive to view domains as unrelated areas of development.

Infant interventionists must be able to assess infants, using strategies from their own discipline, as well as obtain assessment information through observation while another professional conducts assessments. This type of assessment is called **arena assessment** and is discussed in Chapter 2. Interventionists need to be skilled in providing services to a vast range of at-risk and disabled children. Generally, early intervention services are **noncategorical**; services are not grouped by handicapping conditions. Noncategorical services require interventionists to possess an expansive knowledge base.

Family-related Competencies

Families are now seen as collaborators in infant services in the assessment, planning, and intervention processes. Infant interventionists must possess an array of personal and professional skills that permit them to increase family strengths, instead of focusing on family deficits or adjustments (Bailey, Farel, O'Donnell, Simeonsson, & Miller, 1986). To achieve this, infant interventionists must commit to a family-focused approach and understand the family systems approach to serving families (Turnbull & Turnbull, 1990). The **family systems approach** considers the roles of different family members, the role of the family on larger social networks, and the impact of family and social networks on intervention (Geik, Gilkerson, & Sponseller, 1982; Turnbull & Turnbull, 1990). Interventionists must develop multicultural knowledge so they can serve families from culturally diverse backgrounds effectively. Chapter 12 discusses the family systems approach and developing multicultural sensitivity.

A family-focused approach requires infant interventionists to be skilled in working *through* families, as well as working directly with infants. This process necessitates competencies in **intervention coaching**, assisting parents and family members in identifying and promoting interactions which appear to facilitate learning in the at-risk or special needs child. Appendix B provides a list of resources to which professionals may direct families for additional support.

Team-related Competencies

Infant and toddler intervention is characterized by cross-disciplinary service delivery models. Infant interventionists must be able to share their discipline expertise, learn from other team members, and collaborate with team members (which includes the family) to develop integrated assessment and planning. To serve effectively as a consultant to other members of a team, team members must actively practice team building and develop team communication skills. Despite the obvious importance of collaboration in quality infant services, team processing continues to be ignored by many programs training infant interventionists (Bruder & McLean, 1988). Chapter 2 discusses strategies for successful team building and functioning.

Interagency and Advocacy-related Competencies

Most infant services have indicated a need to improve their interagency coordination skills (Trohanis, 1988). Interagency collaboration necessitates skills in understanding the larger service delivery context and knowing the range of services available for families. Interagency collaboration may require infant interventionists to serve as advocates for families while making efforts to secure or expand services. Because P.L. 99–457, Part H, permits a spectrum of services, interventionists may be involved with a number of services. In addition to infant education programs, it is likely that infant interventionists will work with child care centers and hospital-based services.

In addition to these basic skill areas, infant interventionists must be flexible, mature, independent, tenacious, and tolerant (Garland & Linder, 1988). Because infant interventionists go into families' homes, they must have good listening skills and possess the ability to communicate that they can be trusted. See Appendix C for a list of national professional associations and volunteer organizations that may assist professionals in their roles as advocates for very young children and their families.

Although infant service providers are expected to be knowledgeable, skillful, and provide a variety of services to families, most tend to be modestly paid. The gap between what personnel are expected to do, and what they are paid, is an issue which must be addressed (Healy, Keesee, & Smith, 1989). The following chapters of this book are organized around these major competency areas and are designed to provide both knowledge and applied skills for infant interventionists.

SUMMARY

This chapter discussed the key legislation that has shaped the United States' commitment to its youngest at-risk and handicapped children. Federal incentive programs for children younger than 3 years of age have slowly emerged over the past 3 decades. The most significant legislation influencing services for children from birth through age 2, P.L. 99–457, Part H, was passed in 1986. This law has created expectations in professionals and families alike that infant and toddler services will be offered to all children and families who deserve them. Although federal legislation has increased the number of services available to young children with special needs, it continues to be the responsibility of professionals in the field to ensure that the quality of programs increases as well (Smith & Strain, 1988). Quality infant and toddler services appear to be linked to quality personnel training and interagency coordination.

A summary of some of the key concepts of this chapter follows:

1. Most infant services have one or more of these three principal objectives:
   □ to provide information, support, and assistance to families
   □ to build parental confidence as the primary facilitator of their child's development
   □ to foster effective interactions between parent(s), family members, and child to promote mutual feelings of competence and enjoyment
2. Infant intervention is often the beginning of a long relationship with a series of professionals during a handicapped child's life. A family-focused approach allows parents to be parents, and to be informed so they can assist and direct, as much as each individual family may elect, what happens to them and their family. Early intervention services should increase feelings of competence and self-sufficiency.
3. The efficacy of infant intervention studies should be judged not by changes in the development of the child alone, but also by the success of the support offered the family in their adaptation to life with the child who is at risk or who has special needs.
4. Cost-benefit investigations suggest that for every $1 invested in early intervention services, there is the potential for a $3 reduction in long-term, public special education costs.
5. Although many models of infant and toddler intervention are promoted, there is not sufficient research to make decisions about which model is most effective, or most cost-effective, with different children and different families.
6. Part H of P.L. 99–457 is the first national initiative to provide full services to all eligible at-risk and handicapped infants. This law does not require states to serve infants and toddlers. It merely provides financial incentives and federal guidance for providing infant services.
7. At present, there is little uniformity between states in policy and programs for at-risk and handicapped infants and their families.
8. As of 1987, more than 80% of all states had some form of entitlement to services for children prior to school age. Only a few states had entitlements for services for the birth to 3-year-old population.
9. Many professionals in infant programs indicate the need to improve in the area of interagency coordination which is expanded by P.L. 99–457, Part H.
10. The shortage of trained infant interventionists, physical and occupational therapists, and speech therapists is expected to continue into the next decade.

As the upcoming chapters reveal, infant and toddler intervention is unique in its history, philosophy, instructional priorities, and professional responsibilities. Infant interventionists must possess broad-based child-related, family-related, team-related, and interagency/advocacy-related competencies in order to effectively facilitate the development of young children and their families.

DISCUSSION QUESTIONS

1. What skills, besides those mentioned in this chapter, should infant interventionists possess to maximize their facilitative role with young children and their families?
2. Why is it difficult to establish the efficacy of infant intervention research?
3. How should infant intervention personnel shortages be handled in the next decade? Explain the effect of each suggestion on the quality and availability of services.

APPLIED ACTIVITIES/PROJECTS

1. Contact your local lead agency and interview a case manager. Ask for the case manager's view of the advantages and disadvantages of interagency collaboration and coordination in infant and toddler services.
2. Interview a local infant service provider. Without breaking confidentiality, discuss some of the issues that may have arisen while resolving a family's conflicts about their intervention services.
3. Contact infant interventionists in three settings (home, center, and hospital). Ask these professionals to list their present concerns about the implementation of P.L. 99–457, Part H. Next to each concern, devise at least two means to handle the issue.

SUGGESTED READINGS

Ballard, J., Ramirez, B., & Zantal-Wiener, K. (1987). *Public Law 94–142, section 504, and Public Law 99–457: Understanding what they are and are not*. Reston, VA: The Council for Exceptional Children.

Cunningham, K., Cunningham, K., & O'Connell, J. (Undated). *Cultural perceptions and their impact on special education service delivery*. Flagstaff, AZ: Native American Research and Training Center, Northern Arizona University.

Garwood, S. G., & Fewell, R. K. (Eds.). (1983). *Educating handicapped infants: Issues in development and intervention*. Rockville, MD: Aspen.

Hochman, J. (1987). *Planning programs for infants, II*. Edison, NJ: INTERACT, Pediatric Rehabilitation Dept., John F. Kennedy Medical Center, 2050 Oak Tree Road, Edison, NJ 08820.

Meisels, S., & Shonkoff, J. (Eds.). (1989). *Handbook of early intervention*. New York: Cambridge University Press.

REFERENCES

Allen, D. A. (1980, September). *Relationship-focused intervention with high-risk infants: First year findings*. Paper presented at the Annual Meeting of the American Psychological Association, Montreal, Canada.

Bagnato, S., & Neisworth, J. (1985). Efficacy of interdisciplinary assessment and treatment for infants and preschoolers with congenital and acquired brain injury. *Analysis and Intervention in Developmental Disabilities, 5*, 107–128.

Bailey, D., Farel, A., O'Donnell, K., Simeonsson, R., & Miller, C. (1986). Preparing infant interventionists: Interdisciplinary training in special education and maternal child health. *Journal of the Division for Early Childhood, 11*(1), 67–77.

Ballard, J., Ramirez, B., & Zantal-Wiener, K. (1987). *Public Law 94–142, section 504, and Public Law 99–457: Understanding what they are and are not.* Reston, VA: The Council for Exceptional Children.

Bendell, R., Culbertson, J., Shelton, T., & Carter, B. (1986). Interrupted infantile apnea: Impact on early development, temperament, and maternal stress. *Journal of Clinical Child Psychology, 15,* 304–310.

Bennett, F. C. (1982). The pediatrician and the interdisciplinary process. *Exceptional Children, 48,* 306–314.

Berrueter-Clement, J., Schweinhart, L., Barnett, W., Epstein, A., & Weikart, D. (1984). *Changed lives: The effects of the Perry Preschool Program on youths through age 19* (Monograph No. 8). Ypsilanti, MI: High/Scope Educational Research Foundation.

Bricker, D. (1986). *Early education of at-risk and handicapped infants, toddlers, and preschool children.* Glenview, IL: Scott, Foresman.

Bricker, D., Bailey, E., & Bruder, M. (1984). The efficacy of early intervention and the handicapped infant: A wise or wasted resource? In M. Wolraich & D. Routh (Eds.), *Advances in developmental and behavioral pediatrics, Vol. 5* (pp. 373–423). Greenwich, CT: JAI Press.

Bruder, M., & McLean, M. (1988). Personnel preparation for infant interventionists: A review of federally funded projects. *Journal for the Division for Early Childhood, 12*(4), 299–305.

Burke, P., McLaughlin, M., & Valdivieso, S. (1988). Preparing professionals to educate handicapped infants and young children: Some policy considerations. *Topics in Early Childhood Special Education, 8*(1), 73–80.

Campbell, P., Bellamy, G., & Bishop, K. (1988). Statewide intervention systems: An overview of the new federal program for infants and toddlers with handicaps. *Journal of Special Education, 22*(1), 25–40.

Clarke, A., & Clarke, A. (1976). *Early experience: Myth and evidence.* New York: The Free Press.

The Council for Exceptional Children (1988). *Preschool services for children with handicaps* (ERIC Digest #450). Reston, VA: Author.

Dunst, C., Trivette, C., & Deal, A. (1988). *Enabling and empowering families: Principles and guidelines for practice.* Cambridge, MA: Brookline Books.

Edgar, E. (1988). Policy factors influencing research in early childhood special education. In S. Odom & M. Karnes (Eds.), *Early intervention for infants and children with handicaps: An empirical base* (pp. 63–74). Baltimore, MD: Paul H. Brookes.

Field, T., Goldberg, S., Stern, D., & Sostek, A. (1980). *High-risk infants and children: Adult and peer interaction.* New York: Academic Press.

Fraas, C. J. (1986). *Summary of the Education of the Handicapped Act Amendments of 1986, P.L. 99–457.* Washington, DC: The Library of Congress, Research Service.

Garland, C. W., & Linder, T. W. (1988). Administrative challenges in early intervention. In J. B. Jordan, J. J. Gallagher, P. L. Hutinger, & M. B. Karnes (Eds.), *Early childhood special education: Birth to three* (pp. 5–28). Reston, VA: The Council for Exceptional Children.

Garwood, S. G., & Sheehan, R. (1989). *Designing a comprehensive early intervention system: The challenge of Public Law 99–457.* Austin, TX: PRO-ED.

Geik, I., Gilkerson, L., & Sponseller, D. (1982). An early intervention training model. *Journal of the Division for Early Childhood, 5,* 42–52.

Gilkerson, L., Hilliard, A., Schrag, E., & Shonkoff, J. (1987). Point of view: Commenting on P.L. 99–457. *Zero to Three, 7*(3), 13–17.

Greer, J. (1990). The drug babies. *Exceptional Children, 56,* 382–384.

Guralnick, M., & Bennett, F. C. (Eds.). (1987). *The effectiveness of early intervention for at-risk and handicapped children.* Orlando, FL: Academic Press.

Hanson, M. (1985). An analysis of the effects of early intervention services for infants and toddlers with moderate and severe handicaps. *Topics in Early Childhood Special Education Quarterly, 5,* 36–51.

Healy, A., Keesee, P., & Smith, B. (1989). *Early services for children with special needs: Transactions for family support.* Baltimore, MD: Paul H. Brookes.

Karnes, M. B., & Stayton, V. D. (1988). Model programs for infants and toddlers with handicaps. In J. B. Jordan, J. J. Gallagher, P. L. Hutinger, & M. B. Karnes (Eds.), *Early childhood special education: Birth to three* (pp. 67–108). Reston, VA: The Council for Exceptional Children.

Kochanek, T. T., Friedman, D. H., Bagnall, P., & Fazzio, P. (1988). *Incorporating family assessment and Individualized Family Service Plans into early intervention programs: A developmental, decision making process.* Providence: Rhode Island College.

Lally, J., Mangione, P., Honig, A., & Wittmer, D. (1988). More pride, less delinquency: Findings from the 10-year follow-up study of the Syracuse University Family Development Research Program. *Zero to Three, 8*(4), 13–18.

Lamb, M., Garn, S., & Keating, M. (1981). Correlation between sociability and cognitive performance among 8-month-olds. *Child Development, 52,* 711–713.

McCollum, J. (1987). Early interventionists in infant and early childhood programs: A comparison of preservice training needs. *Topics in Early Childhood Special Education, 7*(3), 24–35.

Meisels, S. J., Harbin, G., Modigliani, K., & Olson, K. (1987). Formulating optimal state early childhood intervention policies. *Exceptional Children, 55*(2), 159–165.

Moxley-Haegert, L., & Serbin, L. (1983). Developmental education for parents of delayed infants: Effects on parental motivation and children's development. *Child Development, 54,* 1324–1331.

National Center for Clinical Infant Programs (1985, July). *Training and manpower issues in services to disabled and at-risk infants, toddlers, and their families.* Unpublished report of a national meeting on training needs. Washington, DC: Author.

National Center for Clinical Infant Programs (1986). *Infants can't wait.* Washington, DC: Author.

Odom, S., Yoder, P., & Hill, G. (1988). Developmental intervention for infants with handicaps: Purposes and programs. *The Journal of Special Education, 1*(1), 11–24.

Ottenbacher, K. J. (1989). Statistical conclusion validity of early intervention research with handicapped children. *Exceptional Children, 55,* 534–540.

Peterson, N. (1987). *Early intervention for handicapped and at-risk children.* Denver: Love Publishing.

Piaget, J. (1952). *The origins of intelligence in children.* New York: International Universities Press.

Public Law 99–457. (1986). Washington, DC: 99th Congress, October 8, 1986.

Safford, P., Gregg, L., Schneider, G., & Sewell, J. (1976). A stimulation program for young sensory-impaired, multihandicapped children. *Education and Treatment of the Mentally Retarded, 11,* 12–17.

Shonkoff, J., Hauser-Cram, D., Krauss, M., & Upshur, C. (1988). Early intervention efficacy research: What have we learned and where do we go from here? *Topics in Early Childhood Special Education, 8*(1), 81–93.

Simeonsson, R. (1985). Efficacy of early intervention: Issues and evidence. *Analysis and Intervention in Developmental Disabilities, 5,* 203–209.

Smith, B. (1988a). Early intervention public policy: Past, present, and future. In J. B. Jordan, J. J. Gallagher, P. L. Hutinger, & M. B. Karnes (Eds.), *Early childhood special education: Birth to three* (pp. 213–228). Reston, VA: The Council for Exceptional Children.

Smith, B. (Ed.). (1988b) *Mapping the future of children with special needs*. Iowa City: University of Iowa Press.

Smith, B., & Strain, P. (1988). Early childhood special education in the next decade: Implementing and expanding P.L. 99–457. *Topics in Early Childhood Special Education, 8*(1), 37–47.

Suarez, T., Hurth, J., & Prestridge, S. (1987, November). *Innovation in early childhood special education: An analysis of the Handicapped Children's Early Education Program projects funded from 1982–1986*. Paper presented at the Annual Meeting of the American Education Research Association, Washington, DC.

Thorp, E., & McCollum, J. (1988). Defining the infancy specialization in early childhood special education. In J. B. Jordan, J. J. Gallagher, P. L. Hutinger, & M. B. Karnes (Eds.), *Early childhood special education: Birth to three* (pp. 147–161). Reston, VA: The Council for Exceptional Children.

Trohanis, P. L. (1988). Preparing for change: The implementation of Public Law 99–457. In J. B. Jordan, J. J. Gallagher, P. L. Hutinger, & M. B. Karnes (Eds.), *Early childhood special education: Birth to three* (pp. 229–240). Reston, VA: The Council for Exceptional Children.

Turnbull, A., & Turnbull, H. (1990). *Families, professionals, and exceptionality: A special partnership* (2nd ed.). Columbus, OH: Merrill.

U. S. Department of Education. (1987). *Ninth annual report to Congress on the implementation of the Education of the Handicapped Act*. Washington, DC: U. S. Government Printing Office.

U. S. Department of Health and Human Services. (1986). *The status of handicapped children in Head Start programs*. Washington, DC: U. S. Government Printing Office.

U. S. House of Representatives. (1986). *Education of the Handicapped Act Amendments of 1986; Report 99–860*. Washington, DC: U. S. Congress.

Weiner, R., & Koppelman, J. (1987). *From birth to 5: Serving the youngest handicapped children*. Alexandria, VA: Capital Publications.

White, K. R. (1986). Efficacy of early intervention. *Journal of Special Education, 19,* 401–416.

Widerstrom, A., & Goodwin, L. (1987). Effects of an infant stimulation program on the child and the family. *Journal of the Division for Early Childhood, 11,* 143–153.

Yarrow, L. J., Rubenstein, J. L., & Pedersen, F. A. (1975). *Infant and environment: Early cognitive and motivation development*. New York: Wiley.

2

Transdisciplinary Approach to Infant and Toddler Intervention

Sharon A. Raver

OVERVIEW

This chapter discusses issues relating to the transdisciplinary model of providing services to infants and toddlers and their families, including:

□ service delivery models of intervention
□ comparison of unidisciplinary, multidisciplinary, interdisciplinary teaming, and transdisciplinary models
□ techniques for increasing the efficiency of transdisciplinary services
□ personal, professional, and administrative characteristics that enhance the effectiveness of transdisciplinary teaming

The types of services a family receives depend on the range of service options available in the community in which a family lives. Services also depend on the severity of the child's handicapping condition or the nature of the suspected delay.

SERVICE DELIVERY MODELS OF INTERVENTION

For infants and toddlers service delivery models tend to be a combination of two settings—home and center programs. The most common models are

□ home participation only
□ home participation followed by center participation
□ combination of home and center participation
□ center participation only
□ monitored infants and toddlers

Home-based Programs

In home-based programs an infant interventionist travels to a family's home to work directly with the family and child in their own environment. The interventionist views both the parent *and* the child as the focus of the intervention. That is, the service provider is concerned with advancing the developmental progress of the child, as well as enhancing the sense of well-being and competence of family members. Generally, this is achieved by working directly with the child, and in addition, working directly with any family member present during a home visit.

The interventionist's presence in a home can arouse strong feelings in family members regarding their attitudes toward the handicapped child, their living circumstances, and parental competence. Families' reactions to home visitation may range from feelings of gratitude to feelings of resentfulness. There is no single best way to handle the range of emotions family members may express. Usually some balance between empathy and objectivity is best for most families.

Home-based programs offer the advantage of continuous contact with the child and family in their own environment, flexibility of time and intensity of service, increased contact with all family members, and a relatively low cost of implementation. Disadvantages of this model include inconsistency in training and experience among service providers, and limited opportunities to coordinate additional services such as therapies and contact with other children with or without disabilities.

Center-based Programs

In center-based programs children are brought to a central location to receive direct services. The majority of infant and toddler centers also offer services for family members, usually while children participate at the center. The range of services varies depending on the number of staff. In some programs, parents are guided through intervention activities with their children with professionals acting as facilitators or models. Other programs offer parent information, training, or social sessions for families that may involve siblings and/or extended family members. Center-based programs tend to have variable attendance schedules, with few requiring daily attendance.

Center-based programs provide distinct advantages for families. These programs tend to provide consistent, prearranged programs and, in some cases, transportation. A potential lack of flexibility to accommodate the needs of individual children and their families, limited interaction with nonhandicapped children, and, at times, a gap in services during the summer are considered disadvantages of the center-based model.

Monitored Infants and Toddlers

Generally, children with mild handicaps, those who are at risk for mild developmental delays, and those from home- or center-based programs involved in transitions to **least restrictive environments** (LRE) such as community child care programs are

Center-based infant and toddler programs provide opportunities for regular play sessions with other children.

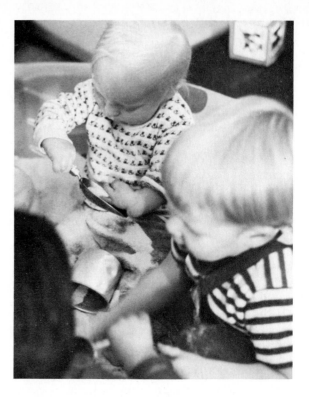

placed on monitoring programs. When a child is being monitored, the family regularly meets with team members to have their child assessed and to discuss their child's progress in the least restrictive environment. Decisions focus on the type of support necessary in the setting in which the child is being monitored. Unfortunately, due to limited services for at-risk children and those with developmental delays, some children whose needs may be best served by home-based or center-based programs may be placed on monitoring programs rather than offered no services at all. Chapter 8 discusses monitoring and tracking in detail.

Increased community awareness of early intervention, and increased awareness of community-based infant and toddler workers of the needs of at-risk and handicapped young children and their families are viewed as advantages of monitoring in least restrictive environments. The increased demand for inservice training for personnel by specialized interventionists who are already overburdened with responsibilities, and the potential for poorly coordinated and monitored interventions are recognized as disadvantages of monitoring systems.

Financial considerations and location often dictate whether a center- or home-based program is available to a family. Interestingly, Tingey (1986) reports that half-day programs for handicapped children produce as many gains as full-day programs, and programs that expect parent involvement do not tend to be more effective than programs that do not. Nonetheless, as stated in Chapter 1, children and families respond differently to each program model. It is quite possible that neither the cheapest nor the most effective program is the most cost-effective (Smith, 1988).

APPROACHES TO INTERVENTION

Family-focused Approach

As indicated in Chapter 1, infant and toddler intervention programs must support—not supplant—the family's role. A family's needs and priorities, not those of the professionals serving the family, nor the professionals' perceptions of a family's needs, are the basis for all decision making. Every effort must be made to match services to a family's unique style and goals. Traditionally, family involvement models have focused on individual parents through counseling, or by training the parent-child dyad as in the case of parent-mediated behavior management interventions. However, in the family-focused approach, families are seen as interdependent systems and services are designed for families, not for parents or individual children. It is now accepted that what happens to one member of a family affects all other members of that family (Turnbull & Turnbull, 1990).

Despite the philosophical acceptance of the family-focused approach, evidence suggests some discrepancies arise between what professionals consider best practice and what occurs in programs. Karnes and Stayton (1988) found that most HCEEP programs offer services for parents rather than the entire family, despite the fact that 38% of the HCEEP programs surveyed indicate that they adhere to a family systems approach to designing intervention programs.

Team Approach

The provisions of P.L. 99–457 made significant changes in the staffing of infant and toddler programs. This act requires that services include a multidisciplinary assessment and a written **Individualized Family Service Plan (IFSP)** developed by a multidisciplinary team that includes parents. Several team structures for providing services to at-risk and handicapped children and their families have been used. These team approaches differ in philosophy and operation. Table 2–1 outlines the differences in the multidisciplinary, interdisciplinary, and transdisciplinary team approaches to intervention.

With the passage of P.L. 99–457, the **unidisciplinary approach**, independent evaluation and planning by a single professional without input or consultation from other child development disciplines (Bennett, 1982), is no longer tenable. Although the most common approach to infant intervention until the mid-1980s, best practice today agrees that a strict unidisciplinary approach is increasingly inappropriate as cases become more complex.

The term **multidisciplinary approach** to providing services is frequently used to describe an evaluation and management process in which numerous individual

TABLE 2–1
Three approaches to infant intervention.

	Multidisciplinary	Interdisciplinary	Transdisciplinary
Assessment	Separate assessments by team members	Separate assessments by team members	Team members and family conduct a comprehensive developmental assessment together
Parent participation	Parents meet with individual team members	Parents meet with team or team representative	Parents are full, active, and participating members of the team
Service plan development	Team members develop separate plans for their discipline	Team members share their separate plans with one another	Team members and the parents develop a service plan based upon family priorities, needs, and resources
Service plan responsibility	Team members are responsible for implementing their section of the plan	Team members are responsible for sharing information with one another as well as for implementing their section of the plan	Team members are responsible and accountable for how the primary service provider implements the plan
Service plan implementation	Team members implement the part of the service plan related to their discipline	Team members implement their section of the plan and incorporate other sections where possible	A primary service provider is assigned to implement the plan with the family
Lines of communication	Informal lines	Periodic case-specific team meetings	Regular team meeting where continuous transfer of information, knowledge, and skills are shared among team members
Guiding philosophy	Team members recognize the importance of contributions from other disciplines	Team members are willing and able to develop, share, and be responsible for providing services that are a part of the total service plan	Team members make a commitment to teach, learn, and work together across discipline boundaries to implement unified service plan
Staff development	Independent and within their discipline	Independent within as well as outside of their discipline	An integral component of team meetings for learning across disciplines and team building

Source: From "Early Intervention Team Approaches: The Transdisciplinary Model" by G. Woodruff & M. J. McGonigel. In *Early Childhood Special Education: Birth to Three* (p. 166) edited by J. B. Jordan, J. J. Gallagher, P. L. Hutinger, & M. L. Karnes, 1988, Reston, VA: The Council for Exceptional Children. Reprinted by permission.

consultations from different disciplines are obtained, but in which the various evaluations are carried out independently of each other with little opportunity for professional interaction, comparison, debate, or integrated planning (Bennett, 1982). This process omits the potential benefits of group synthesis and has resulted in duplicate services for families.

The **interdisciplinary approach** defines a process in which professionals from different, but related, disciplines work together to assess and manage problems by actively participating in mutual decision making. Team members share information with one another but independently implement their section of a plan.

In contrast, the term **transdisciplinary approach** describes what some believe to be the ideal type of interdisciplinary team functioning. The transdisciplinary approach not only involves the mutual sharing of assessment results, but dictates professional involvement and participation that crosses traditional discipline boundaries (Bennett, 1982). This approach was originally used by programs needing to provide comprehensive services with limited staff and facilities. Professionals from child development, counseling, early childhood, family life studies, health and recreation, nursing, nutrition, psychology, social work, special education, and speech and hearing science are natural choices for transdisciplinary team membership. With this approach professionals work together, with the direct guidance of a family, to develop a unified and integrated plan for the child and the family (McCollum & Hughes, 1988).

RATIONALE FOR THE TRANSDISCIPLINARY APPROACH

The principal rationale for the transdisciplinary approach for serving young handicapped children is the desire for fewer people to work directly with the family and child, improved continuity in programming, maximum consistency of services in the home and center, and improved integration of parent participation.

The transdisciplinary approach is an attempt to meet the needs of the child and family by avoiding compartmentalization and fragmentation of planning and services. It works to consolidate medical and educational services through coherent programming and consistent handling of the family plan by all the professionals involved. Transdisciplinary dialogue makes it difficult to view children as segregated areas of need. For example, a speech pathologist can no longer view only communicative and cognitive deficits, nor can a physical therapist be concerned only with the motor needs of a child. Interaction across discipline lines permits professionals to get a more balanced picture of the whole child.

The architects of P.L. 94–142 obviously believed that group decisions provide safeguards against individual errors in judgment, while recognizing that only a group of specialists from different professions could deal effectively with the increasingly complex problems facing special education today (Pfeiffer, 1982). Although many acknowledge the transdisciplinary approach as best practice, it is also becoming increasingly understood that the same team approach may not be necessary for all program functions. In other words, transdisciplinary teaming may be appropriate for assessments, and yet may not be as feasible or desirable for plan implementation (McCollum & Hughes, 1988).

Despite the merits of the transdisciplinary approach, transdisciplinary teaming is not universally applied. This may be due to a philosophical agreement with transdisciplinary teaming but limited access to other child professionals. Needless to say, the shared responsibilities of transdisciplinary teamwork is not easily achieved. The approach demands flexibility, tolerance, and understanding among and between those involved (Garland, Woodruff, & Buck, 1988).

Role of Transdisciplinary Team Members

Members of a transdisciplinary team systematically cross traditional discipline boundaries to develop an in-depth understanding of other disciplines so they are able to provide services to families who require skills outside their own discipline when it is appropriate or necessary. The exact way this is handled varies from program to program, and from family to family. The goal is to provide services to families that might not be available if there were strict disciplinary divisions.

Transdisciplinary team members have many responsibilities. They conduct assessments as a team, with the guidance of families. They develop service plans as a team, again with the direct collaboration of families, using the families' priorities. And each team member is accountable for how the **primary service provider**, a team member authorized by the team to work directly with the family, implements the plan with the family. Frequent meetings are used to discuss assessment, diagnosis and goal setting, planning and program implementation, and evaluation of the program and child. (Chapter 13 discusses the development of Individualized Family Service Plans.)

Further, team members are responsible for organizing regular staff development meetings for teaching their discipline skills to team members as well as sharing discipline-specific information. An integral component of transdisciplinary team meetings is learning across discipline lines. For example, a physical therapist might be selected from a team to work directly with a family to improve tone and balance in a cerebral palsied child, and also to develop better social interactions, improve communicative skills, and improve feeding. The program the physical therapist implements is created by the full transdisciplinary team and is monitored by the team at periodic meetings (Healy, Keesee, & Smith, 1989).

The more severe a handicapping condition, and the more specialized the needed interventions, the greater the chances of limited cross-discipline responsibility sharing. Each discipline, particularly medically-oriented fields, has standards of professional responsibility that limit sharing of disciplinary roles. It is the responsibility of each professional to clearly state when it is inadvisable to share professional skills.

Role release.   The process of **role release** is what separates transdisciplinary teaming from interdisciplinary teaming. Role release, or role sharing, is the sharing of responsibilities and roles, usually across disciplines, by more than one team member. Intervention in infancy demands that personnel function as generalists as well as specialists (McCollum & Hughes, 1988). Often there is insufficient staff to provide the full range of services families deserve. For this reason, role release allows professionals to teach discipline-specific skills to other professionals on their team from different discipline backgrounds. For instance, a physical therapist may teach a speech pathologist appropriate handling techniques for a motor-involved infant. This type of interaction creates a system that trains interventionists to work not only as professionals within their own disciplines, but also as team members who acknowledge, respect, and rely on the expertise of their colleagues and of families (Woodruff, 1980).

The process of role release demands continuous professional and personal change. Since the professional releasing skills is ultimately responsible for the quality of services given to families, role release involves continuous dialogue between team members. When problems arise, they must be handled swiftly. Properly implemented role release requires the use of **limit setting**. Limit setting occurs when team members—collaboratively—work out a procedure or make a decision that will reduce the chances of the same or similar conflict with role release occurring in the future. For example, if shared assessments created conflict, an agreement could be made that assessment information would be shared only after implementation. Naturally, limit setting is most productive when approached in a supportive, not accusatory, style. Infant interventionists must be continually expanding their professional knowledge while openly acknowledging legitimate limits to different areas of expertise.

Most disciplines have codes of ethics or standards that guide their professional activities. In the transdisciplinary model it is usually left to each professional to interpret to what extent role sharing jeopardizes these professional standards (Drew & Turnbull, 1987). Professionals must be clear on both the strengths and weaknesses of role release, and establish explicit guidelines for skills that can be shared, as well as clear mechanisms for follow-up on released skills.

Despite the need for safeguards, role sharing can be a fulfilling activity. A physical therapist who worked with infants for 5 years commented: "I know I am doing a good job when my colleagues ask me questions. I demonstrate the handling techniques I want a family to use so my team members can teach the family. However, I never release a skill that I am not absolutely certain a team member or the family member can do accurately. Not everyone on my team decides to do therapies. Some just don't feel comfortable and some just don't want to. My team members help me do my job. They don't do my job for me."

Arena assessment. Transdisciplinary teams often use a process assessment called **arena assessment**. In arena assessment one professional does the testing while the other team members, including the family, observe (Wolery & Dyk, 1984). The professionals sit on the floor around the child and parent(s), and observe while one professional acts as the facilitator. The role of the facilitator is to engage the child in activities that demonstrate the child's developmental strengths and weaknesses (Woodruff, 1980).

Before an arena assessment, team members meet and identify for the facilitator behaviors they would like to see for their individual evaluations. Following the assessment, if the professionals in the arena did not observe all they needed, parent

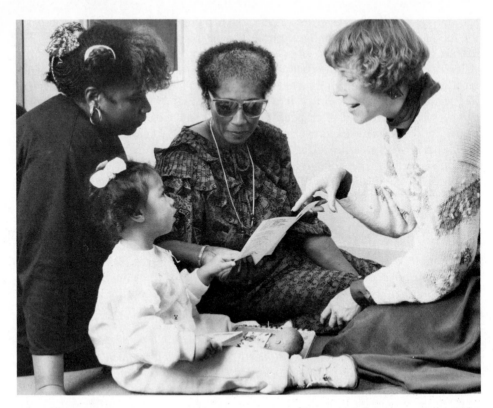

The transdisciplinary team approach is an attempt to meet the family's needs while limiting the number of professionals the family encounters regularly.

report items are used or another assessment time is arranged. Professionals who use arena assessment report it saves time, and that with training they can see what they need for their discipline-specific evaluations while also seeing the whole child.

Arena assessment offers advantages for families, the child, and the team (Woodruff, 1980). The advantages for the family are that it

- communicates to parents that they are fully functioning members of the team
- prevents different service providers from asking the same questions
- communicates that efforts to assist the child are a series of problem-solving experiences

Some advantages for the child are that

- only one assessment time is needed, instead of separate domain-specific assessments
- the child demonstrates strengths in a natural situation

Advantages for the team are

- it provides comprehensive, integrated assessment of the child

□ the team shares knowledge of child's development based on the same observation of the child, leading to easier consensus

□ it expands knowledge of all team members because all see the child from
their discipline and simultaneously receive a perception of the child from
another discipline

Following arena assessments, the team meets so the sharing of intervention
practices becomes natural and continuous. Transdisciplinary arena assessment forces
team members to seek integrated strategies and interventions because the intervention plan is written as a group, not by professionals individually. It also may work to
develop cohesiveness in teams. Cohesiveness is a sense of oneness team members
experience that results in their willingness to work harder toward the group's goals
and their desire to remain part of the group. Often, however, cohesiveness does not
occur spontaneously.

Effectiveness of the Transdisciplinary Approach

It should not be concluded that highly trained and specialized professionals find it
easy to work collaboratively. Problems with the transdisciplinary process have been
well delineated. The most common complaints are

□ differing levels of participation by different professional groups (Gilliam &
Coleman, 1981)

□ a lack of meaningful discussion in team meetings (Bailey, DeWert, Thiele, &
Ware, 1983)

□ a lack of training and guidance in the team process (Crisler, 1979)

□ the inability of professionals to work together in a truly integrative fashion
(Fordyce, 1982)

Problems with interdisciplinary and transdisciplinary teaming have been recorded in all disciplines, not just education. The forming of a successful team is a
continuous process. It is unrealistic to expect a team to work well together immediately or to expect a team to operate smoothly indefinitely. Bailey (1984) developed
a conceptual model for pinpointing different interactional difficulties teams may
experience. Figure 2–1 portrays examples of some of the more common team
dysfunctions that may arise as a team operates. At any point, a team may become
overstructured, disorganized, and/or develop ambiguous roles. Remediation of
difficulties lies in the ability to recognize conflicts, and to improve team communication.

Team communication techniques.   Problems arise when staff and administrators
do not share similar perceptions. Effective transdisciplinary teams *actively* create a
climate supporting open communication. Teams are made, not born (Fewell, 1983).
Interacting teams are characterized by relaxed, direct communication; coacting teams
are characterized by communication that all flows through a central person (Spencer
& Coye, 1988). Obviously, interacting communication produces more successful
teamwork.

FIGURE 2–1
Interactional difficulties teams may experience. (From "A Triaxial Model of the Interdisciplinary Team and Group Process" by D. B. Bailey, *Exceptional Children, 51,* 1984, p. 21. Copyright © 1984 by The Council for Exceptional Children. Reprinted by permission.)

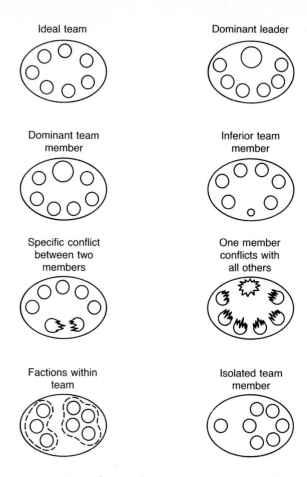

Two methods used to create a positive climate for team operations and to improve communication are conflict resolution strategies and team building skills. First, **conflict resolution strategies** are essential for handling disputes. Team members state the conflict as explicitly as possible, generate several means of resolving the conflict, and then conscientiously follow agreed-upon solutions. For conflict to have positive outcomes, it must be actively managed by the team leader and team members. It is best to confront conflicts immediately. In fact, before conflicts are experienced, teams should devise a system for decision making and handling disputes so conflicts are never handled in a haphazard manner. Spencer and Coye (1988) suggest a five step decision-making process for teams.

1. *Problem definition and information gathering.* State the problem clearly in terms of the discrepancy between the present situation and the desired situation. Do not seek solutions at this point. If the conflict involves family goal setting, families should be involved in the process.
2. *Alternative generation.* List all potential good ideas, even those that are not possible due to budget constraints. Keep ideas separate from an evaluation of their potential usefulness.

3. *Alternative selection.* Systematically evaluate benefits of each alternative and correlate alternatives with the group's or family's needs.
4. *Implementation.* Follow agreed-upon plan exactly. Failure to follow it precisely will create new conflicts.
5. *Monitoring.* Evaluate whether the decision achieved what it was intended to achieve. If desired objectives were not accomplished, the decision-making process is recycled from the first step.

The process of conflict resolution is improved when team members have a common language. If discipline-specific jargon is used, it must be defined so all members can communicate openly. It is not uncommon for members from different disciplines to be trained in different missions. Different missions result in different goals and solutions.

At times, a third party may be needed to mediate conflicts that are not resolved quickly. Interestingly, some programs report that involving families as full members of the transdisciplinary team lessens professional conflicts and discipline loyalties because the team is unified by the family members' objectives.

Second, team building skills can also improve team functioning. **Team building** refers to the process of helping a team engage in continuous self-examination, gathering information about themselves as individuals and as a group, and using that data to make decisions (Garland & Linder, 1988). Figure 2–2 presents common team-

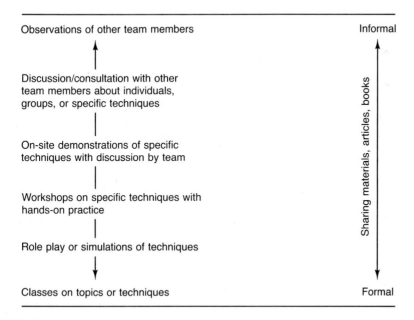

FIGURE 2–2
Models for team building. (From "Administrative Challenges in Early Intervention" by C. W. Garland & T. W. Linder in *Early Childhood Special Education: Birth to Three* [p. 19] edited by J. B. Jordan, J. J. Gallagher, P. L. Hutinger, & M. B. Karnes, 1988, Reston, VA: The Council for Exceptional Children. Reprinted by permission.)

building activities that range from informal observations of other team members to more formal activities such as classes on topics and/or techniques. The team-building process can only occur when the team leader encourages self-examination and systematically creates a climate supportive of change (Garland & Linder, 1988). Assessment tools such as the *Skills Inventory for Teachers (SIFT)* (Garland, 1979) are useful in averting difficulties that interfere with optimal teamwork. The SIFT has 150 items to assess the efficiency of team functioning and to examine attitudes affecting team dynamics.

Successful transdisciplinary teams acknowledge that rewarding teamwork is not a given, but is the result of good problem solving and team-building skills. As a consequence, more personnel preparation programs in intervention are providing systematic training in crossing discipline boundaries and team process skills.

A speech therapist with training in pediatrics cautioned, "I never let anyone do my evaluations or re-evaluations. I am very careful about what task I release to others. I never lose sight of the fact that the bottom line is that I am responsible for the quality of services a family gets. Transdisciplinary teaming works for me because I am very careful about what I am willing to release." Successful transdisciplinary teams invest hard work, practice, and trust. Additionally, certain personal, professional, and administrative characteristics seem to enhance successful teamwork.

Personal Characteristics

Personalities described as open, cooperative, and with a willingness to share and listen are necessary personal characteristics of transdisciplinary team members (McCollum & Hughes, 1988). A willingness to take risks also enhances an individual's ability to make changes often demanded by transdisciplinary teaming (Garland & Linder, 1988). The temperaments involved in a team are as important as the professional expertise each team member contributes to team decision making. Team members must acknowledge that they need each other to accomplish their goals.

An infant interventionist with a background in nursing and early childhood remarked, "I was afraid to talk (in the team meetings) in the beginning. I was used to doing 'my own thing' and not having anyone quiz me about why I was doing it. I had to really work at it. I think I have become a better person because of transdisciplinary teamwork. I am more open—less defensive—with everyone now. Even my husband!"

To actively control personal variables that may interfere with rewarding teamwork, members must re-examine their personal views of the validity of other disciplines' contributions, and how families are to be involved in service delivery. Differences in individual beliefs about the mission of a program will spill over into team dynamics and ultimately lead to interpersonal tensions.

Professional Characteristics

The objective is not to come to staffings to merely endorse what other professionals suggest from their area of expertise, nor is it to defend one's professional perspective. Protection of professional turf is a common conflict in transdisciplinary teaming. At times, disciplines overlap in both assessment and management, and this may strain transdisciplinary work. For example, the child psychiatrist, social worker, special educator, and behaviorally trained pediatrician may all feel capable of managing an acting-out toddler and working directly with a family. But when solutions differ, teamwork is stressed.

Other times, due to different discipline orientations, there may be a tendency to resist strong leadership by one discipline. Professionals from some disciplines may feel that some disciplines are not as important in serving families as others. Nonetheless, these attitudes are sometimes altered when professionals face the multiple demands placed on them by families.

As one occupational therapist noted: "I would find myself in a home with a family and the mother would start crying and telling me about the troubles she was having with her in-laws ignoring her C. P. (cerebral palsied) child and I would just feel panicked. I didn't know how to handle it. If she wanted to talk about her son's motor skills, I was ready to go but this end of intervention was all new to me. My team members taught me some communication techniques that have saved my life. I can see now how I can help the whole family now if I have to. I am learning a lot. Mostly I am getting real good at saying (to my team), 'Help me. What should I do?'"

Although professional differences or biases may never be eliminated completely, nor should they be, input from as wide a variety of professionals as possible still offers the best potential for meeting the needs of young handicapped children.

Administrative Characteristics

Through hiring practices, administrators can often control both personal and professional characteristics that encourage the success of the transdisciplinary approach to service delivery. Administrators must allow time for the team to plan, practice, and critique their work together. Administrators should regard teaming time as part of a strategy that ensures quality services. One infant program director commented, "It may look like a coffee break to someone from the outside, but my staff is working on teaming skills. They have to trust one another to put their ideas out for everyone to agree or attack, as the case may be. Administrators have to give time for this."

Ambiguous roles can introduce team conflict and tension. Administrators need to openly clarify team members' roles, duties, and responsibilities (Garland & Linder, 1988). In some programs, administrators serve as team leaders. In others, team leaders are selected from the team membership. Still others rotate the role of team leader by caseload. Whatever the case, strong leadership is essential for transdisciplinary teaming. Professionals must have experience and maturity to function both as team leaders in some circumstances and as equal partners in others. Team leaders must have the ability to foster a climate of mutual trust, in addition to the following abilities (Woodruff & McGonigel, 1988):

- □ communicate their belief in the transdisciplinary model and their commitment to making the model work
- □ listen and analyze what is being said
- □ participate in and manage a group

TRANSDISCIPLINARY CASES

A PARENT SPEAKS OUT

At 32 months of age, Rachel was referred to an infant intervention program by the family's pediatrician. She was the ninth of 11 children. Rachel's divorced mother was unemployed and did not marry Rachel's father. An arena assessment revealed delayed verbal comprehension (receptive language), limited single word speech (expressive language), and awkward fine motor coordination. Generally, Rachel's receptive and expressive language functioning were at about the 22-month-old level and fine motor skills were at about the 23-month-old level. Interviews with Rachel's mother revealed that Rachel was 6 weeks premature, and had experienced chaotic early sensory stimulation because her mother separated from her husband around the time of Rachel's birth. They divorced when Rachel was 20 months old.

The transdisciplinary team consisted of a psychologist, a speech therapist, an occupational therapist, and a special educator. All but the special educator were employed part-time by the program. The team nominated Bill, the psychologist, to be case manager for Rachel and her family, and team leader for the team, because he had room on his caseload. The psychologist also provided direct services to the family. At the time of intake, Rachel's mother was job searching and desiring child care

for her two other preschool children and after-school care for the school-aged children in the home. Rachel's mother appeared uncomfortable taking a decisive role in Rachel's arena assessment and first IFSP.

Because of the mother's occupational plans, intervention consisted of assisting Rachel's enrollment in a child care program (for nonhandicapped children) in which the other preschool children were also eventually placed. The plan involved training sessions for the child care staff in conjunction with evening home visits with Rachel's mother. After training and consultation from the speech therapist and the occupational therapist, the psychologist conducted the home visits to implement the plan the team and Rachel's mother had collaboratively written. Because the psychologist was new to infant intervention, he requested weekly training sessions with the therapists. On two occasions, the occupational therapist also came on home visits to follow up on techniques that had been released.

After 7 weeks in the program, Rachel's mother revealed, "I knew something was wrong with Rachel but I am glad that someone else thinks so too. I couldn't believe they helped me find child care for my kids and sends Bill to work with me on Thursday nights. Sometimes, Rachel's father will try to be there too. Sometimes, he can't get

- □ organize and conduct meetings
- □ manage the team's time efficiently
- □ supervise staff, regardless of their disciplinary backgrounds
- □ facilitate decision making
- □ include families as equal team members

Also, administrators can control the size of a team. As a group increases in size, the potential for information sharing and discussion from each member decreases (Spencer & Coye, 1988).

SUMMARY OF PROCEDURES

The transdisciplinary approach to infant intervention demands particular personal, professional, and administrative characteristics to function optimally. Skills in role release, arena assessment, group communication techniques, decision-making strate-

off work. I was afraid when I went in for them evaluations. Rachel was afraid too. I didn't know what to say when they asked me what I wanted for Rachel. All I want is for her to talk right."

PROFESSIONALS SPEAK OUT

Ricky, 22 months, suffered severe malnutrition and maternal deprivation during the first year of life due to his mother's drug addiction. At 14 months Ricky was removed from the home, placed in foster care, and referred for infant services. Ricky's foster care mother had two other school-aged foster children, as well as two school-aged birthchildren. Ricky had no access to children his own age and his foster mother reported that because he was especially small for his age, everyone in the family tended to baby him. After an arena assessment and an interview with Ricky's foster mother (his birth mother was unavailable), the team and the foster mother concluded that language development (receptive and expressive) and planned experiences with other young children were needed. Ricky manifested mild to moderate delays across most developmental domains.

Because of Ricky's placement in foster care, his social worker was selected by the transdisciplinary team as the case manager. The social worker had never served as a case manager, nor participated in a transdisciplinary team. Consequently, he had mixed feelings about handling the case, particularly because three agencies were involved. The social worker reported, "I've worked in bureaucracies all my professional life so when they told me I was going to be case manager of a transdisciplinary team, I first said, 'Great, what's that?' Then I said, 'Why me?' Reluctant? Yes, I was reluctant! I thought, 'Oh, boy, here we go again!' I mean, how could three different agencies cooperate; much less find a time to meet? But, after some stalling, it worked out, and I learned a lot. The team and his foster mother decided it was best for Ricky to be in a center-based infant program and have occasional home visits. Not everyone agreed though. The infant program person wanted an immediate placement in the early intervention program while his pediatrician wanted more of a wait-and-see kind of plan. The compromise was to go with the center program and hold off on home visits right now. His foster mother and his natural mother—who wants to regain custody—attend [training] sessions there [the infant program]. The team will meet at least once a year. I can see some progress in Ricky. The team just held my hand and got me through the intake and assessments. . . . I can see how this will reduce the messages Ricky's foster mom and real mother get. The teamwork stuff will probably get easier next time."

gies, and team building are not commonly demanded of child development professionals. Yet a lack of training in team dynamics and experience may contribute to poorly functioning teams. Although transdisciplinary teaming is not considered the easiest approach to intervention, many contend the benefits to the child and the family make the effort worthwhile. A summary of key procedures from this chapter follows:

1. Use professionals representing a variety of disciplines, offering a variety of services, to meet the complex demands of at-risk and handicapped children and their families.
2. Use the transdisciplinary approach to infant and toddler services to increase chances of unified services to families.
3. Employ team-building strategies to improve cross-discipline communication. Use program time for meetings to share formal and informal cross-discipline information and for follow-up to improve transdisciplinary teaming.

4. Include families as fully functioning members of teams. This entails professionals accepting families' expectations and limits on the degree to which they care to be involved. It also involves allowing parents to be parents.
5. Use arena assessments and role release for shared program planning and implementation, to increase opportunities for truly integrated services for families.
6. Establish explicit guidelines for skills that can be shared, in addition to well-delineated procedures for follow-up of released skills, to control the quality of services.
7. Alter interpersonal and team dynamics to improve the effectiveness and satisfaction of transdisciplinary teamwork.
8. Develop a plan for conflict resolution before disputes arise to ensure smoother team functioning. Handle team dysfunction swiftly by improving communication skills, and developing conflict resolution, decision-making, and team-building skills.

SUMMARY

The quality of the transdisciplinary approach is no better than the quality of the disciplinary expertise, mutual respect, and group process skills of the participants. Differences and tension among team members must be combatted for the good of the child and the family. Although conceptual models for identifying team dysfunctions are available, research is needed to identify better techniques to improve team functioning. Further, research examining the efficacy of the transdisciplinary approach of intervention is needed. The transdisciplinary team approach only provides general guidelines for forming teams and encouraging effectiveness. It is up to team leaders and members to create an atmosphere conducive to effective team operation. Because of its structure, the transdisciplinary approach establishes high standards for communication and collaboration. However, when this approach works well, professionals have the chance to expand their skills through role release and parents have the chance to feel truly invested in a program.

DISCUSSION QUESTIONS

1. How do the multidisciplinary and transdisciplinary approaches to infant intervention differ?
2. What are the strengths and weaknesses of using arena assessments?
3. What are some of the potential liabilities of role release? How does a professional handle limit setting with another professional who does not share the same perspective?

APPLIED ACTIVITIES/PROJECTS

1. Interview infant interventionists on their views of multidisciplinary versus transdisciplinary services for families. Ask for a detailed defense of the approach seen as most productive for their program.

2. Assume you are working in a home-based program for infants who are at risk for delayed development. You have a colleague who has difficulty with the concept of role release. Using the communication techniques discussed in this chapter, role play a staff meeting in which the issue is brought up, and bring it to a resolution.

3. Role play a transdisciplinary staff meeting with professionals from nursing, special education, early childhood, speech therapy, and physical therapy. Select a team leader and case manager for a hypothetical family. Identify a conflict you assume you might encounter in the field and work toward a resolution as a team. Limit decision making to 30 minutes.

SUGGESTED READINGS

Infants and Young Children. Frederick, MD: Aspen. This is a quarterly professional journal concerned with early identification and treatment for the birth to 3 group and directed toward an interdisciplinary audience.

Jordan, J. B., Gallagher, J. J., Hutinger, P. L., & Karnes, M. B. (Eds.). (1988). *Early childhood special education: Birth to three.* Reston, VA: The Council for Exceptional Children.

Journal of Early Intervention. Reston, VA: The Council for Exceptional Children; Division of Early Childhood. This professional journal, formerly called *Journal of the Division for Early Childhood,* publishes articles about at-risk and handicapped children from birth to preschool, and their families.

Peterson, N. (1987). *Early intervention for handicapped and at-risk children: An introduction to early childhood special education.* Denver, CO: Love Publishing.

Topics in Early Childhood Special Education. Austin, TX: PRO-ED. This topical professional journal addresses issues and treatment of infant and preschool at-risk and handicapped children.

Zero to Three. Washington, DC: National Center for Clinical Infant Programs (NCCIP). NCCIP is a national clearinghouse offering services and information to professionals and families involved in infant services. Articles in its journal are timely and from a transdisciplinary orientation.

REFERENCES

Bailey, D. B. (1984). A triaxial model of the interdisciplinary team and group process. *Exceptional Children, 51,* 17–25.

Bailey, D., DeWert, M., Thiele, J., & Ware, W. (1983). Measuring individual participation on the interdisciplinary team. *American Journal of Mental Deficiency, 88,* 247–254.

Bennett, F. C. (1982). The pediatrician and the interdisciplinary process. *Exceptional Children, 48,* 306–314.

Crisler, J. R. (1979). Utilization of a team approach in implementing Public Law 94–142. *Journal of Research and Development in Education, 12,* 101–108.

Drew, C. J., & Turnbull, H. R. (1987). Whose ethics, whose code: An analysis of problems in interdisciplinary intervention. *Mental Retardation, 25,* 113–117.

Fewell, R. (1983). The team approach to infant education. In S. Garwood & R. Fewell (Eds.), *Educating handicapped infants: Issues in development* (pp. 299–322). Rockville, MD: Aspen.

Fordyce, W. (1982). Interdisciplinary process: Implications for rehabilitation psychology. *Rehabilitation Psychology, 27,* 5–11.

Garland, C. W. (1979). *Skills inventory for teachers.* Lightfoot, VA: Child Development Resources.

Garland, C. W., & Linder, T. W. (1988). Administrative challenges in early intervention. In J. B. Jordan, J. J. Gallagher, P. L. Hutinger, & M. B. Karnes (Eds.). *Early childhood special education: Birth to three* (pp. 5–28). Reston, VA: The Council for Exceptional Children.

Garland, C., Woodruff, G., & Buck, D. (1988). *Case management.* (Division for Early Childhood White Paper). Reston, VA: The Council for Exceptional Children.

Gilliam, J. E., & Coleman, M. (1981). Who influences IEP committee decisions? *Exceptional Children, 47,* 642–644.

Healy, A., Keesee, P., & Smith, B. (1989). *Early services for children with special needs: Transactions for family support.* Baltimore, MD: Paul H. Brookes.

Karnes, M. B., & Stayton, V. D. (1988). Model programs for infants and toddlers with handicaps. In J. B. Jordan, J. J. Gallagher, P. L. Hutinger, & M. B. Karnes (Eds.), *Early childhood special education: Birth to three* (pp. 67–108). Reston, VA: The Council for Exceptional Children.

McCollum, J. A., & Hughes, M. (1988). Staffing patterns and team models in infancy programs. In J. B. Jordan, J. J. Gallagher, P. L. Hutinger, & M. B. Karnes (Eds.), *Early childhood special education: Birth to three* (pp. 129–146). Reston, VA: The Council for Exceptional Children.

Pfeiffer, S. I. (1982). The superiority of team decision making. *Exceptional Children, 49,* 68–69.

Smith, B. (Ed.). (1988). *Mapping the future for children with special needs: P.L. 99–457.* Iowa City: University of Iowa Press.

Spencer, P., & Coye, R. (1988). Project BRIDGE: A team approach to decision making for early services. *Infants and Young Children, 1*(1), 82–92.

Tingey, C. (1986). Early intervention: Learning what works. *Exceptional Parent, 16,* 32–37.

Turnbull, A. P., & Turnbull, H. R. (1990). *Families, professionals, and exceptionality: A special partnership.* (2nd ed.). Columbus, OH: Merrill.

Wolery, M., & Dyk, L. (1984). Arena assessment: Description and preliminary social validity data. *The Journal of the Association for the Severely Handicapped, 9,* 231–235.

Woodruff, G. (1980). Transdisciplinary approach for preschool children and parents. *The Exceptional Parent, 10*(1), 13–16.

Woodruff, G., & McGonigel, M. J. (1988). Early intervention team approaches: The transdisciplinary model. In J. B. Jordan, J. J. Gallagher, P. L. Hutinger, & M. B. Karnes (Eds.), *Early childhood special education: Birth to three* (pp. 164–181). Reston, VA: The Council for Exceptional Children.

PART II

INTERVENTION STRATEGIES FOR DEVELOPMENTAL DOMAINS

3

Neuromotor Development in Infants and Toddlers

Toby M. Long and Sharon A. Raver

OVERVIEW

This chapter discusses early motor development and the role of the developmental therapist on the transdisciplinary team with infants and toddlers who have neuromotor dysfunctions. It includes:

- □ terminology used to describe central nervous system dysfunctions
- □ major neurodevelopmental treatment models
- □ management of feeding problems
- □ appropriate handling and positioning techniques
- □ use of adaptive equipment

The development of efficient motor skills is an important prerequisite to normal cognitive, social, and communication development (Malpass, 1963). Environmental exploration, through controlled movement, is basic to the child's learning because early motor experiences form the groundwork for later learning. Many infants and toddlers who are developmentally delayed, disabled, or at risk have difficulty organizing their sensory and motor systems in ways that allow for successful interaction with objects and people.

Because of the adaptability and plasticity of the infant's brain, the first 18 months of life are seen as a particularly crucial time for motor intervention (Bobath & Bobath, 1964). Intervention during this period attempts to maximize the potential of children with diagnosed or suspected motor deficits. Traditionally, developmental therapists provide therapeutic intervention directly to the child, often in one-to-one situations. Today, however, more developmental therapists recognize the value of working in teams.

ROLE OF THE DEVELOPMENTAL THERAPIST IN TEAMS

The term **developmental therapist** was first used by Banus and colleagues (1971) and now is used to describe the overlapping roles of occupational and physical therapists in their work with very young children with special needs. Developmental therapists play a significant role in facilitating motor control, improving muscle strength, increasing range of motion, and enhancing physical endurance. Since the passage of P.L. 94–142, the Education of the Handicapped Act, providers of related services, such as developmental therapists, have struggled to define their role in early intervention.

Now with the focus on teamwork mandated in P.L. 99–457, many developmental therapists participate with other professionals on teams to design and implement Individualized Family Service Plans (IFSP) with families. Although multidisciplinary and interdisciplinary teams are common approaches, the transdisciplinary team model is frequently recommended because it facilitates the free exchange of information, skills, and knowledge among disciplines (Woodruff & McGonigel, 1988).

As discussed in Chapter 2, the transdisciplinary approach streamlines intervention efforts through the process of role release (United Cerebral Palsy National Collaborative Infant Project, 1978). Developmental therapists teach other team members, including the family, intervention strategies that traditionally have been part of their role responsibilities. Today, developmental therapists may not be the professionals providing direct services to the child. Consequently, they must train the assigned primary service provider in techniques necessary for the child's motor management. Therapists decide which skills are appropriate to be released and which are not. Generally, only therapeutic techniques, not evaluation, assessment, or accountability, are released (Giangreco, York, & Rainforth, 1989). Table 3–1 compares the roles of developmental therapists on interdisciplinary and transdisciplinary teams.

Additionally, therapists are responsible for ensuring that those trained have some basic understanding of why certain strategies facilitate normal tone and movement. A regular schedule for training and monitoring released skills is imperative to support team members and the child's family. When skills are released in this way, there can be a blending of therapeutic and developmental strategies that significantly promotes generalization by the child.

Communication between developmental therapists and professionals from other disciplines is essential for effective transdisciplinary teaming. When the child's primary need is in the motor area, developmental therapists may be selected by the team to act as the family's primary service provider and/or case manager. Although this is common, it is not always the case because of the inconsistent availability of staff, parental requests, and caseload limitations. In general, the role of the developmental therapist is to

- collaborate with the other team members in designing the child's program
- embed therapeutic intervention into all program activities
- provide role support through training and monitoring of the primary service provider, the family, and other team members as needed

TABLE 3–1

Comparison of developmental therapist's roles in interdisciplinary and transdisciplinary team models.

Case: Jenny, 18-month-old child, with a diagnosis of right hemiplegia, is beginning to ambulate. She prefers to use her left arm because movement in her right arm is difficult. She does not cross midline, transfer objects, or reach above her head with her right arm. Her range of motion is limited in her shoulders, making dressing difficult.

Interdisciplinary Team Model		Transdisciplinary Team Model	
Education goal:	Jenny will reach out and grab a doll from the toy shelf, in 7 out of 10 trials with her right arm.	Goal:	Jenny will be able to push both arms through her jacket or into an over-the-head shirt during dressing in all settings.
Physical therapy goal:	Jenny will increase the range of motion of right shoulder flexion by 10°.		

Activities	Activities
A. Jenny will be requested and encouraged to reach up and grap her doll from the shelf with her right arm (setting: infant program).	A. During circle time, one teacher-directed activity will be chosen that requires the children to reach above their heads to carry an object or clap, etc. During the activity, the primary service provider will passively move Jenny's arm through full range of motion, incorporating gentle shoulder joint mobilization. (Developmental therapist [DT] will instruct primary service provider in proper range-of-motion and mobilization techniques. DT will monitor these activities weekly.)
B. Jenny will receive passive range-of-motion exercises with mobilization to her right shoulder (setting: physical therapy room twice weekly for ½ hour sessions).	
C. Parents will be taught range-of-motion exercises to be done each evening prior to bed (setting: home).	B. Similar routines will be carried out prior to and as needed throughout table top activities and prior to feeding; home and center.
	C. Jenny will be positioned in prone with arms over a wedge or roll encouraging full shoulder forward flexion during a fine motor or art activity. Prior to the activity, the primary service provider will provide gentle passive range-of-motion and inhibition techniques to decrease synergistic posturing. (DT will monitor and train primary service provider and family weekly, and as needed.)

Transdisciplinary teamwork can be challenging. All team members must be committed to this perspective for services to be integrated, interactive, and family-focused. Ultimately, the quality of services families receive continues to rest with the quality of training and follow-up developmental therapists offer the primary service providers.

TERMINOLOGY

Certain terms are necessary in forming a shared vocabulary with developmental therapists. It is important to understand terms used to describe different types of movement, **tone,** and concerns about children with atypical motor development.

Supine refers to lying on the back; **prone** refers to lying on the stomach. **Flexion** refers to the bending of a part of the body at a joint. **Extension,** the opposite of flexion, means to straighten out. **Hyperextension** pertains to straightening out a part of the body beyond the range considered typical. **Hypertonia** is increased muscle tone; **hypotonia** is decreased muscle tone. **Extensor posturing** refers to the maintenance of the extremities or trunk in a straightened or extended position. It is usually seen in children with increased tone in the extensor muscles. The **labyrinthine reflex** is a primitive reflex that usually is lost by 3 months of age in nonhandicapped children. If the child is lying in a supine position, the posture is characterized by legs straightening out, shoulders retracted, neck arched, and head pressed against the surface. **Disassociation** is the ability to move one segment of the body while holding another segment still, or moving in the opposite direction. **Midline** refers to the middle segment of the body. **Proprioceptive** is a term to describe the sensory receptors found in joints that sense where the body is in space. **Nonprogressive** means that a condition does not worsen over time. **Orthotics** are orthopedic appliances used to support, align, prevent, or correct deformities or to improve the functioning of movable body parts. **Apgar scores** measure the effect of loss of oxygen and damage to the circulation of newborns. Scores higher than 6 are associated with an adequate prognosis; scores of 3 to 5 have a 20% incidence of neurodevelopmental problems (Batshaw & Perret, 1981).

CENTRAL NERVOUS SYSTEM DYSFUNCTION

The central nervous system consists of the brain and the spinal cord. Many developmental disabilities result from damage to some portion of the central nervous system that causes the individual's motor repertoire to be reflexive and stereotyped (Batshaw & Perrett, 1981). Epilepsy, mental retardation, and cerebral palsy are common examples of central nervous system dysfunction. Children who manifest a motor disability with no known cause may also have a central nervous system dysfunction.

Although individual intervention strategies need not depend on the specific diagnosis (Harris & Tada, 1983), it is important for team members to have a basic understanding of the common conditions typically referred to developmental therapists for treatment. Table 3–2 describes the **etiology,** or cause, and motor characteristics of some common handicapping conditions. The motor disabilities of children with cerebral palsy, spina bifida, and Down Syndrome influence their ability to explore the environment efficiently.

Cerebral Palsy

Cerebral palsy (CP) is the term used to describe a nonprogressive disorder of movement or posture caused by a lesion to the immature brain. Handicaps associated with

TABLE 3–2
Motor characteristics of common handicapping conditions.

Condition	Etiology	Characteristics	Associated Conditions (Present in some but not all cases)
Arthrogryposis multiplex congenita	Unknown; disease begins prenatally	Fixed limbs, joint deformities, muscle atrophy, normal intelligence	Congenital heart disease, respiratory disorders
Cerebral palsy	Multiple prenatal, perinatal, and postnatal causes that lead to anoxia or brain hemorrhage	Nonprogressive disorder of movement or posture with abnormalities of muscle tone and in coordination	Mental retardation, speech disorders, visual deficits, hearing loss, seizure disorders, perceptual problems
Myelomenigocele	Embryonic neural tube defect of multifactorial (genetic and environmental)	Varying degrees of lower extremity paralysis due to protrusion of spinal cord through opening in vertebrae	Hydrocephalus, bowel and bladder incontinence, loss of sensation, mental retardation, visual-perceptual deficits
Spinal muscle atrophy	Autosomal recessive or autosomal dominant inheritance	Progressive weakness and atrophy of proximal muscles (hips, shoulders, and trunk) appearing in early infancy; normal intelligence	Respiratory disorders and joint contractures secondary to muscle weakness
Osteogenesis imperfecta	Autosomal dominant inheritance	Brittle bone disease with multiple skeletal deformities and frequent fractures; normal intelligence	Deafness, respiratory deficits secondary to bony deformities of rib cage
Juvenile rheumatoid arthritis	Unknown	Autoimmune disease characterized by painful, swollen joints and limited movement; normal intelligence	Joint contractures and deformities

Source: Reprinted from *Educating Handicapped Infants: Issues in Development and Intervention* by S. G. Garwood and R. R. Fewell, p. 346, with permission of Aspen Publishers, Inc., © 1983.

TABLE 3–3
Classification of cerebral palsy.

Movement Disorder	Characteristics
Spasticity	Hypertonic, increased muscle tone, diminished voluntary muscle control, associated with birth asphyxia
Athetosis	Slow, writhing, extraneous movements of the extremities, upper extremities more often affected, frequent oral-motor involvement, associated with kernicterus
Ataxia	Diminished balance, lack of proximal muscle control, lower extremities more often affected, very unstable gait, associated with cerebellum insult

Topographical Distribution	Characteristics
Hemiplegia	One side of the body affected, upper extremities more affected than lower, upper extremity hypotonia, associated with birth trauma
Diplegia	All extremities affected, lower extremities significantly more affected, spasticity most often present, associated with problems of prematurity
Quadriplegia	All extremities affected, upper extremities more affected than lower, mental retardation common, associated with problems with asphyxia and PVL (penventricular leukomalacia)

cerebral palsy are sensory impairment, visual impairment, seizure disorders, learning disabilities, communication disorders, mental retardation, and behavior disorders.

The more severe the neuromotor dysfunction, the greater the likelihood of multiple handicaps (Molnar, 1985). Because of motor handicaps, it is difficult to accurately assess the cognitive functioning of children with more involved forms of cerebral palsy such as quadriplegic cerebral palsy (all extremities affected). In spite of this, the incidence of mental retardation is reported to be between 40 to 60% (Shotick, 1978).

The incidence of cerebral palsy has remained relatively constant during the last 40 years. Although there appeared to be a decrease in the incidence of certain types of CP during the 1960s (Kudjavcer, Schoenberg, Kurland, & Grover, 1984), the general incidence remains about 2 per 1,000 live births (Paneth, 1986). Some suggest there may be a rise in the incidence of spastic diplegic CP (involvement in all extremities, with lower extremities more affected) due to the survival rates of very low birthweight infants.

Classification systems have been developed that describe cerebral palsy according to the type of the movement disorder. The most widely accepted system was developed by the American Academy of Cerebral Palsy and Developmental Medicine (Minear, 1956). Table 3–3 shows this classification system.

The etiology of CP is usually divided into prenatal, perinatal, and postnatal categories. Prenatal factors include those related to heredity, infections, Rh incompatibility, metabolic disorders, fetal anoxia, and developmental deficits of the brain. Unfortunately, unknown causes account for about 30% of all cerebral palsy cases in the prenatal category (Bleck & Nagel, 1975). Perinatal factors are those that happen around the time of birth and include brain trauma or injury, asphyxia, and problems related to a premature delivery. Problems associated with prematurity account for 33 to 60% of all cases of cerebral palsy. Postnatal factors include brain injury due to trauma, toxicity, anoxia, tumors and brain infections including bacterial and viral encephalopathies.

It is very difficult to predict the course of a child's development from descriptive information about the type of cerebral palsy. The data from The National Collaborative Perinatal Study (Nelson & Ellenberg, 1984), which collected data on 54,000 pregnancies and deliveries, found that low birthweight and clinical asphyxia were factors most associated with cerebral palsy. Nonetheless, no one factor definitively predicts cerebral palsy.

Spina Bifida

Myelomeningocele, meningocele, spina bifida occulta, and anencephaly are conditions caused by **neural tube defects**. With an incidence of 0.4 to 1.0 in every 1,000 live births, neural tube defects are among the most common birth defects (Anderson, 1989).

These defects are caused by abnormal fetal development which results in a lack of bony closure around the spinal cord. **Myelomeningocele** involves a protrusion of the spinal cord. In **meningocele** only the coverings of the cord (meninges) are protruding. **Spina bifida occulta** is a bony defect in which there is failure of the posterior bones of the spinal column to form. **Anencephaly**, the most serious of the neural tube defects, is a lack of closure of the part of the nervous system that would form the cerebral hemispheres and is considered fatal (Melnick & Myrianthopoulos, 1987).

These spinal defects require immediate surgical repair, which damages the spinal cord. Handicaps associated with spinal defects are **hydrocephalus**, lack of bowel and bladder control, learning disabilities, mental retardation, and bony abnormalities of the back and lower extremities.

The incidence of neural tube defects is higher in females, mid-spring conceptions, and in families of low socioeconomic status (Badell-Ribera, 1985). The incidence in the United States has been reduced to 0.50 per 1,000 births (Windham & Edmunds, 1982). The etiology of these defects is still uncertain, but generally it is assumed they are related to a number of factors such as familial predilection and influence by unknown environmental agents.

The motor disability seen in children with myelomeningocele is characterized by flaccid paralysis in those muscles that receive innervation from the nerves at the level of the protrusion. As meningoceles and spina bifida occulta do not involve nerves, paralysis is not common.

Down Syndrome

Down Syndrome, the most common chromosomal abnormality in humans (Kozma, 1986), is caused when the child has extra chromosome material. The nondisabled child has 46 chromosomes. The child with Down Syndrome has 47. The most common type of Down Syndrome is characterized by an extra chromosome on the 21st chromosome pair and is called **trisomy 21**. Trisomy 21 develops as a result of non-disjunction of two homologous chromosomes upon conception.

There are two other forms of Down Syndrome. The translocation type is due to breakage of chromosome 21 during cell division. This broken piece of chromosomal material attaches to another chromosome, providing extra chromosomal material. The third type of Down Syndrome, Mosaicism, accounts for only 1 to 2% of all cases and is caused by some cells being affected while others remain normal. The percentage of affected cells varies from child to child.

Congenital heart defects are present in about 40 to 60% of all cases of Down Syndrome (Kozma, 1986), and approximately 40 to 60% have hearing losses (Pueschel, 1984). Physical features include marked hypotonia, a flat nasal bridge, epicanthal folds, small mouth, and low-set ears. Additionally, a child with Down Syndrome may have intestinal problems, respiratory infections, thyroid problems, vertebral instability, and present a range of mental retardation (Kozma, 1986).

The majority of children with Down Syndrome fall in the moderately retarded range. Harris (1981) found that young children with Down Syndrome perform significantly higher on cognitive than motor testing. Hypotonia and joint hyperextensibility influence the child's ability to develop muscular stability which in turn influences motor milestones.

OTHER CONDITIONS THAT INHIBIT NEUROMOTOR DEVELOPMENT

Many developmental disabilities are difficult, if not impossible, to diagnose in the first 2 years of life. Generally, infants and toddlers who manifest atypical motor development or motor difficulties do not have an identified diagnosis. These children are often first suspected of having a developmental problem because of a delay in achieving gross motor milestones. After the child is assessed, a general delay in most areas of development is discovered and the child is categorized as developmentally delayed.

At-risk children often have conditions that increase the likelihood of motor difficulties, such as blindness or low birthweight. Certain characteristics seem related to increased risk (Sweeney, 1985). For instance, the infant with a **hypertonic profile** tends to be irritable, tolerates only minimal handling, shows disorganized movements and extensor posturing, and may have decreased mobility of oral musculature. The infant with a **hypotonic profile** tends to be difficult to arouse, molds easily, fixates at the shoulders and hips (stiffens the muscles around the joints), and may have a weak suck or poorly coordinated suck-swallow mechanism. Children with hypotonia, decreased anti-gravity movement, hyperextension of the neck, elevated and retracted shoulders, decreased midline arm movements, excessively extended trunk, immobile pelvis, and weight bearing on toes when held in standing tend to be at high risk for motor problems.

TREATMENT MODELS

Although many treatment or therapeutic intervention programs are used, there are three approaches that are commonly associated with treatment of infants and toddlers with central nervous system dysfunctions. These approaches are the neurodevelopmental treatment approach (NDT), the proprioceptive neuromuscular facilitation (PNF) approach, and the sensorimotor approach. Each approach focuses on facilitating the coordination of movement, centers on normal sensorimotor development, and incorporates sensory stimulation in its treatment strategies. Additionally, these approaches stress the importance of caregiver follow-through in regular home routines. Similarities and differences in these theoretical approaches are presented in Table 3–4. Typically, most developmental therapists use a combination of these approaches, or the holistic approach.

Neurodevelopmental Therapy

The neurodevelopmental treatment approach (NDT) was developed by Karel and Berta Bobath more than 40 years ago for the treatment of individuals with cerebral palsy (Bobath & Bobath, 1952). Over the years it has become one of the most widely

TABLE 3–4
Theoretical approaches to intervention strategies.

Case:	Phillip, an 8-month-old infant with Down Syndrome, is functioning at the 4-month level in gross-motor skills as measured by an age equivalent on the Bayley Motor Scales.
Goal:	Improve developmental activities in prone position.
Objective:	Phillip will maintain a prone-on-elbows position for 5 seconds, 3 of 4 trials, for 5 consecutive days.

Neurodevelopmental Treatment Approach	Proprioceptive Neuromuscular Facilitation	Sensorimotor Approach to Treatment
1. Inhibit tonic labyrinthine reflex in prone position. 2. Facilitate equilibrium responses in prone position over large therapy ball. 3. Facilitate protective extension in prone position over large therapy ball.	1. Place infant in prone-on-elbows position and encourage head-raising with visual or auditory stimuli. Provide resistance to head-raising by pushing down into flexion. 2. Provide joint compression through head and spine in prone position. 3. Provide joint approximation through shoulders into elbows.	With child in prone position on mat: 1. Apply joint compression through head and spine. 2. Provide fast brushing to posterior neck and upper trunk muscles. 3. Apply joint compression through shoulders to elbows.

Source: Adapted from *Educating Handicapped Infants: Issues in Development and Intervention* by S. G. Garwood and R. R. Fewell, p. 352, with permission of Aspen Publishers, Inc., © 1983.

accepted treatments and is often used as the basis of treatment for other neuromotor disabilities (Harris, 1981; Stern & Gorga, 1988). Unlike the other two treatment strategies, a therapist can obtain certification in this approach by attending an 8-week training program. However, certification is not required to incorporate NDT principles and strategies into a holistic treatment plan.

The goals of the NDT approach are to

☐ facilitate normal muscle tone to allow normal movement patterns to occur
☐ facilitate automatic postural responses
☐ prevent secondary complications such as contractures (irreversible shortening of muscle fibers that causes decreased joint mobility) and deformity (Bobath, 1980)

It is believed that in reaching these goals the child's neurological system is available to learn efficient and functional motor skills.

The goals of NDT are reached through specific handling of the child. Treatment techniques attempt to inhibit abnormal movement patterns and facilitate automatic and volitional movements. The NDT approach stresses the importance of facilitating automatic responses rather than teaching specific exercises. Because the infant develops movement patterns in all positions, the child is handled in a variety of positions. Proponents of NDT stress early treatment (Köng, 1966; Bobath, 1980) because early treatment is believed to influence the development of basic movement patterns that develop during the first years of life. Although the NDT approach is commonly used, the empirical data on the effectiveness of neuromotor programming neither supports nor refutes the value of NDT (Horn, 1989).

Proprioceptive Neuromuscular Facilitation

Proprioceptive neuromuscular facilitation (PNF) is another intervention strategy that is based on the concepts of normal neuromotor development. PNF, like NDT, uses sensory stimulation to facilitate movement. Specific patterns of movements that incorporate spiral and diagonal movement components are the hallmark of PNF techniques. The originators of the technique, Knott and Voss (Voss, 1972), emphasize the importance of motor learning that incorporates both volitional control and automatic reaction to specific stimulation.

Additionally, resistance is applied when handling the child because it is believed that resistance will produce a strong muscle action contributing to stronger sensory feedback. PNF stresses auditory feedback as one of its primary sensory modalities. The tone of the therapists voice can facilitate or inhibit the child's progress. Extremely loud voices are not recommended for infants and young children because they may produce a negative effect (Harris & Tada, 1983).

Sensorimotor Approach

Margaret Rood's treatment approach is based on the duality of sensorimotor functions (Stockmeyer, 1972). This duality includes mechanisms that allow for movement to occur and mechanisms that allow for the maintenance of body posture. These two mechanisms form the basis for four general stages of neuromotor function that, in turn, lay the groundwork for normal motor development. These stages include

□ mobility (movement of the arms and legs, as seen in the first few months of life)
□ stability (the infant's ability to prop up on both arms)
□ mobility in a weight-bearing pattern (unilateral reaching in the prone position)
□ mobility in a non-weight-bearing position (manipulation)

Various sensory modalities are used to facilitate mobility and stability. Besides handling the child, this treatment approach utilizes modalities such as icing, brushing, and vibration to produce a muscle contraction. A holistic program of intervention is stressed through the interplay of motor, language, and cognition. It is believed that attainment of high level skills is dependent upon the child's ability to process all environmental input. Just a few studies, addressing only isolated techniques, have been conducted using sensory stimulation procedures, so it is difficult to quantify the empirical effectiveness of this approach (Horn, 1989). Nonetheless, there is widespread clinical acceptance of this approach.

Other Treatment Models

Although the treatment models just discussed are the most frequently used in therapeutic programs, patterning, myofascial release, craniosacral therapy, reflex therapy, sensory integrative therapy, and neurorehabilitation are other approaches used. Some of these approaches, such as patterning and myofascial release, are controversial. Patterning, or neuromuscular reflex therapy, is based on promoting motor development through the recapitulation of primitive patterns of movement and requires significant time commitments from caregivers. Other models, such as sensory integrative therapy and neurorehabilitation, are respected in the therapeutic community and are often part of a holistic therapy program.

Adjuncts to Therapy

Because of the complexity of neuromotor dysfunctions, it is not enough to provide only therapeutic handling. A holistic developmental therapy program is also concerned with orthopedic and functional impairments. Adaptive equipment and orthotics, such as tone reducing casts or ankle foot orthosis, are often used. Children with spina bifida tend to be fitted with appropriate orthotics around 8 to 12 months of age when they are ready to begin standing and make attempts at ambulation. Neuromuscular stimulation in the form of biofeedback or functional electrical stimulation and orthopedic surgery to lengthen tendons are other treatments used with toddlers after 2 years of age. A relatively new neurosurgical procedure—selective dorsal rhizotomy, involving the cutting of some of the sensory nerves in the spinal cord—is becoming popular as an alternative treatment for certain children with spastic cerebral palsy.

FEEDING TECHNIQUES

Infants and young children with central nervous system dysfunction frequently have oral motor problems which lead to feeding difficulties. Infants may have problems sucking, coordinating a suck-swallow pattern, or maintaining a seal on a nipple. These difficulties are typically seen in preterm infants and may be due to immaturity of the neuromotor mechanism that controls these skills. Abnormal motor patterns controlling the lips, tongue, and facial musculature may also be responsible for these problems. Further, persistence of primitive oral reflexes can influence the efficiency of movement during feeding.

Morris and Klein (1987) divide feeding problems into three categories:

☐ problems with function of individual oral structures
☐ problems with sensory processes
☐ problems with the feeding processes

Many children with neuromotor dysfunction have a combination of these problems.

Guidelines for the Treatment of Oral Motor Dysfunction

To improve oral motor functioning, team members must

☐ rule out any medical complications that could influence feeding function
☐ collaborate with the family and other team members to determine feeding needs
☐ collaboratively design a functional oral motor intervention plan
☐ provide intervention within a whole body context

Treatment of oral structures and feeding skills can only be effective when combined with intervention involving the extremities and trunk because of the strong interplay between oral mechanisms and the body.

When oral motor difficulties are present, feeding can be a stressful time for the child as well as the family. Parents indicate that feeding problems are one of the most persistent, stress-related experiences they share with their children. Low cheek tone and lip retraction are common feeding problems. Suggested intervention for these problems follows.

Problem 1: Low cheek tone and decreased strength in the cheeks, which reduce the infant's ability to maintain an adequate suck on a nipple.

Intervention: Provide tactile and proprioceptive input to the infant's cheek by stroking each cheek from the jaw line out toward the temporomandibular joint (the joint that connects the jaw to the cheek bone). Use firm yet gentle pressure. This may be needed intermittently throughout the feeding session and may be done during breastfeeding.

Problem 2: Due to hypertonia, lips are pulled back over the mouth (lip retraction), making it difficult to suck.

Intervention: Feed in a quiet environment, making sure the child is in a well-supported position with the extremities flexed and in toward the midline of the body.

Because of the interplay between oral mechanisms and the body, improvement of feeding skills involves intervention with the extremities and trunk.

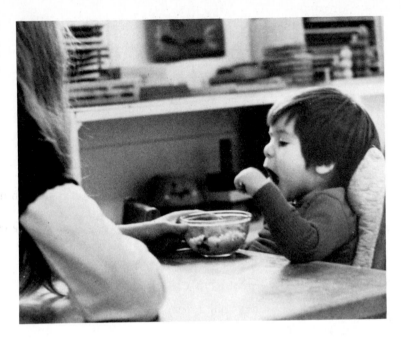

Prior to feeding, and throughout the meal as needed, wipe the child's face in toward the lips with a cloth or fingers. Use firm but gentle and consistent pressure.

Difficulty processing sensory input is another common problem in feeding. Hypersensitivity, long-term tube feedings, and choking and/or gagging are frequently observed in children with neuromotor dysfunctions. A suggested intervention for each follows.

Problem 1: Hypersensitivity, resistance to touch, may be caused by overstimulation to the oral area due to long-term tube feedings or intubation.
  Intervention: Feed in a quiet environment with few distractions. Using firm yet gentle pressure, slide finger around the outer surface of the lips, move from the midline out to the corner of the mouth, doing top and bottom lips. Do this prior to feeding as well as throughout feeding as needed.

Problem 2: Long-term need for nasogastric or gastrostomy tube feedings.
  Intervention: During each tube feeding provide a pacifier for the infant to suck. This will help the infant practice sucking and associate sucking with satiation.

Problem 3: Choking and gagging.
  Intervention: Assess to determine if the swallow reflex is active. Assess the infant's breathing pattern, making sure it is rhythmic and regular. Assess which types of foods tend to prompt choking in the older infant or toddler. If any of these problems are present, follow guidelines specific to the problem.

These are only a few of the problems that interfere with a positive feeding experience for the child and caregivers. Successful intervention must consider the unique characteristics of the child (e.g., oral motor strengths and weaknesses, food preferences), the environment (e.g., distractions during feeding, time of day), the caregiver (e.g., level of anxiety, preparation), and the feeding equipment (e.g., adapted bottle, chair).

THERAPY DECISIONS

In deciding to provide developmental therapy to handicapped or at-risk infants and toddlers, teams must make a series of decisions that affect the child, the family, and intervention staff. Traditionally, in the **direct service delivery model**, children demonstrating atypical motor development are recommended to receive therapy directly from physical or occupational therapists. This individualized therapy may be part of a center- or home-based program or may be provided in a clinic. The number of sessions per week varies, but typically two to three times per week is recommended. Depending on the setting, a home program and/or a classroom positioning schedule may be established.

In contrast, developmental therapists in the **consultative service delivery model** evaluate the child and provide therapy suggestions for the child's caregivers and intervention professionals. Suggestions include handling, position changes, and/or specific exercise programs. It is the responsibility of the consulting developmental therapist to monitor the program, and frequently reevaluate the therapeutic plan.

In the **transdisciplinary team service delivery model**, however, it is unnecessary to make decisions regarding direct versus consultative services. Motor assessment is part of a comprehensive evaluation conducted by all members of the team. Based on the team's findings and the family's needs and priorities, goals are generated that view the child's motor needs as just one significant component of the child's developmental needs. Therapeutic motor activities are embedded into developmental areas so the complete child profits from interventions. Because motor development is crucial during the first years of life, it is common for developmental therapists to be asked to serve as the primary service provider when motor delays are the major developmental concern for the child.

The process of role release inherent in the transdisciplinary team model also means that other team members release their skills to developmental therapists. As this teaming approach grows in acceptance, it is becoming increasingly clear that formal training among team members, usually consisting of weekly sessions, produces the highest quality of services for families. Unfortunately, decisions about which service delivery model to use are often based on the availability of therapists and funding resources rather than which model would most benefit the child and family.

Play

Infancy and toddlerhood are also critical times for social development and the emergence of play skills. It is generally agreed that learning and development take place within the context of the child's transactions with the environment. Transactions, or social interplays—between the child, environmental demands often placed by the caregiver, and the caregiver—provide a natural structure for intervention for infants with special needs (Williamson, 1988). Play for infants or toddlers with disabilities or who are at risk should be designed to

□ enhance normalization
□ develop enjoyable leisure activities
□ facilitate specific areas of development
□ reduce undesirable behaviors
□ train for necessary skills (Musselwhite, 1986).

Within a therapeutic framework, play can be a natural vehicle for facilitating motor skills and may motivate the child during motor activities. Toys should be selected that are appropriate for the child's age and ability level. Children with atypical motor development need toys that can be easily manipulated and adapted. Williams, Briggs, and Williams (1979) suggest basic adaptations to increase the appropriateness of play materials for children with motor limitations. For example, they suggest that play materials may need to be stabilized, enlarged, prosthetized, or made more familiar or concrete. Manipulations required may need to be minimized by changing switch mechanisms. Toys may need to be less distracting by removing extraneous cues (e.g., taping sections of the toy) or made more inviting by enhancing cues (e.g., adding sounds to the action). Some materials may need to be made more durable or safe.

Finally, they suggest that materials may need to be made physically and mechanically accessible, a special concern for the child with movement dysfunctions. **Physical accessibility** entails changing the position of the toy or material, or the position of the child, to allow the child better access to the material. Play gyms, which allow toys to be suspended, increase the child's involvement with materials. Placing the child in a sidelying position or in a supported sitting position could also allow the child better accessibility. **Mechanical adaptation** refers to making changes to the switches of mechanical toys to allow the child to control the toy independently (Musselwhite, 1986). Adding a push switch to a wind-up toy makes it easier for the child to play with the toy without assistance.

In addition to adapting toys or using toys as therapeutic equipment, play is an excellent form of movement exploration. Creative movement experiences may be designed to meet therapeutic goals. For example, facilitating equilibrium reactions in an 18-month-old could easily be enhanced by dancing rhythmically to music or waving streamers either while sitting or standing. Play-oriented transactions have the additional benefit of increasing child and caregiver pleasure and, consequently, involvement.

Prespeech

The development of speech involves the complex coordination of oral musculature, oral reflexes, and respiration. This coordination begins at birth and continues to develop and refine during the first years of life. The time between birth and the utterance of a child's first meaningful words is considered the prespeech period (O'Conner, Williamson, & Siepp, 1983). During this period, the coordination necessary for voice production and speech are developed through oral reflex maturation and the oral motor control used in feeding and oral play (vocalizations).

The child's oral reflex maturation and the ability to drink, suck, swallow, and take solid foods are related to later skill in speech. In addition, prespeech development depends on the coordination of breathing and phonation. The child must be able to breathe in a regular rhythmical pattern. Abnormal trunk tone or an inability to stabilize the trunk inhibits smooth breathing. Infants at risk for speech production dysfunction often demonstrate a pattern of shallow and irregular breathing.

Guidelines for the treatment of breathing and phonation dysfunction. As with feeding, it is important to first rule out any medical complications that might contribute to respiratory problems. Prior to initiating a prespeech program, consultation with the speech-language pathologist is also advised. Commonly, breathing and phonation problems are handled by placing the child in a position in which breathing, and consequently phonation, are easier for the child. For example, the interventionist might consider one or more of the following:

- □ place the infant in a sidelying position (to decrease hyperextension or hyperflexion of the trunk) to facilitate rhythmical breathing
- □ stimulate phonation by applying gentle pressure to the ribcage while at the same time vocalizing a vowel such as "ooooo"
- □ decrease tone in the trunk during sitting by rotating and turning the trunk while vocalizing rudimentary vowel-consonant combinations such as "baaabaaabaa"

As with all intervention, such activities are best when they are incorporated into the child's regular routines.

ASSESSMENT

Assessment of children with atypical or delayed motor development may be done for screening, diagnosis, and program planning purposes.

Screening

Screening is the first step in identifying infants and toddlers requiring developmental support. Two popular screening tools are the Denver Developmental Screening Test (Frankenburg, Dodds, Fandal, Kazuk, & Cohrs, 1975) and the Milani-Comparetti Motor Development Screening Test (Kliewer, Bruce, & Trembath, 1977). The Denver Developmental Screening Test assesses gross- and fine-motor, language, and personal-social skills. Results are classified as normal, abnormal, or questionable, based on the number of passed items at a certain age. This test is often used by physicians as a part of well-baby visits. The Milani-Comparetti Motor Development Screening Test attempts to correlate functional motor achievement with underlying neurological functioning. It assesses the maturity of neuromotor reflexes, automatic reactions, and protective and equilibrium reactions. Both tests are considered fairly reliable in identifying children at risk and are easy to administer.

Diagnosis

Diagnostic tools provide information regarding how the child compares with children of the same age. Many general diagnostic instruments, such as the Bayley Motor Scale, part of the Bayley Scales of Infant Development (Bayley, 1969), give information about motor development as well as functioning in other developmental domains. Standardized tools such as this allow interventionists to determine whether the child has achieved motor milestones, but do not provide information about the quality of the child's movement.

A standardized motor evaluation tool that provides information about the quality of movement is the Peabody Developmental Motor Scales (Folio & Fewell, 1980). This tool assesses both fine- and gross-motor skills from birth through 7 years of age. A variety of normed scores can be derived including percentile rank, motor age equivalent, and a developmental motor quotient. A developmental profile, which outlines the child's strengths and weaknesses, can be generated.

Standardized tools are not sufficient for planning purposes and must be supplemented with nonstandardized assessment instruments. The Movement Assessment of Infants (MAI) (Chandler, Andrews, Swanson, and Larson, 1980) is a nonstandardized tool popular with developmental therapists. It was developed to identify motor dysfunction, establish a basis for early intervention, and monitor the effects of therapy when motor behavior is below the 12-month level. The MAI also provides guidelines for making clinical observations of movement quality. It assesses reflex maturation, muscle tone, and volitional movement. A high-risk score can be obtained on children 4 months of age or older.

Program Planning

Using the information gained from standardized or nonstandardized diagnostic instruments, interventionists design strategies that use the child's strengths and minimize or ameliorate deficits and abnormalities. Functional skills, rather than developmental milestones, are stressed. To ensure that intervention focuses on the whole child, criterion-referenced curricula are often used by developmental therapists to identify skills in areas other than motor. For programming purposes, items should be adapted, when possible, to permit the child's best performance. Interpretation of test results should consider the degree of prematurity, the quality of movement patterns, muscle tone, and functional skill performance.

PROGRAMMING

As team members, developmental therapists attempt to integrate neurodevelopmental strategies for enhancing posture and movement into the child's total developmental plan. To accomplish this, therapists must adapt curricula, recommend appropriate handling and sensorimotor activities, and design adaptive equipment.

Adapt Curricula

Fewell and Sandal (1983) describe several guidelines for adapting curricula. They recommend the following to better meet the needs of children with movement dysfunctions:

- □ use proper handling prior to an activity to diminish detrimental effects of abnormal posturing and tone
- □ use appropriate positioning to assist the child in maintaining neutral postures
- □ increase access to programming materials and activities
- □ arrange activities in a manner that minimizes movements required by the infant to accomplish the tasks

To facilitate motor development, goals must be clearly delineated; activities must facilitate automatic reactions, protective responses, and equilibrium reactions; and suggestions for generalizing skills must be stated. Positioning and handling suggestions are helpful in adapting instruction.

Determine Positioning

Proper positioning, integrated into the infant's daily routine, can greatly affect the muscular imbalance often seen in infants and toddlers with atypical motor development. **Positioning** is placing the child in certain postures that attempt to promote symmetrical body alignment, normalize muscle tone, and promote functional skills. For instance, when placed in the supine position, the hypotonic baby often "fixes" against gravity (the child stiffens the muscles around the hips and shoulders to maintain a posture). But placing the child in prone and sidelying positions enhances flexion and counteracts shoulder retraction and neck hyperextension so the child has a more normalized posture. Demonstrations of common handling and positioning techniques are shown in Figures 3–1 and 3–2.

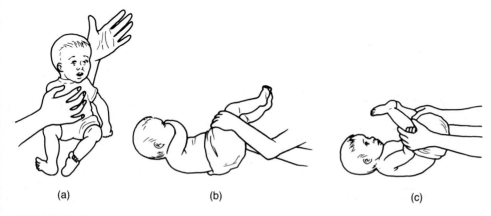

(a)   (b)   (c)

FIGURE 3–1
Sensorimotor activities during routine caregiving. (a) Facilitate head lifting when burping. (b) Decrease lower extremity hypertonicity during diaper change. (c) Inhibit shoulder retraction during diaper change.

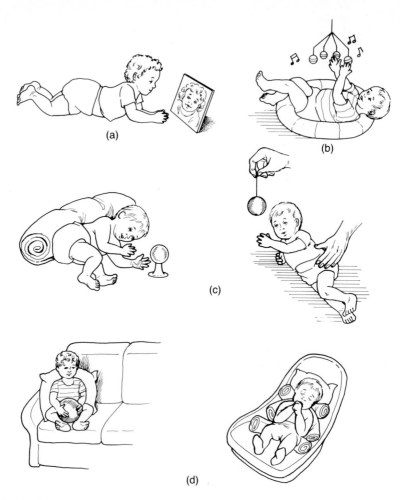

FIGURE 3–2

Activities for promoting symmetrical body alignment, normalized muscle tone, and functional skills in infants and toddlers. (a) To increase weight bearing on upper extremities, place toys near child to encourage reaching and shifting of weight from arm to arm. (b) To increase head alignment with body, and movement of arms and legs in front of child, place child supine in a small inflatable swim ring and dangle toy 8 to 12 inches from child's chest. (c) To increase manipulation of toys, and bringing hands together and to the mouth, place child in a supported sidelying position. (d) To increase the chances of hands being brought together in front of face with the shoulders rounded, place the child in an infant seat using rolled blankets under each shoulder. (From *Tips from Tots: A Resource Guide for Your Infant and Toddler. Mighty Movements 1, 2* [pp. 1–2] by C. Baker and T. Long, 1989, Palo Alto, CA: VORT. Copyright © 1989 by Toby Long. Reprinted by permission.)

The creative use of blankets, diapers, and/or towel rolls in prone, sidelying, and supine positions with head support can help increase flexion. The flexed position is also helpful in decreasing **disorganized** (random and uncoordinated) **movements**. All positioning should be done so the child is placed in the center of family activity and, when appropriate, with another child nearby to encourage child-to-child play.

To increase weight bearing on the upper extremities, place a rolled towel, diaper, or small blanket under the child's arms. This encourages the child to lift the head and take weight on the forearms. A bright toy or mirror placed in front of the child encourages head lifting.

The supine position should only be used when adaptations are made for proper body alignment. To facilitate a chin tuck and prevent shoulder retraction, place a small roll or wedge under the child's head. To facilitate hip flexion and foot-to-mouth action, place a small wedge under the child's hips. Suspend toys from an activity gym to encourage swiping.

A supported sidelying position encourages midline activity with the hands and promotes hand activity without movement of the legs. The trunk should remain symmetrical and the head should be supported so it is aligned with the trunk.

The goal of supported sitting is to maintain a straight trunk with the pelvis placed directly under the hips. A small wedge under the hips facilitates erect sitting. Many children have difficulty maintaining an upright posture in a high chair for feeding. A small wedge placed at the back may be helpful. The seat belt of the high chair should be around the hips, not the waist. Modification of the infant seat or vehicle safety seat may be needed for small or preterm infants. Place small rolls behind the shoulders to decrease retraction and facilitate a midline orientation so hands are free to manipulate materials.

Select Sensorimotor Activities

As described in the treatment models section, sensory input though tactile, vestibular, proprioceptive, visual, and auditory stimuli is used to assist the infant in achieving quality interaction with caregivers and normal posture and movement. Swaddling is a form of tactile stimulation that is valuable in promoting flexion and midline orientation in the very young infant. Swaddling also helps to decrease irritability, especially in preterm infants (Figure 3–3).

Vestibular movement, such as rocking and swinging, is helpful for some children. Slow, repetitive movement in a vertical direction can soothe the irritable infant. Quicker movements or more abrupt movements in the horizontal plane are arousing. Swaddling during movement provides additional tactile input to assist in calming the infant. It is important to maintain a flexed position during movement. Older infants or toddlers may tolerate more vigorous movement such as rhythmical bouncing when held at a therapist's shoulder or being rocked horizontally.

Sensorimotor activities are easily built into caregiving routines. To facilitate head lifting, for example, sit the infant up for burping during feeding. Decrease hypertonicity in the legs during diaper changes by gently rocking the infant's pelvis.

FIGURE 3–3
Common position and sensorimotor activity for preterm infants.
Small blanket rolls behind the
shoulders decrease retraction;
swaddling prevents flexion and
may decrease irritability in preterm infants.

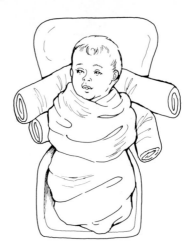

Shoulder retraction can be inhibited by providing weight bearing on the shoulders during diapering.

Appropriate carrying of the infant can also assist to normalize muscle tone and promote body alignment. Carry the child in a sitting position, with the adult's forearm under the thighs, using the adult's trunk for support. Face the child away from the adult to vary the child's visual experience. Carry the child by holding the infant facing out diagonally across the adult's body, with the adult's arm through the child's legs to promote trunk rotation, disassociation, and improve phonation. Support the infant under the axilla, the armpit, on the side of the body closest to the ground.

Adapt Equipment

Adaptive equipment is used to enhance functional skills in children with abnormal muscle tone, limited range of motion, decreased strength, and poor muscle control. **Adaptive equipment** is any device or material that enhances the independence of the child by controlling for abnormal postural responses. A towel roll is considered a piece of adaptive equipment when used with infants. As children grow the equipment often becomes more complicated and expensive.

For the child with lower extremity hypertonicity, facilitate weight bearing and an upright posture through the use of a prone stander or supine board. Sidelyers, benches, and child-size tables and chairs may also be helpful.

Bolsters and wedges are simple pieces of adaptive equipment often seen in early intervention programs. They are used for trunk support when the child is placed in the prone position. The supported prone position facilitates head lifting and upper extremity weight bearing.

Proper positioning in sitting is important for toddlers. Sitting provides access to table activities, and places children on the same level as their peers. Many children with multiple handicaps need adaptive sitting devices for transportation and inde-pendent mobility. To adapt or design a chair, the child should sit in the chair with

Sensorimotor activities are easily
built into caregiving routines.

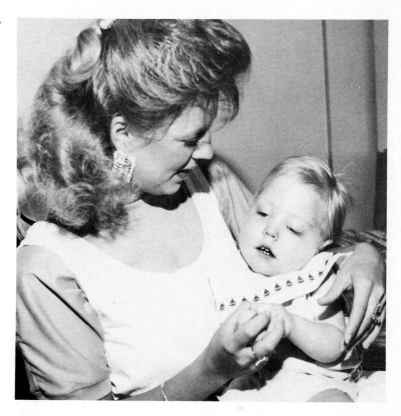

the hips, knees, and ankles maintained at 90° angles. The safety belt should fit at the hips and shoulders, and may need to be supported. The chair should be lightweight and flexible. The chair should be useful for a variety of situations such as table sitting and moving about the room.

Aesthetics are an important consideration in designing adaptive equipment and may influence the child's social integration. Adaptive equipment should only be considered if it increases the child's opportunities for exploration, socialization, and community involvement.

In summary, appropriate therapeutic programming for young children with neuromotor dysfunctions requires the collaborative effort of all team members. A consistent plan of intervention with all staff members is necessary. Today, motor dysfunction is viewed as part of the total developmental needs of the child, not as a separate area of concern. Emphasizing the use of therapeutic strategies throughout all daily activities produces the most satisfying results. The following case studies illustrate the often enormous demands placed on families with children with neuromotor dysfunctions and the potential for changes in the child and family when intervention is begun early.

TRANSDISCIPLINARY CASES

THE GREEN FAMILY

Danny Green, a 22-month-old boy, was born at 25 weeks gestation weighing 580 g (about 1.5 pounds). He is the firstborn in a two-parent, professional family. His Apgar scores were 4 at 1 minute, and 5 at 5 and 10 minutes. Neonatal complications included respiratory distress syndrome, bronchopulmonary dysplasia, hyperbilirubinemia, and grade II and III intraventricular hemorrhage (refer to Chapter 6 and the Glossary for descriptions of these conditions). Danny had a stormy hospitalization. He had difficulty fighting infections and became septic on three separate occasions. He also underwent surgery for necrotizing enterocolitis and was diagnosed as having stage III retinopathy of prematurity.

While in the hospital he was enrolled in The Chronically Ill Infant Intervention Project (C–III). This special project provides interdisciplinary team services (special education, occupational therapy, nurse practitioner) in the hospital and home setting until the child is 2 years of age. When discharged from the hospital at 4 months, Danny was at significant risk for developmental problems. He required oxygen therapy through a nasal cannula until 8 months. He developed significant feeding problems requiring multiple changes in his formula and feeding routine. He was followed closely by a nutritionist and was readmitted to the hospital twice for failure to thrive.

Danny received weekly developmental support from an educator and an occupational therapist. For the first 6 months after discharge, the nurse also made weekly home visits. Danny's parents'

flexible work schedules allowed them to be integrally involved in his developmental program. Danny was also followed regularly by a hospital-based clinic that provides follow-up services for infants until 24 months of age.

At 12 months, Danny scored significantly below average on the Bayley Scales of Infant Development, even when scores were adjusted for his degree of prematurity. His motor development was influenced by severe hypotonia and weakness. The hospital clinic team recommended a center-based early intervention program. However, the family chose to add the services of a private physical therapist and educational specialist to complement the C–III program instead. The private interventionists worked closely with the C–III team to provide a well-coordinated program and became part of the family's Individualized Family Service Plan.

Although Danny is at high risk for severe developmental problems, it appears he may have only minor motor delays. He began walking at 18 months of age. Feeding problems have diminished and he now tolerates a variety of foods in increasing quantities. Because of his progress and parental agreement, C–III team home visits have been reduced to biweekly. The family reports they continue to feel comfortable with their decision to initiate private therapy in lieu of a center-based program. Danny is now involved in a weekly mother's day out group as well as attending an out of home child care arrangement.

The Greens remain pivotal members of the intervention team. They appear to accept the possibility that Danny will need special help throughout

SUMMARY OF PROCEDURES

The developmental therapist is a principal resource for assessment and intervention strategies for transdisciplinary team members. Developmental therapists train other professionals on their team, including families, to carry out therapeutic activities with children with motor deficits. They assume responsibility for systematically training and monitoring skills that have been released. Additionally, they learn skills outside their discipline from team members so they are able to provide comprehensive, integrated services to families. A summary of the key concepts of this chapter follows.

his school years and indicate they are pleased with how far he has come in only 22 months.

THE BOLLE FAMILY

Michael Bolle, 20 months old, was born at 25 weeks gestation weighing 920 g (a little more than 2 pounds). Michael is the third child of a two-parent, professional family. Apgar scores were 1 at 1 minute and 6 at 5 minutes. Neonatal complications included respiratory distress syndrome, bronchopulmonary dysplasia, stage I retinopathy of prematurity, and periventricular leukomalacia (see Chapter 6 and the Glossary for definitions). Michael had a difficult hospitalization. He was intubated, breathing through a tube connected to a respirator, for several months. He was irritable and difficult to console because he tolerated only minimal handling.

The Bolles had difficulty communicating their concerns to the hospital neonatal intensive care unit (NICU) staff. They expressed anger at physicians for painting such a bleak developmental picture of their son. The family experienced extreme stress that eventually led to Michael's father's slow withdrawal from involvement in Michael's care.

Michael was discharged from the hospital at 6 months of age, requiring 24-hour oxygen therapy and 24-hour nursing services. At 10 months, Michael was referred to a home-based infant education program where he receives weekly developmental services. He also receives private physical therapy twice weekly and private infant education services weekly.

Michael has always demonstrated significant delays and an atypical pattern of development. He is severely hypertonic in all extremities and hypotonic in his trunk. Primitive reflexes persist, interfering with the attainment of motor skills. At 12 months, he was evaluated by a pediatric orthopedist and a pediatric physician who diagnosed cerebral palsy. Although Mrs. Bolle suspected this diagnosis, she still found it difficult to accept. She provides Michael with the best services she can obtain and follows through with all medical and developmental appointments.

At 16 months, Michael no longer required the use of oxygen, but he remains medically fragile because of his respiratory condition. He receives nursing services 18 hours a day and continues with multiple home visits from various specialists. The specialists communicate regularly through the use of a communication book left in his home. Slowly, the Bolles are beginning to become more involved with Michael's care. They now include Michael in family outings and he spends more time with the family in the kitchen and family room. Mr. Bolle is also spending more time with Michael.

Since Michael's birth, the family has been consumed with stress and uncertainty. Although one cannot predict the future, it appears that Michael's motor handicaps may influence his development in all skill areas. The family has begun to differentiate Michael's strengths from his weaknesses. This continues to be a difficult process for the family. Supporting each family member is a major focus of intervention with this family, in the hope that the stress and feelings of helplessness will become more manageable.

1. Use consultation and shared observations between the developmental therapist, the family, and other professionals to identify the quality of motor performance so individually tailored intervention plans may be developed.
2. Use tactile and proprioceptive experiences to reduce oral structure problems and problems in sensory processing that interfere with feeding.
3. Use physical accessibility and mechanical adaptation to enhance materials manipulation in infants and toddlers with movement dysfunction.
4. Use proper positioning and tactile stimulation to facilitate breathing and phonation necessary for prespeech development.

5. Embed appropriate handling, positioning, and therapeutic activities into all developmental interventions and into daily caregiving routines.
6. Use adaptive equipment to enhance independence and to control for movement and posture abnormalities in infants and toddlers.

SUMMARY

Although infants are born with most basic movements, they must develop postural control and coordination of movement in order to manage their world efficiently. Infants and toddlers with disabilities, and those at risk for disabilities often have barriers to the development of functional movement that limit their ability to explore and learn. The role of the developmental therapist as a team member serving such children is currently in transition. Today, therapy services may be offered by the direct service model, the consultative model, or the transdisciplinary team model. Through the process of role release, developmental therapists assume the responsibility to teach families and other professionals the correct physical management of the child with neuromotor dysfunctions. In addition, they learn skills from their team members from education, nursing, social work, and child development (Harris & Tada, 1983). Whatever the model of teamwork or the choice of service delivery, the goal of developmental therapists continues to be to assist families in their efforts to facilitate an effective system of movement in their children.

DISCUSSION QUESTIONS

1. Some developmental therapists are uncomfortable with the transdisciplinary team approach. What reasons may have prompted these feelings and how can they be reconciled?
2. A 2-year-old child with cerebral palsy "walks" with a walker, but she walks on her toes and is flexed over the walker. Her parents are pleased and would like her to practice walking so she can be the flower girl in her uncle's wedding. They request that ambulation training be part of her IFSP. The developmental therapist disagrees with this, stating that the child is not ready to walk as she needs to decrease her muscle tone and improve lower extremity weight bearing. Using a family-centered approach, how can this dilemma be resolved?

APPLIED ACTIVITIES/PROJECTS

1. Select a partner for a role play in which one of you is a parent and the other is an infant interventionist. Explain to the parent the following terms and how they are involved with a child's motor functioning: flexion/extension, hypotonia/hypertonia, handling/positioning, neurodevelopmental treatment, adaptive equipment. Avoid the use of jargon.
2. Interview two parents with children about the same age with similar family compositions. One parent should have an infant born prematurely and the other an infant born at fullterm. Make an adjustment in the child's age for prematurity. Gather information regarding caregiving activities (schedules for feeding, sleeping, and daily activities), development of the infant (all domains and temperament), and parent opinions regarding their relationship with their child, their concerns, and needs. Write a comparison of the two families. In what ways do the families' needs differ?

SUGGESTED READINGS

Finnie, N. (1974). *Handling the young cerebral palsied child at home*. New York: Dutton.

Hanson, M. J., & Harris, S. R. (1986). *Teaching the young child with motor delays: A guide for parents and professionals*. Austin, TX: PRO-ED.

Katz, K. S., Pokorni, J. L., & Long, T. M. (1989). *Chronically ill and at-risk infants: Family-centered intervention from hospital to home*. Palo Alto, CA: Vort.

Occupational Therapy Practice. A quarterly journal for developmental therapists. Available from Aspen Publishers. Frederick, MD 21701–9782.

Penso, D. E. (1987). *Occupational therapy for children with disabilities*. Frederick, MD: Aspen.

Sweeney, J. (Ed.). (1986). *Physical and occupational therapy in pediatrics*. New York: Haworth Press.

REFERENCES

Anderson, S. M. (1989). Secondary neurologic disability in myelomeningocele. *Infants and Young Children: An Interdisciplinary Journal of Special Care Practices, 1,* 9–21.

Badell-Ribera, A. (1985) Cerebral palsy: Postural-locomotor prognosis in spastic diplegia. *Archives of Physical Medicine and Rehabilitation, 66,* 614–619.

Banus, B. S., Hayes, M., Kent, C. B., Komick, M. P., & Sukiennicki, D. C. (1971). *The developmental therapist: A prototype of the pediatric occupational therapist*. Thorofare, NJ: Slack.

Batshaw, M., & Perret, Y. (1981). *Children with handicaps: A medical primer*. Baltimore, MD: Paul H. Brookes.

Bayley, N. (1969). *Bayley scales of infant development manual*. New York: Psychological Corporation.

Bleck, E. E., & Nagel, D. A. (Eds.). (1975). *Physically handicapped children: A medical atlas for teachers*. New York: Grune & Stratton.

Bobath, K. (1980). *A neurophysical basis for the treatment of cerebral palsy* (2nd ed.). Philadelphia: Lippincott.

Bobath, K., & Bobath, B. (1952). A treatment of cerebral palsy based on the analysis of the patient's motor behavior. *The British Journal of Physical Medicine, 15*(5), 107–117.

Bobath, K., & Bobath, B. (1964). The facilitation of normal postural reactions and movements in cerebral palsy. *Physiotherapy, 50,* 526–532.

Chandler L. S., Andrews, M. S., Swanson, M. W., & Larson, A. H. (1980). *Movement assessment of infants: A manual*. Rolling Bay, WA: Movement Assessment of Infants.

Fewell, R. R., & Sandall, S. R. (1983). Curricula adaptations for young children: Visually impaired, hearing impaired and physically impaired. *Curricula in Early Childhood Special Education, 2*(4), 51–66.

Folio, M., & Fewell, R. (1980). *Peabody Developmental Motor Scales and activity cards*. Allen, TX: Teaching Resources.

Frankenburg, W. K., Dodds, J. B., Fandal, A. W., Kazuk, E., & Cohrs, M. (1975). *Denver Developmental Screening Test: Reference manual* (Revised 1975 ed.). Denver: LADOCA Project and Publishing Foundation.

Giangreco, M. F., York, J., & Rainforth, B. (1989). Providing related services to learners with severe handicaps in educational settings: Pursuing the least restrictive option. *Pediatric Physical Therapy, 1,* 55–63.

Harris, S. R. (1981). Effects of neurodevelopmental therapy on improving motor performance in Down's syndrome infants. *Developmental Medicine and Child Neurology, 23,* 477–483.

Harris, S. R., & Tada, W. L. (1983). Providing developmental therapy services. In S. G. Garwood & R. R. Fewell (Eds.), *Educating handicapped infants: Issues in development and intervention* (pp. 343–368). Rockville, MD: Aspen.

Horn, E. (1989). Motor skills intervention for children with neuromotor deficits: Two decades of research. *DEC Communicator, 15,* 2.

Kliewer, D., Bruce, W., & Trembath, J. (1977). *The Milani-Comparetti Motor Development Screening Test.* Omaha, NE: Meyer Children's Rehabilitation Institute, University of Nebraska Medical Center.

Köng, E. (1966). Very early treatment of cerebral palsy. *Developmental Medicine and Child Neurology, 8,* 198–202.

Kozma, C. (1986). Down Syndrome—What is it? In K. Stray-Gundersen (Ed.), *Babies with Down Syndrome: A new parent's guide,* (pp. 1–25). Kensington, MD: Woodbine House.

Kudjavcer, T., Schoenberg, B. S., Kurland, L. T., & Grover, R. V. (1984). Cerebral palsy: Trends in incidence and changes in concurrent neonatal mortality: Rochester, MN, 1950–1976. *Neurology, 33,* 1433.

Malpass, L. (1963). Motor skills in mental deficiency. In N. R. Ellis (Ed.), *Handbook of mental deficiency: Psychological theory and research.* New York: McGraw-Hill.

Melnick, M., & Myrianthopoulos, N. C. (1987). Studies in neural tube defects: Pathologic finding in a prospectively collected series of anencephalics. *American Journal of Medical Genetics, 26,* 797–810.

Minear, W. L. (1956). A classification of cerebral palsy. *Pediatrics, 18,* 841.

Molnar, G. E. (1985). Cerebral palsy. In G. E. Molnar (Ed.), *Pediatric rehabilitation* (pp. 420–467). Baltimore: Williams & Wilkins.

Morris, S. E., & Klein, M. D. (1987). *Pre-feeding skills: A comprehensive resource for feeding development.* Tucson, AZ: Therapy Skill Builders.

Musselwhite, C. R. (1986). *Adaptive play for special needs children: Strategies to enhance communication and learning.* San Diego: College-Hill Press.

Nelson, K., & Ellenberg, J. L. (1984). Obstetric complications as risk factors for cerebral palsy or seizure disorders. *Journal of the American Medical Association, 251,* 1843–1848.

O'Connor, F. P., Williamson, G. G., & Siepp, J. M. (1983). Pre-speech. In F. P. O'Connor, G. G. Williamson, & J. M. Siepp (Eds.), *Program guide for infants and toddlers with neuromotor and other developmental disabilities* (pp. 183–205). New York: Teachers College Press.

Paneth, N. (1986). Etiologic factors in cerebral palsy. *Pediatric Annals, 15,* 141–201.

Pueschel, S. M. (Ed.). (1984). *The young child with Down Syndrome.* New York: Human Sciences Press.

Shotick, A. L. (1978). Mental retardation. In W. M. Cruickshank (Ed.), *Cerebral palsy: A developmental disability.* Syracuse, NY: Syracuse University Press.

Stern, F. M., & Gorga, D. (1988). Neurodevelopmental treatment (NDT): Therapeutic intervention and its efficacy. *Infants and Young Children: An Interdisciplinary Journal of Special Care Practices, 1,* 22–32.

Stockmeyer, S. A. (1972). A sensorimotor approach to treatment. In P. H. Pearson & C. E. Williams (Eds.), *Physical therapy services in the developmental disabilities* (pp. 186–222). Springfield, IL: Charles C. Thomas.

Sweeney, J. K. (1985). Neonates at developmental risk. In D. A. Umphred (Ed.), *Neurological rehabilitation* (pp. 137–164). St. Louis, MO: C. V. Mosby.

United Cerebral Palsy National Collaborative Infant Project (1978). *Staff development handbook: A resource for the transdisciplinary process.* New York: United Cerebral Palsy Associations of America.

Voss, D. E. (1972). Proprioceptive neuromuscular facilitation: The PNF method. In P. H. Pearson & C. E. Williams (Eds.), *Physical therapy services in the developmental disabilities* (pp. 223–282). Springfield, IL: Charles C. Thomas.

Williams, B., Briggs, N., & Williams, R. (1979). Selecting, adapting, and understanding toys and recreation materials. In P. Wehman (Ed.), *Recreation programming for developmentally disabled persons* (pp. 15–36). Baltimore: University Park Press.

Williamson, G. G. (1988). Motor control as a resource for adaptive coping. *Zero to Three, 9,* 1–7.

Windham, G. C., & Edmunds, L. D. (1982). Current trends in the incidence of neural tube defects. *Pediatrics, 70, 333–337.*

Woodruff, G., & McGonigel, M. J. (1988). Early intervention team approaches: The transdisciplinary model. In J. B. Jordan, J. J. Gallagher, P. L. Hutinger, & M. B. Karnes (Eds.), *Early childhood special education: Birth to three* (pp. 163–181). Reston, VA: The Council for Exceptional Children.

4

Cognitive Development in Infants and Toddlers

Sharon A. Raver

OVERVIEW

This chapter discusses intellectual development in infants and toddlers, including:

- □ major assumptions regarding normal cognitive development
- □ effects of early experience on cognitive development
- □ Piagetian theory of early intelligence
- □ procedures for assessing cognitive development
- □ strategies for enhancing cognitive development

Infants are no longer viewed as passive recipients of care. The past 35 years of research in child development reveal that infants learn, respond, and interact from the moment they are born (Ambron, 1975). It is now believed that infants develop intellectually through a continuing interaction between their inborn abilities and the stimulation they receive from their environment (Anastasiow, 1986).

ASSUMPTIONS OF NORMAL COGNITIVE DEVELOPMENT

Generally, **cognitive development** is described as the progressive change in internal mental processes such as thinking, reasoning, and remembering, or as the ability to function adaptively in the world by receiving information from the environment, understanding the meaning of this information, and using it to plan appropriate actions (Dunst, 1981; Piaget, 1952). Early cognitive development is expressed by skills in communication, social, and motor development (Bayley, 1969; Dunst, 1981).

In infant and toddler intervention, efforts to facilitate cognitive development tend to focus on the child's ability to exert some control over the physical and social aspects of the environment. This control is critical for the development and motivation of all learning. Contemporary thinking about typical cognitive development in infants and toddlers may be summarized by the following four major assumptions.

The infant's capacity to learn is present from birth.   Studies of infant **perception** (the ability to learn or receive environmental information by using the senses of sight, hearing, smell, and/or touch) clearly indicate that the senses are the starting point for the infant's expanding understanding of the world (Lockman, 1983).

Attention to visual stimuli is developed in fullterm newborns, but in general, preterm infants have significantly less differential attentiveness to novel visual stimuli (Rose, Feldman, McCarton, & Wolfson, 1988). This lack of visual alertness may have implications for later development. A study of 100 preterm infants, from various social class and ethnic backgrounds, found that developmental functioning at age 5 could be predicted moderately well from infant visual attention evaluated as early as the term date (Cohen & Parmelee, 1983).

By contrast, research on infant visual acuity (how well the infant visually resolves patterned information) suggests that visual acuity is relatively immature at birth, although the newborn sees well at 8 to 12 inches (about the distance from the mother's arms to her face during feeding) (Neifert, 1986). By 4 months of age the normal infant can recognize internal and external parts of a compound figure; by 6 months of age, visual acuity is close to adult levels.

Research on hearing indicates that newborns hear well and respond well to their mother's voice or similarly pitched voices (Neifert, 1986). By the first month, normal infants will look in the direction of a sound in some circumstances and are able to perceive some speech sounds. By 4 months, infants turn their heads in the direction of a sound. However, differences in early experience, such as those created by very low birthweight and prematurity, can place children at a disadvantage for learning about their environment. For example, Lawson and colleagues (1984) compared the response of preterm and fullterm infants to moving objects presented with or without accompanying sound. They found differences in attention and recognition between fullterm and preterm infants at 3 months of age. At 6 months of age, the high-risk preterm infants continued to show responses different from the fullterm infants.

In some cases, disadvantages imposed by risk conditions may persist into early childhood. Gilbride (1983) evaluated 22 premature infants who experienced asphyxia or chronic lung disease (CLD) but who had no gross developmental abnormalities. Twenty-one age-matched fullterm children, with no complications, were used as the comparison group. The children who had been premature were found to be significantly inferior to the comparison group in discriminating auditory tones, perceiving rapid auditory sequences, and exhibiting receptive language skills when they were later assessed between the ages of 4 to 8 years. Similarly, profoundly handicapped infants have been found to display more reflexive than attentive behaviors and to exhibit fewer behaviors in response to auditory signals than normal infants (Flexer & Gans, 1986).

Normal infants experience a steady refinement of their perceptual and cognitive capabilities through early childhood (Yarrow, Rubenstein, & Pedersen, 1975). However, infants and toddlers with atypical early experiences and/or identified risk or handicapping conditions need to be monitored, even in the absence of gross developmental delays, so their true potential may be realized.

The infant learns through social contact.   Infants learn largely from their interactions with caregivers and their environment. In some cases, social interaction may need to be increased, modified, or regulated to facilitate the development of the child with disabilities or with at-risk conditions. For instance, Kilgo and colleagues (1988) found that preterm infants in a neonatal intensive care unit had more weight gain, and higher scores on the Neonatal Behavioral Assessment Scales, than a matching control group when the infants were provided with additional tactile-kinesthetic stimulation. Tactile-kinesthetic stimulation in this study consisted of three, 15-minute periods per day for 10 days.

Parents' perceptions of their child may influence the quality of social interaction their child receives. Infants with interrupted infantile apnea (brief absence of breathing), for example, have been reported as more active during sleep and as less acceptable by their mothers (i.e., failing to match parental expectations and hopes), than control infants (Bendell, Culbertson, Shelton, & Carter, 1986). These perceptions appeared to increase parental stress and social isolation. Although there were apparently no other developmental issues for the infants in this study, the mothers' perceptions could easily interfere with a positive parent-child relationship.

A relationship has been reported between parent interaction style and later cognitive development with preterm infants (Beckwith, 1984), and organically impaired, mentally retarded children (Mahoney, Finger, & Powell, 1985). Although research reveals a wide variation in developmental outcomes in children at risk, increasing pleasurable interactions between parents and their child seems to increase the chances of enhanced cognitive development (Beckwith, 1984).

The infant is an active learner.   Intelligence and other human capacities are not fixed at birth, but are shaped by environmental influences and experiences. Normal infants actively seek information from their surroundings, and act on it. Infants enjoy influencing people and objects. Children with special needs may appear passive and have fewer exploratory skills, so their social contact with adults and their environment may be reduced or altered. In fact, sick and/or malnourished children tend to reduce activity to decrease energy expenditure, which places them at increased developmental risk (Pollitt, 1983). Infants with severe developmental delays may need systematic assistance from caregivers to learn to actively impact their world (Dunst, 1981).

The infant affects caregivers, just as caregivers affect the infant.   Careful observation of social interaction reveals that caregivers' attention, affection, requests, physical interactions, and warmth trigger a response by the infant. The infant's response then affects caregivers in ways that may encourage or discourage further interactions. In other words, aspects of the environment interact with the infant's personal temperament and behavioral patterns and contribute to new outcomes (Dunst, 1981). Sociable infants are capable of eliciting more stimulation from caregivers; this higher social competence seems to lead to accelerated cognitive development (Lamb, Garn, & Keating, 1981).

Certain characteristics of parents' style of interaction and communication seem to influence children's developmental progress. For example, an analysis of maternal language in lower SES mothers found the proportion of imperatives (commands to the child) to be positively correlated with the child's risk status (Adams & Ramey, 1980). **Intervention coaching**, systematic training in ways to promote positive adult-child interactions, has been found to increase the frequency and duration of positive caregiver behaviors (Kelly, 1982).

Effects of Early Experience on Cognitive Development

Early experiences can affect development and learning and influence the degree to which the child's full potential is realized. Handicapping conditions may interfere with development and learning to such an extent that original disabilities become more severe and secondary handicapping conditions may develop (Peterson, 1987). Research with at-risk and handicapped infants indicates that early experiences may either facilitate or hinder the child's cognitive development.

At-risk infants. It is difficult to discuss at-risk children as a group because there are so many variables that may place their development at risk. Each risk category, such as biological risk or environmental risk, may present a unique set of circumstances. Nonetheless, research with one at-risk group, preterm infants, suggests that they are more vulnerable to environmental insufficiencies than fullterm infants. For instance, 45 newborns, weighing 1,500 g or less at birth, monitored by an annual postneonatal intensive care service until the age of 36 months, were found to function at higher levels than nonmonitored infants (Slater, Naqvi, Andrew, & Haynes, 1987). The monitored infants had a 14-point general cognitive index advantage over the nonmonitored controls. Apparently, the continued support the monitored group received was responsible for the differences noted. The researchers found mother-infant behaviors and the quality of the home environment to be most predictive of 3-year-old intellectual development for their population.

Results of longitudinal experiments designed to prevent mild mental deficits in infants in high-risk families indicate that risk frequently takes its toll by the second year of life (Ramey & Gowen, 1984). Escalona (1982) measured the cognitive development of 114 low-birthweight premature infants from primarily low-income, non-White urban families. Although the group showed normal cognitive development through age 15 months, by 28 months of age, and thereafter, a severe decline in cognitive development was associated with low SES. In addition, serious behavioral maladjustments in some children seemed to repress their cognitive development. Prevention programs have been able to reverse this effect on mental development in many at-risk children and have facilitated more positive caregiver-child interactions (Resnick, Armstrong, & Carter, 1988).

Handicapped infants. By using systematic manipulation of the environment, the cognitive functioning of handicapped infants and toddlers may be facilitated (Dunst, 1981). White (1967) demonstrated that by providing institutionalized infants with appropriate environmental experiences to coordinate eye and hand behavior, reaching could be accelerated. The control group, without the benefit of these arranged experiences but in the same setting, developed the ability to reach more than a month later. Research on parent-infant intervention with biologically handicapped infants suggests that **maternal locus of control** (how much control the mother feels she has over what happens to her) has an influence on child developmental gains following intervention (Maisto & German, 1981). The pattern seems to be particularly true for cognitive and language development.

As discussed in Chapter 1, early stimulation/intervention research has produced varied results, with some studies reporting impressive results and others reporting modest changes. Nevertheless, systematic intervention in infancy and toddlerhood appears to create opportunities for positively altering cognitive functioning. Although little uniformity in the philosophical orientation of intervention services exists, many employ Piaget's conceptual framework for stimulating early thinking, reasoning, and problem-solving skills.

PIAGETIAN THEORY OF INTELLIGENCE

Piaget's cognitive-developmental theory is an attempt to map how thinking is acquired and organized (Piaget, 1951; 1952). Piaget outlines four major cognitive stages, to about 11 years of age, characterized by the acquisition of more differentiated mental skills. In Piaget's view, intelligence develops from early motor patterns that are transformed into symbolic thought patterns at later stages, assisted by the process of maturation. Piaget's emphasis on *active* child participation in the construction of knowledge has been embraced by professionals in their efforts to stimulate the cognitive development of young children exhibiting delayed or atypical sensory and motor development.

According to Piaget's construct of intellectual development, infants between birth to 3 years of age experience two significant intellectual periods. They first pass through the sensorimotor period and then begin their passage into the preoperational period (Piaget & Inhelder, 1969).

Sensorimotor Period

The first period of intellectual development, birth to about 2 years of age, is called the **sensorimotor stage**. The sensorimotor period is seen as a crucial time for establishing future intellectual functioning. In this stage, reflexes enable infants to interact with the environment. Patterns, or *schemas* as Piaget called them, link with other behaviors and, if they produce certain results, are repeated (Piaget, 1952). Infants develop and refine intellectual concepts through play, especially play with objects.

During the sensorimotor stage, infants construct reality through looking, listening, and manipulating to combine, modify, and invent new schemes. In the beginning of this stage, infants' interactions are characterized by trial and error. But by the end of the period, toddlers have developed internal symbolic thought. They can quickly solve problems mentally without relying on sensory and motor actions (Piaget & Inhelder, 1969).

Infants' strengths and weaknesses in sensorimotor development influence their evolution of symbolic behavior, reasoning, and later adaptive skills because the skills learned in this period are the foundation for communication, social, self-help, and later reasoning skills (Langley, 1989). Table 4–1 presents examples of sensorimotor goals and sample behaviors for intervention planning. Visual pursuit and object permanence, means-ends relationships, causality, construction of objects in space, imitation, and behaviors relating to objects are concepts that develop simultaneously during the sensorimotor period (Piaget & Inhelder, 1969).

Visual pursuit and object permanence.   These two concepts involve the ability to attend to critical events in the environment and the ability to develop systematic searching, organization, and memory skills. **Auditory localization** (turning head toward sound) and **visual pursuit** (visually following objects) are precursors to object permanence. **Object permanence** is the understanding that an object out of view still exists somewhere else. When the child has developed object permanence, the child searches for an object seen hidden, pulls a cloth from the face or the face of others, and uncovers partially hidden and then later, fully hidden objects (Langley, 1989). Instructional objectives for facilitating development of object permanence might involve developing activities to facilitate persistence, organizing the child's search efforts, increasing the number of events the child must hold in memory, and facilitating the child's ability to deduce appropriate responses. The use of hide and seek and searching games encourages object permanence.

Some handicapping conditions affect the development of object permanence. For instance, visual deficits may slow down the emergence of this concept, but usually do not preclude its development, especially when direct teaching is provided. In other cases, it may be difficult to assess the presence of object permanence. Children with severe motor disabilities, for example, may be difficult to evaluate. However, Fetters (1981) found that when a nontraditional assessment protocol of heart rate and visual tracking was employed with 13- to 29-month-old multihandicapped infants, it appeared that object permanence skills were developed at expected ages.

Means-end relationships.   This concept, often called problem solving, refers to the ability to use insight to solve problems (Piaget, 1952). The child learns to chain together behaviors to accomplish desired goals. Tasks representative of this concept include reaching for interesting objects, moving objects from hand to hand, using tools to get desired objects (e.g., extends reach with a stick, or height with a stool), and playing with toys in a variety of ways. This scheme is seen as the emergence of reasoning.

Causality.   This concept involves the ability to search for the source or the relationship behind a solution of a problem. As the child learns that the environment can be controlled, random body movements lead to more complex actions. Increasing activity in anticipation of an event, shaking a toy, searching objects to discover what makes them work, and learning to direct adults' actions are tasks learned in this scheme (Langley, 1989).

Construction of objects in space.   This concept describes the ability to explore objects, perform several activities with objects, and use objects in an appropriate way. This scheme involves developing an understanding of the three-dimensionality of

TABLE 4–1
Sensorimotor goals for instructional planning (pp. 80–82).

Domain	Goals	Sample Behaviors
Object permanence	1. The development of efficient visual, auditory, and tactile/kinesthetic attending behaviors. 2. Extension of children's persistence in searching for displaced objects. 3. The development of efficient and organized search behaviors. 4. Expansion of the length and number of variables with which children can retain events in their memory. 5. The development of the ability to deduce logically the locale of familiar and preferred objects and activities.	1. Child visually, auditorily, and tactually-kinesthetically manipulates a rattle. 2. Child searches for adult when adult peeks from behind a sofa, calls child's name, and then hides again. 3. Child reaches for toy protruding (partially hidden) from adult's shirt pocket. 4. Child retrieves toy seen hidden under sand in sand box. 5. Child finds a toy hidden first in a shirt pocket and then in a pants pocket.
Means-ends relationships	1. Development of a wide range of behaviors for acting on the environment. 2. Development of the understanding of tool use. 3. Development of the ability to chain behaviors to accomplish a goal. 4. Development of goal-directed behavior. 5. Development of representational problem-solving skills.	1. Child interacts differently with different toys and different people. 2. Child pushes a milk carton aside to get a favorite toy, or uses a drumstick to reach a drum out of reach. 3. Child pulls on blanket to bring favorite toy placed on the blanket within reach. 4. Child brings a box to an adult to have it opened. 5. Child opens coffee can by rubbing the top against a coffee table edge although the child has not observed someone else do this.
Causality	1. Development of behaviors that can be used to create and maintain pleasurable events. 2. Development of the child's understanding of ability to direct an adult's actions. 3. Development of strategies for searching and deducing causal sources or relationships for solving novel problems.	1. Child smiles and coos to maintain eye contact with caregiver to prolong social interaction. 2. Child puts adult's hand on a top after it stops spinning. 3. Child pushes all the buttons on a radio to turn it on when the child has not observed how the radio is activated.

Construction of objects in space

1. Development of the ability to orient to environmental stimuli.
2. Development of the ability to discriminate objects and activities in the foreground relative to children and from objects and activities in the background.
3. Development of the appreciation of the functional side or end of objects.
4. Development of the concept of three-dimensionality and form constancy.
5. Development of the ability to relate objects to each other and combine them in logical spatial orientations for purposeful activity.
6. Development of an understanding of the influence of gravity.
7. Development of the ability to make judgments about spatial relationships.

1. Child looks in the direction of a ringing phone.
2. Child visually follows ball as it is rolled back and forth between children in the same room.
3. Child pretends to drink from a cup with the cup right side up.
4. Child puts blocks into a can or makes a tower with blocks.
5. Child moves car over a picture of a roadway.
6. Child looks down when objects are dropped or fall.
7. Child reaches hand behind a door to retrieve a partially visible toy.

Imitation

1. Facilitation of an increase in the range and extent of complexity of behaviors available for interacting with the environment.
2. Facilitation of an increase in attention to other people.
3. Facilitation of an increase in the extent and quality of observation powers of environmental events.
4. Facilitation of the extent of the ability to replicate observed actions that children can see themselves perform.
5. Facilitation of the extent of the ability to replicate observed actions that children cannot see themselves perform.
6. Facilitation of the extent of the ability to replicate actions observed on previous occasions and in other contexts.

1. Child bangs on high chair tray again after adult imitates child's banging.
2. Child vocalizes again after adult imitates child's initial sound.
3. Child claps hands following adult's model.
4. Child vocalizes a sound already in the child's repertoire (e.g., da-da) following adult's model.
5. Child approximates a word for a common object following adult's model (e.g., ba for ball).
6. Child claps hands to Patty-Cake when no adult model is given.

TABLE 4–1
continued

Domain	Goals	Sample Behaviors
Behaviors relating to objects	1. Development of an increase in the extent and range of behaviors used to manipulate objects.	1. Child mouths, bangs, and throws a rattle.
	2. Development of the ability to discriminate and apply actions dictated by the attributes of objects.	2. Child shakes a rattle but does not shake a bottle.
	3. Development of an understanding of the functional use of objects.	3. Child puts a spoon to the mouth even when it is empty or tries to put a shoe on a foot.
	4. Development of the ability to instigate social interaction with objects.	4. Child brings blocks to adult to initiate play.
	5. Development of the ability to engage in representational play with objects and miniature toy sets.	5. Child places a doll in a bed, covers it, and pretends it is sleeping.
	6. Development of symbolic behavior.	6. Child shows adult a toy horse, makes the horse walk, and says "horsie."

Sources: Reprinted with permission of Merrill, an imprint of Macmillan Publishing Company, from *Assessing Infants and Preschoolers with Handicaps,* edited by Donald B. Bailey and Mark Wolery. Copyright © 1989 by Merrill Publishing Company. Some sample behaviors adapted from Dunst, C. J. (1981). *Infant Learning: A Cognitive-linguistic Intervention Strategy.* Hingham, MA: Teaching Resources Corporation.

objects and using reasoning to solve problems that involve objects. Releasing objects into containers, imitating the use of materials, and using materials appropriately are tasks involved in this concept (Dunst, 1981). Mirror play, stacking rings, formboards, rattles, and blocks are good materials for stimulating this concept.

Because this concept relies strongly on experimentation and persistence, some young children with special needs may experience difficulty with its development. Schwethelm and Mahoney (1986) examined the goal-directed persistence of 44 mentally retarded children, ages 12 to 36 months, on tasks involving objects. Their results indicated differences between persistence on tasks that could be solved quickly, and persistence on tasks that were slightly difficult. Ways of experimenting with objects may need to be taught with direct instruction to some exceptional infants and toddlers (Brassell & Dunst, 1978).

Imitation.   Imitation is the ability to attend to other people, observe events, reproduce observed actions, and eventually reproduce events and actions seen at previous times and in other contexts (Piaget, 1952). Imitation may be **immediate**, as when the child reproduces an action or sound after observing it, or imitation may be deferred. Piaget suggests the process of **deferred imitation** occurs when the child reproduces an action or sound some time after observing it performed (Piaget, 1951; 1952). Imitation is a major achievement for any child because most learning of new behaviors comes from imitation. Eventually, imitation leads to representational play behaviors or imaginative play.

Tasks such as playing Patty-Cake, **cooperative scribbling**, and doll play assist the development of motor imitation. The development of motor/gestural and vocal/verbal imitation is related to communication abilities in developmentally delayed children.

Development of schemes for relating to objects.   This concept refers to the ability to understand that objects produce different reactions, to use objects to attract adult attention, and to use objects for pretend play (Piaget, 1952). In mastering schemes that relate to objects, the child develops strategies for adaptive behaviors such as self-help skills and imaginative play. Tasks that aid in the development of this concept include mouthing, using objects functionally, learning about the attributes of objects, and using objects as symbols of other objects.

Appropriate experiences with objects are necessary for infants to refine their exploration skills. A relationship between object manipulation and social skills with later cognitive functioning has been reported (Seibert, Hogan, & Mundy, 1986). For example, high-risk preterm infants have been reported to manipulate objects less than fullterm infants (Ruff, McCarton, Kurtzberg, & Vaughan, 1984). Early intervention clearly can foster the development of object constructs in developmentally delayed infants (Brassell & Dunst, 1978).

In most children, the beginning indicators of reasoning and speech occur sometime between 18 and 24 months of age. Although Piaget considered the sensorimotor stage to continue until approximately the toddler's second birthday, sensorimotor thinking does not abruptly stop at that time but continues to be refined as the child moves into the next major phase of cognition, the preoperational period (Piaget & Inhelder, 1969).

Preoperational Period

Piaget (1951; 1952) suggested that from about 2 to 7 years of age children experience another phase of cognitive development that has an important new dimension: imagination. The child in the sensorimotor period is primarily interested in the surface characteristics of objects. During the **preoperational period**, the child is more interested in what objects do or what they may represent for the child.

The preoperational period may be divided into the **preconceptual stage** (roughly 2 to 4 years of age), and the **intuitive stage** (roughly 4 to 7 years of age) (Ambron, 1975). The preconceptual stage is characterized by the first appearance of **symbolic representation**, the substitution of a mental image, word, or object for something that is not immediately present. At the beginning of this stage the child's thinking is still immature and often misled by perceptions. During the preoperational stage the child engages in symbolic thinking and makes novel responses, but cognition is still characterized by four major qualities (Ambron, 1975).

Centration.   The child focuses attention on one aspect of a situation and disregards the others. The child is unable to consider multiple attributes simultaneously (e.g., size and texture). This affects the child's ability to successfully problem solve when multiple attributes of the whole must be considered.

Transductive reasoning.   Logical reasoning requires induction and deduction. Inductive reasoning requires the child to generalize from specific cases. Deductive reasoning requires the child to apply general rules to specific cases. Piaget believed that the preoperational child was not capable of inductive or deductive reasoning (Flavel, 1963).

Egocentrism.   The egocentric child is unable to view things from another's perspective. The child appears to have difficulty recognizing that someone else may have a different viewpoint. The young child's language (which expands rapidly during this stage), play, and game-playing skills tend to reflect this egocentric view.

Irreversibility and focus on successive states.   Young children have difficulty seeing that some actions can be easily reversed. For instance, if the child sees clay rolled to form a snake, the child may not believe it can be returned to its original form (Fallen & Umansky, 1985). The child may have difficulty arranging pictures to show successive actions such as an apple in three or four stages of being eaten.

Representational thought in the preoperational period differs from cognitive functioning in the sensorimotor period in several ways (Ambron, 1975). First, representational thought is faster and more flexible. The older toddler is able to plan ahead and anticipate how actions or events may unfold. Second, representational thought is not limited to concrete actions. The child can reflect upon and learn from past experiences. Third, the child can deal intellectually with qualities of objects. The child can purposely consider the features of objects and change them. And finally, representational thought can be socialized and communicated to others. Toddlers enjoy sharing imagined aspects of objects with playmates.

Additionally, during the preconceptual stage early indicators of concept development are demonstrated. The child begins to put things and events in some order.

The child begins to identify similarities and differences in objects' physical attributes, functions, and relationships. Simple sorting, ordering objects by one property, and beginning classification are developed (Piaget & Inhelder, 1969).

Although Piaget's intellectual paradigm is not applicable for all at-risk and developmentally delayed children, his developmental view of cognitive development continues to be used by professionals to organize relationships between development and cognitive processes (Dunst, 1981). His work has presented a starting point to assess and plan for children's cognitive experiences.

ASSESSMENT

The assessment of cognitive skills provides greater understanding of the child's behavior and development, serves as a basis for preparing an individualized plan for the child and family, and furnishes the means for marking the child's progress. Most cognitive assessment instruments attempt to assess the efficiency with which the child uses motor and sensory skills to solve problems (Langley, 1989). Both formal and curriculum-based measures may be used to assess the effectiveness of intervention choices.

Formal Assessment

There are two categories of assessment instruments for measuring cognitive development: traditional scales and ordinal scales. Traditional scales, whether **norm-referenced** or **criterion-referenced**, outline a sample of behaviors considered characteristic of a specific age range. Ordinal scales are based on the assumption that early cognitive abilities involve movement from lower to higher levels of functioning, and most often do not include age ranges or equivalents.

It must be stressed that not all children can be successfully assessed using traditional assessment instruments. The child with profound sensory, motor, social, or intellectual deficits may exhibit insufficient behavior to be measured by those tools. Such a child warrants the use of nontraditional, **process-oriented assessments** to gain meaningful information for program planning. Chapter 9 discusses process-oriented assessment.

A list of common assessment instruments, ordering information, age range, and area(s) assessed is presented in Table 4–2. The Bayley Scales of Infant Development (Bayley, 1969), the Battelle Developmental Inventory (Newborg, Stock, Wnek, Guidubaldi, & Svinicki, 1984), the Vulpe Assessment Battery (Vulpe, 1977), and the Infant Psychological Development Scales (commonly called the Uzgiris-Hunt Scales) (Uzgiris & Hunt, 1975) are commonly used to evaluate the cognitive functioning of handicapped infants and toddlers.

The Bayley Scales (Bayley, 1969) is a standardized instrument that should be administered by a psychologist experienced with young children, and is not recommended for use with children who have moderate to severe physical impairments. The Battelle Developmental Inventory (BDI) (Newborg et al., 1984) assesses all domains of development and allows observations, interviews, and direct testing to be used for evaluation. The Vulpe Battery (Vulpe, 1977), designed for atypical children,

TABLE 4–2
Assessment instruments for cognition and development.

Instrument Name	Ordering Information	Age Range	Area(s) Assessed
Adaptive Performance Instrument (API)	Project CAPE Special Ed. Dept. U. of Idaho Moscow, ID 83843	Birth–2 yrs	All
Assessment in Infancy: Ordinal Scales of Psychological Development	Harper & Row 345 S. Lincoln Dr. Troy, MI 63379	Birth–2 yrs	Cognition
Battelle Developmental Inventory	DLM Teaching Resources P.O. Box 4000 One DLM Park Allen, TX 75002	Birth–8 yrs	All
Bayley Scales of Infant Development	Psychological Corp. 757 Third Ave. New York, NY 10017	1 week– 30 + mos	Mental Motor
Brazelton Neonatal Behavioral Assessment Scale	J.B. Lippincott Co. E. Washington Sq. Philadelphia, PA 19105	Approx. Birth–28 days	Behavioral
Callier-Azusa Scale	Callier Center for Communication Disorders U. of Texas–Dallas 1966 Inwood Rd. Dallas, TX 75235	Birth–4 yrs	All
Carolina Curriculum for Handicapped Infants and Infants at Risk	Paul H. Brookes P.O. Box 10624 Baltimore, MD 21285–0624	Birth–24 mos	All
Diagnostic Inventory of Early Development	Pratt Educ. Media 200 Third Ave., S.W. Cedar Rapids, IA 32404	Birth–7 yrs	All
Early Intervention Developmental Profile	U. of Michigan Press 615 E. University Ann Arbor, MI 48109	Birth–3 yrs	All
Early Learning Accomplishment Profile (E-LAP)	Kaplan School Supply 1310 Lewisville-Clemmons Rd. Lewisville, NC 27023	Birth–36 mos	All
EMI Assessment Scale	EMI Dept. of Pediatrics U. of Virginia Medical Center Box 232 Charlottesville, VA 22908	Birth–24 mos	All

TABLE 4–2
continued

Instrument Name	Ordering Information	Age Range	Area(s) Assessed
Gesell Developmental Scales (Revised)	Psychological Corp. 757 Third Ave. New York, NY 10017	4 wks–36 mos	All
Hawaii Early Learning Profile (HELP)	VORT Corporation P.O. Box 11552–A Palo Alto, CA 94306	Birth–3 yrs	All
Infant Scale of Communicative Intent (ISCI)	Speech & Language Svcs. St. Christopher's Hsptl. 5th & Lehigh Ave. Philadelphia, PA 19133	Birth–18 mos	Receptive/ expressive language
Minnesota Infant Development Inventory (MIDI)	Behavior Science Systems P.O. Box 1108 Minneapolis, MN 55440	1–15 mos	All
Peabody Developmental Motor Scales–Revised	Teaching Resources Corp. 50 Pond Park Road Hingham, MA 02043–4382	Birth–7 yrs	Gross and fine motor
Play Assessment Scale	University of Washington Rebecca R. Fewell, Ph.D. EEU WJ–10 Seattle, WA 98195	Birth–36 mos	All
Receptive-Expressive Emergent Language Scale (REEL)	University Park Press 233 E. Redwood St. Baltimore, MD 21202	Birth–36 mos	Receptive/ expressive lanaguage
Rockford Infant Development Evaluation Scales (RIDES)	Scholastic Testing Svc. 480 Meyer Rd. Bensenville, IL 60106	Birth–4 yrs	All
Sequenced Inventory of Communication Development (SICD)	Western Psych. Services 12031 Wilshire Blvd. Los Angeles, CA 90025	4–48 mos	Receptive/ expressive language
Sewall Early Education Developmental Profiles (SEED)	Sewall Rehab. Center 1360 Vine St. Denver, CO 80206	1–42 mos	All
Uzgiris-Hunt Ordinal Scales of Infant Psychological Development	PRO-ED 5341 Industrial Oaks Blvd. Austin, TX 78735	Birth–2 yrs	Cognition
Vulpe Assessment Battery	National Institute on Mental Retardation 4700 Keele St. Downsview, Ontario M3J 1P3	Birth–72 mos	All

is not standardized and is designed to be used as a diagnostic-prescriptive assessment tool for instructional planning. The Uzgiris-Hunt Scales (Uzgiris & Hunt, 1975), the most frequently used Piagetian-based assessment tool, requires practice and familiarity with Piagetian theory for accurate administration. Dunst's protocol (1980) assists interventionists in successfully developing programs from these scales. Chapters 7 and 8 describe the use of this scale for infants and toddlers with severe disabilities.

Curriculum-based Assessment

Curriculum-based assessment is used to evaluate the effectiveness of intervention activities. A growing number of early intervention programs are moving away from assessment based entirely on developmental milestones and are incorporating curriculum-based assessment, in which each item relates directly to a skill included in the program's curriculum. This type of assessment provides a direct link between testing, teaching, and progress evaluation (Bailey & Wolery, 1989).

Criterion-referenced and curriculum-referenced scales such as the Early Intervention Developmental Profile (Rogers, et al., 1981) and the Hawaii Early Learning Profile (Furuno, O'Reilly, Hosaka, Inatsuka, Allman, & Zeisloft, 1979) have cognitive sections, although they do not provide a thorough assessment of Piaget's sensorimotor concepts (Langley, 1989). The Carolina Curriculum for Handicapped Infants and Infants At Risk (Johnson-Martin, Jens, & Attermeier, 1986), in contrast, covers all developmental domains through 24 months and offers a comprehensive assessment of cognitive skills. This tool has a number of well-organized subsections for assessing Piaget's sensorimotor concepts. The purpose of curriculum-based assessment is to determine the child's level of functioning so that input to the child changes as the child's abilities change.

INTERVENTION

Regardless of the domain, developmental intervention always follows three steps:

- □ assess and identify target behaviors to be achieved
- □ identify methods for teaching and stimulating behaviors
- □ identify steps to achieve target behaviors

Nonhandicapped children seem to follow a fairly predictable sequence of cognitive development. Infants with special needs, on the other hand, may follow normal patterns in some aspects of their cognitive development, and not in others. Because of sensory impairments, at-risk and exceptional infants may need alternative ways to develop or manifest their cognitive competencies.

For example, blind infants do not acquire eye-hand coordination spontaneously. They must learn the nonvisual counterpart of eye-hand coordination that involves learning to locate objects by sound and then learning to reach for them. For this to be accomplished, their environment must be modified to facilitate this type of exploration. Every time a sound is made by an object, the visually impaired child's hand must be manipulated to search for the object in the direction from which the sound came. If such arrangements are not made, the chances of developing eye-hand co-ordination are greatly reduced. As this example illustrates, there are certain techniques that tend to facilitate the development of cognitive skills in very young children.

Strategies for Enhancing Cognitive Development

It is important to remember that developmental scales emphasize the *average* ages for developmental milestones and should only be used as general guidelines for what to expect from infants and toddlers. Most children's development seems to be characterized by spurts of learning. As Murphy, Heider, and Small (1986) state: "Some of the youngest children, like artists, want peace and quiet and time to absorb their experiences, time to let imagination grow" (p. 5). Numerous strategies promote cognitive development. Nine of the most common techniques are discussed here.

Be responsive to the child.   At times, it may be difficult to accurately read the cues of handicapped or seriously ill children. Careful observation is necessary to determine how each child indicates needs, interest, a desire for change, or the wish to continue an interaction. Often subtle signals such as tone of the cry, resistance to eye contact, and increased motor activity are cues that the child desires something (Field, Goldberg, Stern, & Sostek, 1980). The infant who is slow to respond, and not at medical risk, may need to interact more often and continue the activity longer than other infants (Staff, 1988).

The child's responses, needs, capabilities, as well as appearance, evoke reactions from caregivers. One child may be persistent, while another may be difficult to engage in any activity or object. The degree and frequency of frustration the infant or toddler experiences may also influence the child's motivation to learn. Caregivers' responses to the child either support or undermine the child's strengths. To support the child, caregivers must be consistent in their responses to the child's signals so the child is assisted in learning to control the environment, and must adjust their style of interaction to encourage more rewarding interactions (McCollum & Stayton, 1985).

Follow the child's lead and interests.   When one follows the child's lead, there is an opportunity to initiate or maintain interaction with the object or focus of the child's interest. If the child bangs an object instead of inserting it in a can as intended, following the interest in banging may increase the child's length of interaction. After banging has been sufficiently experienced, the adult can try to gradually move the child toward other manipulations of the object. Animated interaction tends to increase the young child's interest and motivation.

Encourage learning through play.   Ideal interactions are pleasurable for everyone involved. Most routine care tasks can be made playful as well as instructive. For instance, allowing the child to taste, smell, and touch the facecloth when it is dry and then again after it is wet may make an ordinary activity special. Such opportunities for stimulation are probably best dispersed throughout the day so parents do not feel pressure to finish an activity even though the child's attention may be strained.

Some families may need to be encouraged to keep the child in areas where most of the activity in the home takes place, as well as to increase playful face-to-face interactions with their child. When mothers are trained to effectively interact with their children, mothers and infants are generally more responsive to each other's behavior and the infants have more self-initiated behavior during interactions (Moran & Whitman, 1985). Family members should always be asked for ideas to facilitate cognitive development during daily routines.

Take turns when interacting with the child.   To promote cognitive skills, caregivers need to balance adult-dominated activities with child-directed play, especially as the child moves into the second year of life. When the child is first learning to take turns, adults can foster the child's initiations and enhance turn-taking by following this sequence:

- □ *wait* for the child to take his/her turn
- □ if the child does not take a turn, *signal* the child to take a turn, and then, if the child still doesn't respond,
- □ *prompt* (physically guide) the child to take a turn. Turn-taking encourages the practice of skills while building on past experiences (Dunst, 1981).

Occasionally, encouraging play sessions between caregivers and the child, without toys, can facilitate spontaneous and creative interactions. This tactic stimulates the use of conventional games (e.g., Peek-A-Boo, This Little Piggy) as well as increases the chance of inventing new games.

Capture the teachable moment.   The teachable moment involves teaching a skill or concept when the child is receptive by creating or taking advantage of a stimulating environment. Simply, this involves matching the infant's readiness to learn with opportunities for learning. The real challenge of intervention is attempting to understand the effects of the handicap on the child's development, designing alternative strategies for minimizing or preventing the effects of the handicapping condition, and recognizing when the infant is *ready* to acquire information from interactions (Langley, 1980).

Observant infant interventionists are alert to indicators of teachable moments. There are also several ways to create teachable moments. For the child who appears ready to begin rolling over, for example, adults may place objects just close enough to the child so that random movements of the child's legs and arms touch or activate the objects. A ball with a bell inside tends to be a good choice because it offers tactile and auditory feedback when touched. As the child's attention to the objects increases, objects need to be gradually moved farther away so the child must move or roll to reach them.

Use naturalistic teaching strategies.   Naturalistic teaching strategies involve embedding teaching and evaluation tactics into routines or activities that are already occurring. These strategies, also referred to as ecological teaching procedures, use an undercurrent of structure so that intended goals are reached but an apparent unstructured playfulness occurs between the adult and the child (Li, 1983).

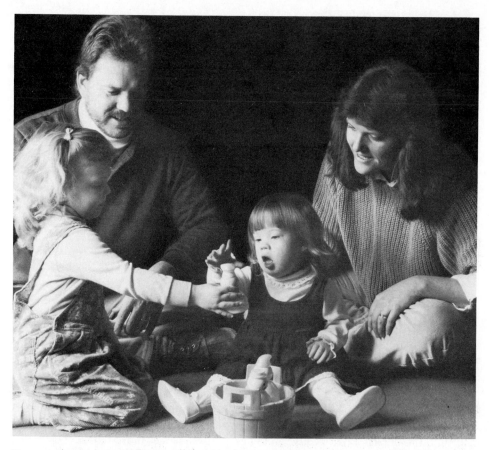

Encouraging learning through play and taking turns with the child are ways to facilitate cognitive development in infants and toddlers.

The most common naturalistic techniques are incidental teaching and naturalistic time-delay. **Incidental teaching** involves the arrangement of the environment so that chances of child-initiated, spontaneous interactions are increased. If the goal is to increase the number of body parts the child points to, for example, a full-length plastic mirror might be placed next to the bathtub during bath time and the child may be asked to wash different body parts. In this way, caregivers can structure opportunities to teach ("You are touching your nose."), prompt ("Show me your nose."), reinforce ("Yes, your nose."), and maintain skills ("Remember where your nose was?"). Yet, instruction occurs during regular routines.

With **naturalistic time-delay**, caregivers withhold assistance from the child in an effort to encourage spontaneous behavior. For example, if the child has trouble operating a toy, the caregiver might go to the child and look at the child expectantly, waiting to see if the child indicates a need for or verbally requests assistance before offering to help (Haring & Innocenti, 1989).

Basically, naturalistic teaching means that everything the child does and everything that is done with the child offers the possibility of teaching, refining, or maintaining skills. There is some evidence that playful experiences that occur during daily routines of diapering, feeding, and dressing may be more effective for teaching the very young child than isolated "learning times" (Dunst, 1981). Nevertheless, naturalistic teaching should not be interpreted as bombarding children with adult-dominated interactions. Children with special needs must also be allowed quiet time to practice skills, play, and learn to entertain themselves without adult direction.

Make consequences count.   Consequences are statements, acts, or events that follow a behavior; they generally either strengthen or weaken the behavior. When the child does something that is followed by a pleasant or interesting action, the child is more likely to repeat or continue the behavior. If the infant swipes at a mobile hanging above the crib and it dances in the air, the child likely will want this action to happen again. On the other hand, when the child does something that is followed by an unpleasant or neutral event, the child is less likely to repeat or continue the behavior. Using the earlier example, if nothing happens each time the child swipes at the mobile, the child will eventually stop trying to reach it.

Natural consequences tend to be more effective in teaching children about their ability to change their environment than artificial consequences. That is, it is more powerful for the mobile to move when the child touches it, than to have an adult move it for the child. The adult cannot be as consistent as the mobile, nor as immediate.

Artificial reinforcers, such as food and toys, are frequently unnecessary and may create a dependency upon tangible rewards. If tangible rewards have been used, **systematic fading** may be necessary before less artificial consequences such as smiles and praise are once again effective (Saunder & Sailor, 1979). Additionally, to enhance the child's understanding of cause and effect, consequences must be tailored to each child and situation, and occur *every time* the behavior occurs.

Encourage predictable routines.   Routines increase the child's ability to predict the environment and therefore improve the child's ability to construct mental representations of reality (Dunst, 1981). Predictability encourages child-initiated responding. Yet within the general structure of predictable routines, children also require some variety. Caregivers must be careful that children do not become dependent on adults to prompt or cue them about appropriate ways to respond. One goal of intervention with cognitive skills is to facilitate spontaneous, and eventually, novel responses.

Use task analysis.   Most cognitive skills are too complex to be acquired at one time by young children. **Task analysis** breaks a skill into small steps that can be taught. For example, to get the child to push a button on a busy box, caregivers might reward the child by pushing a button on the busy box each time the child moves toward the toy. Next, the child's hand could be physically guided to push the button. Gradually, the amount of assistance would be faded until the child could perform the skill independently.

Teaching cognitive goals in sequence from a single developmental curriculum is never adequate. Goals must be functional so they reflect the needs of a particular handicapping condition while enabling the child to increase practical interactions with the environment.

Individualizing Group Intervention

Center-based programs often use some form of small group instruction to promote learning in toddlers. Three or four children might be grouped by chronological age, developmental functioning, domain, need, or interest.

Activity-based instruction involves the process of teaching skills that overlap several domains, within the same age-appropriate activity (Bricker, McDonnell, Trujillo, & Bailey, 1982). Young children learn by doing. Skills to be taught are embedded within common activities for toddlers such as finger painting, water play, and manipulating objects. The objectives of the lesson (i.e., chaining two actions together to complete a desired task and/or object differentiation) are the purpose of the activity, rather than performance in the activity itself. The only requirements for the experiences used in activity-based instruction are that they are engaging and appropriate for the children's level of development.

Focusing on teaching critical skills may enhance generalization of activity-based instruction. **Critical skills** are broad competencies. For example, the critical skill of the objective, "locates objects observed hidden," might be summarized as "organized search behaviors." When interventionists understand critical skills embedded in tasks, they can create opportunities for teaching them during all routines. For example, arrangements might be made for the child to search for hidden cups before snack or socks during dressing. (See Appendix A for a list of critical skills by domains).

Ensuring that individualized cognitive goals—not merely the same goal for each child in the group—are reached through activity-based instruction requires good record keeping and organization. Table 4–3 shows a grid for tracking individualized goals during group activity-based instruction. The grid permits easy access to each child's goals and allows adults to individualize expectations, prompts, and cues. Despite the fact that critical skills are listed by domain on the grid, skills across domains are embedded and reinforced in group activities.

The grid may be placed on a clipboard and used as a data sheet for naturalistic teaching episodes. One way to accomplish this is to observe only a few children each day or only a few children in each activity. Although all children are learning the skills they need, only a few have data collected on their performances. The slashes and circles on the grid in Table 4–3 represent correct and incorrect responses during a teaching episode.

In general, children first should be given the task while the adult observes how the child independently approaches the task. This way the child is permitted to attempt the activity with the least amount of assistance initially. Assistance for cognitive tasks should follow this sequence:

1. child acts independently;

TABLE 4-3

Grid for individual goals for group activity-based instruction.

Individual targets for group activity: _____   Date: _____

Name	Gross motor	Fine motor	Expressive language	Receptive language	Social	Self-help	Sensorimotor
1. Karen	balance sitting 100	pincer grasp	increase frequency and diversity of signals	Functional use of objects 010	turn-taking adult	eating — spoon (physical prompt)	means-end (D vc D) 000
2. Billy	trunk stability |||	eye-hand coordination	speech sound production /d/ /b/	multi-word comprehension (III) 011	functional use of toy (adult-child)	dressing — socks and shoes off (physical prompt)	imitation
3. Shanta	trunk stability	controlled release GMA 011	word production	action word comprehension	turn-taking adult	dressing — assist shirt off	means-end
4. Mike	balance standing	wrist rotation	word production	multi-word comprehension	turn-taking peers	eating — spoon release independently	object differentiation

2. adult uses a gestural cue with words or demonstration of the task, if necessary; and lastly,

3. adult uses physical guidance with words if child does not respond appropriately.

The following scoring key may be used to record the level of assistance the child needed:

Scoring Key

I = **Independent**. Child completes activity independently. Example: Takes and completes 3-piece formboard independently.

VC = **Verbal Command**. Child responds to task when told to do it. Example: "Put the circle in, please."

VA = **Verbal Assistance**. Child responds to task when verbal guidance is given. Example: "Put the circle here, please."

D = **Demonstration**. Child responds to task when given verbal directions while task is performed. Example: "See, the circle goes here," while placing circle in formboard.

GMA = **Graduated Manual Assistance**. Child responds to task when told to do it while being given some degree of physical assistance. Example: "The circle goes here, just like this," while gently guiding child's arm toward the formboard.

IR = **Inappropriate Response**. Child responds in a way not requested. Example: Child mouths formboard.

NR = **No Response**. Child does not react to task in any way. Example: Child stares away from teacher and cries.

Placing copies of the grid in key locations such as the music center, toileting area, and open play area guarantees that opportunities to facilitate or reinforce skills are never overlooked. Data are transferred to individual skill graphs at the end of the day. Although imprecise, this data system requires little adult time and reduces the steps required to collect continuous performance data.

Systematic modification of programming, based on children's responses to activities, is essential for quality intervention. Careful analysis of daily progress provides direction for change and maximizes the efficiency of instruction.

Adapting Commercial Curricula

A curriculum is merely one yardstick against which to measure the child's needs and progress. Selecting goals for intervention from commercial curricula—without adequate observation of the child's skills, the effect of the disability on the child's development, the philosophy of the service option, and the family's desires—must be avoided. A list of some common early intervention curricula, with ordering information, is presented in Table 4-4.

TABLE 4–4
Common curricula for early intervention programs (pp. 96–99).

Curriculum Name	Ordering Information
Activities for Parent-Child Interaction	High/Scope Educational Research Fnd. 600 N. River St. Ypsilanti, MI 48197
Baby Learning Through Baby Play: A Parent's Guide for the First Two Years	St. Martin's Press 175 Fifth Ave. New York, NY 10010
Birth to Three: Developmental Learning and the Handicapped Child	Teaching Resources Corporation 50 Pond Park Rd. Hingham, MA 02043
The Carolina Curriculum for Infants and Infants At-Risk	Brooks Publishing Company P. O. Box 10624 Baltimore, MD 21285–0624
Child Learning Through Child Play (Learning activities for 2 and 3 year olds)	St. Martin's Press 175 Fifth Ave. New York, 10010
CORE: Computer Oriented Record-Keeping Enabler (Designed for use with Macomb 0–3 Core Curriculum)	The Macomb Projects 27 Horrabin Hall Western Illinois University Macomb, IL 61455
Curriculum Guide: Hearing Impaired Children Birth to Three Years and Their Parents	Alexander Graham Bell Association for the Deaf, Inc. 3417 Volta Place, N.W. Washington, DC 20007
Developmental Programming for Infants and Young Children (Volumes 1, 2, 3; Revised Ed.)	University of Michigan Press Department 4B P. O. Box 1104 Ann Arbor, MI 48106
Early Learning Activity Cards—Birth to 36 Months	Kaplan Press P. O. Box 5128 Winston-Salem, NC 27113-5128
Getting Your Baby Ready to Talk	John Tracy Clinic Home Study Plan 806 W. Adams Blvd. Los Angeles, CA 90007
Handling Your Young Premature Baby at Home	R. R. Givens P. O. Box 2922 Alexandria, VA 22301
Hawaii Early Learning Profile (HELP) (Charts and Activity Guide)	VORT Corporation P. O. Box 60880 Palo Alto, CA 94306
HELP . . . at Home	VORT Corporation P. O. Box 60880 Palo Alto, CA 94306

TABLE 4–4
continued

Curriculum Name	Ordering Information
HELP for Parents of Children with Special Needs	VORT Corporation P. O. Box 60880 Palo Alto, CA 94306
HELP—When the Parent is Handicapped	VORT Corporation P. O. Box 60880 Palo Alto, CA 94306
Home Intervention Programming for Sensory Impaired Infants, Preschoolers, and Their Families	SKI*HI Institute Project INSITE UMC ID Utah State University Logan, UT 84322
Home Program Instruction Sheets for Infants and Young Children—Revised	Therapy Skills Builders 3830 E. Bellevue P.O. Box 42050 Tucson, AZ 85733
The Infant and Toddler Handbook (Invitation for Optimum Early Development)	Humanics Limited P.O. Box 7447 Atlanta, GA 30309
Infant Learning: A Cognitive-Linguistic Intervention Strategy	Teaching Resources Corporation 50 Pond Park Rd. Hingham, MA 02043
Learning Games for Infants and Toddlers	New Readers Press Box 131 Syracuse, NY 13210
Learning Through Play: A Resource Manual for Teachers and Parents	Teaching Resources Corporation 50 Pond Park Rd. Hingham, MA 02043
Macomb 0–3 Core Curriculum	The Macomb Projects 27 Horrabin Hall Western Illinois University Macomb, IL 61455
Make Every Step Count: Birth to 1 Year Developmental Parenting Guide	VORT Corporation P. O. Box 60880 Palo Alto, CA 94306
Move with Me (A Parent's Guide to Movement Development for Visually Impaired Babies)	Blind Children's Center 4120 Marathon St. P.O. Box 29159 Los Angeles, CA 90029
Parent-Infant Communication: A Program of Clinical and Home Training for Parents and Hearing Impaired Infants (Revised)	Infant and Hearing Resource Good Samaritan Hospital and Medical Center 1015 22nd Street, N.W. Portland, OR 97210

TABLE 4-4
continued

Curriculum Name	Ordering Information
Position Stickers (Easy-to-use, illustrated stickers to help parents and caregivers implement therapy recommendations) —Developmental Position Stickers —Feeding Position Stickers —Baby Position Stickers —Neonatal Position Stickers	Therapy Skill Builders A Division of Communication Skill Builders 3830 E. Bellevue P.O. Box 42050 Tucson, AZ 85733
Reach Out and Teach: Meeting the Training Needs of Parents of Visually and Multiply Handicapped Young Children	American Foundation for the Blind 15 West 16th St. New York, NY 10011

TRANSDISCIPLINARY CASES

These case studies demonstrate how apparent environmental differences produced different cognitive functioning by the age of 12 months in two children with similar medical histories. Both children received similar medical interventions at comparable facilities in an urban city, received physical therapy services once a week, and were enrolled in the same infant intervention program.

THE WEISS FAMILY

Henry was born at 30 weeks gestation, and had a medical history of chronic lung disease (CLD). He was the first child of Kathy and R. J. Weiss, professionals in their early thirties. After Henry's birth, Kathy took a 2-year leave from her job to devote herself to Henry's care.

When Henry's medical crises stabilized, the nurses in the intensive care nursery trained Kathy to share Henry's daily care until the time of his discharge. R. J. visited the NICU frequently but gave Kathy most of the responsibility for Henry's care. At the time of discharge, the nurses and Kathy trained the early childhood specialist from the local infant intervention program to manage Henry's medical care.

After discharge, Henry received physical therapy and home visits once a week. Although the demands of Henry's care were exhausting, the Weisses had family nearby who provided financial and emotional support, as well as frequent relief with child care. Henry's attachment to his parents was strong. Kathy worked diligently with him to encourage each cognitive milestone, and both parents appeared to delight in Henry's smallest achievement. Kathy boasted to other parents that she had never missed a therapy appointment since Henry's birth despite a succession of noncritical illnesses of her own.

Kathy began personal counseling when Henry was 8 months old. After nearly 2 months of counseling, she concluded that she was "obsessed" with improving Henry's development and decided to return to work part-time. R. J. and their extended family supported the decision. Henry was cared for by an extended family member while his parents worked.

At about this time, the physical therapist began training the family's home visitor in therapeutic intervention skills. Henry's health and developmental progress continued to improve steadily. Sessions with the physical therapist were then reduced to once a month. By a corrected age of 12 months, Henry was assessed as functioning on or above age level in all areas except gross motor. His social and cognitive skills were his strengths. Gross motor skills were about 2 months below expected levels.

TABLE 4–4
continued

Curriculum Name	Ordering Information
Small Wonder —Level I: Birth–18 Months —Level II: 18–36 Months	American Guidance Service Publishers Building Circle Pines, MN 55014–1796
Teaching the Infant with Down Syndrome	EDMARC Corporation P.O. Box 3903 Bellevue, WA 98009
Teaching Your Down Syndrome Infant: A Guide for Parents	University Park Press 233 E. Redwood St. Baltimore, MD 21202
Time to Begin: Early Education for Children with Down Syndrome	Caring, Inc. P.O. Box 400 Milton, WA 98354

THE LOWE FAMILY

Missy was premature (gestation of 31 weeks) with a medical history of chronic lung disease (CLD). She spent 2 weeks less than Henry in the NICU. Missy was the third child of Martha and Fred Lowe, middle-management professionals in their late twenties. Within 8 weeks of Missy's birth, Mrs. Lowe returned to work. Although her variable work schedule made consistent participation in Missy's hospital care difficult, Martha or Fred tried to visit Missy each day. However, the situation placed extreme stress on the family. Missy's two sisters, 7 and 8 years old, seemed especially distressed by the commitments Missy required from their parents.

Even before discharge from the hospital, the Lowes attended support meetings sponsored by the infant intervention program to which the medical team had referred them. The other families and the infant staff offered emotional support to the family. Extended family members were supportive but lived nearly 8 hours away by car, so contact was sporadic. The family appeared to gain significant support from their social circle, however.

At discharge, Missy's attachments and the family's attachments to her were described as good by the case manager (the special educator in the infant intervention program who served as primary service provider). However, child care for all the children was noted as a persistent problem for the family. Child care problems also made it difficult to make physical therapy appointments. For this and other reasons, the home visitor requested additional training from the program's physical therapist for herself and the family so therapy could be more consistently reinforced at home.

Because of the parents' nontraditional work schedules, it was often difficult to set times for home visits that did not overburden the family. The home visitor's records indicated that nearly 40% of scheduled home visits were canceled, often due to unexpected illness of one or more family members or job-related circumstances. Mr. and Mrs. Lowe commented that they had little time or energy left at the end of the day, and often were unable to satisfy their desired goals with Missy. The babysitter (who had three other children under the age of 3 in her care) was also inconsistent in following through with activities designed to increase Missy's responsiveness to her environment.

Three months before Missy's first birthday, her parents separated. At that point, financial stresses increased significantly and all family members evidenced signs of stress and depression. (Mrs. Lowe gained weight and the older children developed school problems.) When Missy was evaluated at 12 months corrected age, moderate to severe developmental delays were revealed. The most severe delays were in the areas of cognitive development and fine and gross motor.

SUMMARY OF PROCEDURES

Infant programs must be flexible to adapt interventions to the changing demands and needs of each child, and those of the child's family. A summary of key procedures discussed in this chapter follows.

1. Use Piagetian development theory to organize learning activities in which children explore objects and the environment.
2. Use naturalistic teaching techniques and naturalistic time-delay to facilitate cognitive development, to increase learning opportunities, and to increase the chances of generalization of skills.
3. Ask family members for suggestions about how cognitive skills might be included in different situations and settings within the child's usual routines.
4. Encourage and plan playful interactions between caregivers and the child with, and then without, materials to facilitate the acquisition, maintenance, and generalization of cognitive skills.
5. Make children's experiences count by using natural consequences and avoiding artificial reinforcers.
6. To facilitate cognitive development in the young child
   □ be responsive to the child
   □ make an effort to follow the child's lead and interests
   □ encourage children to learn skills through social experiences and play
   □ use turn-taking
   □ capture the teachable moment
   □ use naturalistic teaching strategies
   □ make consequences meaningful
   □ provide predictable routines
   □ task analyze complex skills
7. Use grids to facilitate recordkeeping in group activities in center-based toddler intervention programs.
8. Use a continuum of assistance when teaching cognitive skills or any new skill: wait for the child to act independently; use gestures, words, or demonstration; and lastly, if necessary, gently physically guide the child with words.

SUMMARY

Research with nonhandicapped infants demonstrates that the perceptual and cognitive capabilities of infants are well organized, and in some cases, sophisticated (Yarrow, Rubenstein, & Pedersen, 1975). Piaget has strongly influenced how professionals view cognitive development in very young children. His theory emphasizes learning as an active process which relies on appropriate environmental opportunities (Dunst, 1981). Piaget conceptualizes the development of cognition as dependent on both internal and external factors.

Because cognitive development is expressed by skills in the social, language, and fine-motor domains, the strategies discussed in this chapter are appropriate for enhancing several developmental domains. The emotional and physical demands that accompany the birth of an at-risk or special needs child can never be underestimated. For this reason, any technique used with children and their families should focus on the pleasurable aspects of interaction. In that way cognitive functioning may be fostered and an additional coping mechanism is provided for family members.

DISCUSSION QUESTIONS

1. What are some different ways a cup and a spoon could be used to encourage means-end, imitation, and object permanence skills in a child whose cognitive functioning is approximately at the 24-month level?
2. Using information about child development, in what ways might an 18-month-old handicapped child (with cognitive functioning of about 12 months) and a nonhandicapped child of the same chronological age differ in how they manipulate objects?
3. What are the advantages and disadvantages of encouraging family members to use naturalistic teaching strategies with at-risk and/or handicapped children during daily routines?
4. Explain how helping parents learn to play games and enjoy their infants may facilitate cognitive development.

APPLIED ACTIVITIES/PROJECTS

1. Arrange to observe the administration of a standardized infant intelligence test such as the Bayley. Based on your observation, were any Piagetian concepts evaluated? If so, describe the item and explain which concept(s) were assessed.
2. Observe a family with an infant with special needs during meal time. Based on your observation and with the family's input, develop ways to teach, maintain, and/or generalize three cognitive skills using naturalistic teaching strategies.
3. Explain how three cognitive goals for a child operating at Piaget's preoperational stage could be facilitated using incidental teaching strategies while preparing a child for a nap in a center-based program and at home.

SUGGESTED READINGS

Bailey, D. B., & Wolery, M. (Eds.). (1989). *Assessing Infants and Preschoolers with Handicaps.* Columbus, OH: Merrill.

Beadle, M. (1971). *A child's mind: How children learn during the critical years from birth to age five.* Garden City, NY: Anchor Books.

Dunst, C. J. (1980). *A clinical and educational manual for use with the Uzgiris and Hunt Scales of Infant Psychological Development.* Austin, TX: PRO-ED.

Dunst, C. J. (1981). *Infant learning: A cognitive-linguistic intervention strategy.* Hingham, MA: Teaching Resources Corporation.

Exceptional Parent. Magazine for parents of children with disabilities published eight times a year. Exceptional Parent, 605 Commonwealth Ave., Boston, MA 02215.

McConkey, R., & Jaffree, D. (1983). *Making toys for handicapped children: A guide for parents and teachers.* Englewood Cliffs, NJ: Prentice-Hall.

Morris, L. (Ed.). (1986). *Extracting learning styles from social/cultural diversity: Studies of five American minorities*. Norman: University of Oklahoma Press.

Piaget, J. (1952). *The origins of intelligence in children*. New York: International Universities Press.

Yarrow, L. J., Rubenstein, J. L., & Pedersen, F. A. (1975). *Infant and environment: Early cognitive and motivation development*. New York: Wiley.

REFERENCES

Adams, J., & Ramey, C. (1980). Structural aspects of maternal speech to infants reared in poverty. *Child Development, 51,* 1280–1284.

Ambron, S. R. (1975). *Child development*. San Francisco: Rinehart Press.

Anastasiow, N. (1986). *Development and disability: A psychological analysis for special educators*. Baltimore: Paul H. Brookes.

Bailey, D. B., & Wolery, M. (Eds.). (1989). *Assessing infants and preschoolers with handicaps*. Columbus, OH: Merrill.

Bayley, N. (1969). *Bayley Scales of Infant Development*. New York: Psychological Corp.

Beckwith, L. (1984). Parent interaction with their preterm infants and later mental development. *Early Child Development and Care, 16,* 27–40.

Bendell, R., Culbertson, J., Shelton, T., & Carter, B. (1986). Interrupted infantile apnea: Impact on early development, temperament, and maternal stress. *Journal of Clinical Child Psychology, 15,* 304–310.

Brassell, W., & Dunst, C. (1978). Fostering the object construct: Large-scale intervention with handicapped infants. *American Journal of Mental Deficiency, 82,* 507–510.

Bricker, D., McDonnell, A., Trujillo, G., & Bailey, E. (1982). *Early intervention program: Program description and procedural manual*. Eugene: University of Oregon, Center on Human Development.

Cohen, S., & Parmelee, A. (1983). Prediction of 5-year Stanford-Binet scores in preterm infants. *Child Development, 54,* 1242–1253.

Dunst, C. J. (1980). *A clinical and educational manual for use with the Uzgiris and Hunt Scales of Infant Psychological Development*. Austin, TX: PRO-ED.

Dunst, C. J. (1981). *Infant learning: A cognitive-linguistic intervention strategy*. Hingham, MA: Teaching Resources Corporation.

Escalona, S. K. (1982). Babies at double hazard: Early development of infants at biologic and social risk. *Pediatrics, 70,* 670–676.

Fallen, N. H., & Umansky, W. (1985). *Young children with special needs*. Columbus, OH: Merrill.

Fetters, L. (1981). Object permanence development in infants with motor handicaps. *Physical Therapy, 61,* 327–333.

Field, T., Goldberg, S., Stern, D., & Sostek, A. (1980). *High-risk infants and children: Adult and peer interactions*. New York: Academic Press.

Flavell, J. H. (1963). *The developmental psychology of Jean Piaget*. Princeton, NJ: Van Nostrand.

Flexer, C., & Gans, D. (1986). Distribution of auditory response behaviors in normal infants and profoundly multihandicapped children. *Journal of Speech and Hearing Research, 29,* 425–429.

Furuno, S., O'Reilly, A., Hosaka, C., Inatsuka, T., Allman, T., & Zeisloft, B. (1979). *The Hawaii Early Learning Profile and activity guide*. Palo Alto, CA: VORT.

Gilbride, K. E. (1983, August). *High-risk infants: Auditory processing deficits in later childhood*. Paper presented at the annual meeting of the American Psychological Association, Anaheim, CA.

Haring, N., & Innocenti, M. (1989). Managing learning time. In C. Tingey (Ed.), *Implementing early intervention* (pp. 279–302). Baltimore: Paul H. Brookes.

Johnson-Martin, N., Jens, K., & Attermeier, S. (1986). *The Carolina Curriculum for Handicapped Infants and Infants At Risk*. Baltimore: Paul H. Brookes.

Kelly, J. (1982). Effects of intervention on caregiver-infant interaction when the infant is handicapped. *Journal of the Division for Early Childhood, 5,* 53–63.

Kilgo, J., Holder-Brown, L., Johnson, L., & Cook, M. (1988). An examination of the effect of tactile-kinesthetic stimulation on the development of preterm infants. *Journal of the Division for Early Childhood, 12*(4), 320–327.

Lamb, M., Garn, S., & Keating, M. (1981). Correlation between sociability and cognitive performance among 8-month-olds. *Child Development, 52,* 711–713.

Langley, M. B. (1980). *The teachable moment and the handicapped infant*. ERIC Exceptional Child Education Report, Series No. 79–5. Reston, VA: The Council for Exceptional Children.

Langley, M. B. (1989). Assessing infant cognitive development. In D. Bailey & M. Wolery (Eds.), *Assessing infants and preschoolers with handicaps* (pp. 249–274). Columbus, OH: Merrill.

Lawson, K. R., Ruff, H., McCarton-Daum, C., Kurtzberg, D., & Vaughan, H. (1984). Auditory-visual responsiveness in full-term and preterm infants. *Developmental Psychology, 20,* 120–127.

Li, A. K. (1983). Pleasurable aspects of play in enhancing young handicapped children's relationships with parents and peers. *Journal of the Division of Early Childhood, 7*(1), 87–92.

Lockman, J. J. (1983). Infant perception and cognition. In S. G. Garwood & R. R. Fewell (Eds.), *Educating handicapped infants: Issues in development and intervention* (pp. 117–164). Rockville, MD: Aspen.

Mahoney, G., Finger, I., & Powell, A. (1985). Relationship of maternal behavioral style to the development of organically impaired mentally retarded infants. *American Journal of Mental Deficiency, 90,* 296–302.

Maisto, A., & German, M. (1981). Maternal locus of control and developmental gain demonstrated by high-risk infants: A longitudinal analysis. *Journal of Psychology, 109,* 213–221.

McCollum, J., & Stayton, V. (1985). Infant/parent interaction: Studies and intervention guidelines based on the SIAI model. *Journal of the Division for Early Childhood, 9*(2), 125–135.

Moran, D., & Whitman, T. (1985). The multiple effects of a play-oriented parent training program for mothers of developmentally delayed children. *Analysis and Intervention in Developmental Disabilities, 5,* 73–96.

Murphy, L., Heider, G., & Small, C. (1986). Individual differences in infants. *Zero to Three, 2*(2), 1–8.

Neifert, M. (1986). *Dr. mom: A guide to baby and child care*. New York: New American Library.

Newborg, J., Stock, J., Wnek, L., Guidubaldi, J., & Svinicki, J. (1984). *The Battelle Developmental Inventory*. Allen, TX: Developmental Learning Materials.

Peterson, N. (1987). *Early intervention for handicapped and at-risk children*. Denver: Love Publishing.

Piaget, J. (1951). *Play, dreams and imitation in childhood*. New York: Norton.

Piaget, J. (1952). *The origins of intelligence in children*. New York: International Universities Press.

Piaget, J., & Inhelder, B. (1969). *The psychology of the child*. New York: Basic Books.

Pollitt, E. (1983). Morbidity and infant development: A hypothesis. *International Journal of Behavioral Development, 6,* 461–475.

Ramey, C., & Gowen, J. (1984). A general systems approach to modifying risk for retarded development. *Early Child Development and Care, 16,* 9–26.

Resnick, M., Armstrong, S., & Carter, R. (1988). Developmental intervention program for high-risk premature infants: Effects on development and parent-infant interactions. *Journal of Developmental and Behavioral Pediatrics, 9,* 73–78.

Rogers, S., Donovan, C., D'Eugenio, D., Brown, S., Lynch, E., Moersch, M., & Schafer, S. (1981). *Early Intervention Development Profile* (rev. ed.) Ann Arbor: The University of Michigan Press.

Rose, S., Feldman, J., McCarton, C., & Wolfson, J. (1988). Information processing in 7-month-old infants as a function of risk status. *Child Development, 59,* 589–603.

Ruff, H., McCarton, C., Kurtzberg, D., & Vaughan, H. (1984). Preterm infants' manipulative exploration of objects. *Child Development, 55,* 1166–1173.

Saunder, R., & Sailor, W. (1979). A comparison of three strategies of reinforcement on two-choice language problems with severely retarded children. *AAESPH Review, 4,* 323–333.

Schwethelm, B., & Mahoney, G. (1986). Task persistence among organically impaired mentally retarded children. *American Journal of Mental Deficiency, 90,* 432–439.

Seibert, J., Hogan, A., & Mundy, P. (1986). On the specifically cognitive nature of early object and social skill domain associations. *Merrill-Palmer Quarterly, 32,* 21–36.

Slater, M., Naqvi, M., Andrew, L., & Haynes, K. (1987). Neurodevelopment of monitored versus nonmonitored very low birth weight infants: The importance of family interactions. *Journal of Developmental and Behavioral Pediatrics, 8,* 278–285.

Staff. (1988). Early intervention for children birth through 2 years. *NICHCY News Digest, 10.* Washington, DC: National Information Center for Children and Youth with Handicaps.

Uzgiris, I., & Hunt, J. (1975). *Assessment in infancy: Ordinal scales of psychological development.* Urbana: University of Illinois Press.

Vulpe, S. (1977). *Vulpe Assessment Battery.* Toronto: National Institute on Mental Retardation.

White, B. (1967). An experimental approach to the effects of experience on early human behavior. In J. P. Hill (Ed.), *Minnesota Symposium on Child Psychology (Vol. 1)* (pp. 230–255). Minneapolis: University of Minnesota Press.

Yarrow, L. J., Rubenstein, L., & Pedersen, F. A. (1975). *Infant and environment: Early cognitive and motivation development.* New York: Wiley.

5

Social and Communication Development in Infancy

Lou Rossetti

OVERVIEW

This chapter discusses social and communicative development and the role of the speech pathologist on the transdisciplinary team with infants and toddlers, including:

- the influence of prelinguistic factors on later linguistic development
- the relationship between social and early communicative development
- the development and assessment of prelinguistic behaviors
- the development and assessment of language comprehension and language expression

Language is the single best predictor of future cognition in the young child. In addition, language disorders are the best predictor of developmental deficits (Capute, Palmer, & Shapiro, 1987). Infants and toddlers with risk conditions and disabilities often display **socio-communicative** delays (Cogswell & Rossetti, 1987; Largo, Molinari, Pinto, Weber, & Duc, 1986; Rossetti, 1986; 1989). Specifically, socio-communicative skills involve maternal-infant interaction and attachment, as well as the child's overall ability to comprehend and process language. Delays in socio-communicative performance tend to translate into deficiencies in early experience with language, which may set into motion a cycle of delayed development.

Delayed speech and language development is the most common symptom of developmental disability in childhood. Speech and language delays affect approximately 5 to 10% of all children. Sixty-nine percent of all 3 to 5 year olds receiving early intervention services have language disabilities. In populations of children known to be at risk for developmental deficits, such as those with Down Syndrome, the percentage of children who display some form of communicative deficit is substantially higher. In fact, in the course of the regular day a pediatrician will see at least one or two children with communicative deficits (Coplan, 1985). The responsibility to facilitate speech and language in young children with disabilities is no longer the sole domain of speech-language pathologists. As with all auxiliary personnel, the role of the speech pathologist has changed as recognition of the value of teamwork in services for infants, toddlers, and their families has grown.

ROLE OF THE SPEECH-LANGUAGE PATHOLOGIST IN THE TRANSDISCIPLINARY TEAM

The intent of P.L. 99–457 is to provide comprehensive services for infants and toddlers and their families from a team service delivery model. The team approach, however, does not ignore the need for specific interventions provided by professionals trained in a particular discipline.

The primary responsibility of speech-language pathologists is to assist young children and their families in understanding the links between aspects of prelinguistic development and later communicative development, and how each of these areas may be modified by controlling interactions with adults and objects. Speech-language pathologists offer a range of services in hospital-, home-, and center-based programs.

In the Hospital

An increasing number of speech-language pathologists are being asked to provide services to infants in hospital settings, either prior to discharge to the home or during initial or later hospitalizations. Services may include consultation with hospital staff, direct intervention activities with the child, or interaction with parents.

Consultation with hospital staff.   Initially, the primary caregivers for sick or premature infants are hospital personnel. Consequently, speech-language pathologists collaborate with hospital personnel by offering suggestions for activities that might enhance the socio-communicative development of the infants. One typical recommendation is to provide stimulation when infants are alert. However, the opportunities for socio-communicative stimulation in the hospital nursery are controlled, in part, by nursing routines, staffing patterns, and the philosophy of the staff (Jacobson & Wendler, 1988).

Direct service to the infant.   The infant's medical status largely determines which services can be provided directly to the infant in the hospital nursery. As the infant becomes stronger and begins making efforts to interact, speech-language pathologists may become more involved with the child. This involvement may include demonstrating for families how they may recognize and capitalize upon their infant's early interactive attempts. Instruction about the identification and management of oral motor/feeding problems is often shared with developmental therapists. These services integrate oral motor/feeding activities with socio-communicative activities that benefit feeding, attachment, and early interactive behaviors.

Speech-language pathologists tend to use these opportunities as a chance to clarify for families, and other team members, the importance of feeding behaviors to oral motor skills, which translate later into speech and language skills. And, most commonly, speech-language pathologists may be involved in assessing the child before discharge.

Direct service to parents.   Parents of sick or premature infants frequently feel disenfranchised from the parenting process. These feelings have profound implications for the establishment of early interaction patterns and later socio-communicative development. Speech-language pathologists may be involved with parents to strengthen feelings of involvement, provide information regarding future development, and offer support.

In the Home

Encouraging positive adult-infant attachment and interaction are the primary goals for the transition from the hospital to the home setting. Through intervention coaching, speech-language pathologists guide parents and other family members in developing strategies for enhancing quality socio-communicative development. Part of this task involves helping parents recognize how essential their interactions are in shaping their child's communicative skills. For example, Jacobson, Starnes, and Gasser (1988) found that mothers who do not talk frequently to their premature infants generally have infants who score lower on developmental scales than infants whose mothers provide frequent language stimulation. In this study, after some mothers were trained to offer descriptions and praise to their children, the frequency of verbal interactions with the children increased.

In Center-based Programs

One advantage of center-based programs for young children with communicative delays is the accessibility of other members of the transdisciplinary team. The speech pathologists' roles in center-based programs are similar to their roles in other settings. They use input from parents and other team members to enhance children's socio-communication.

Depending on the program, speech pathologists may provide direct services to the child and family, or may train and release skills to other team members who will provide direct services. Specialized assessments tend to be conducted by the speech-language pathologist, often with team members present so results are more easily discussed. Generally, speech pathologists are highly selective about which skills are appropriate for release. Table 5–1 demonstrates the differences in the speech pathologist's role between the interdisciplinary and transdisciplinary team models.

Additionally, speech pathologists expand their skills beyond their discipline by systematically learning from other team members. This may be useful in many ways because not all speech pathologists are trained to work with infants. Reacting to the team approach to infant intervention, one speech-language pathologist commented: "I have worked it both ways—when I first started [with infants and preschool-aged

TABLE 5–1

Comparison of speech-language pathologist's role in interdisciplinary and transdisciplinary team models.

Child: Jonathon is a 17 month old with a history of prematurity and low birthweight, middle ear pathology, general failure to display adequate socio-communicative development, and an overall lack of interest in using language to interact with people.

Interdisciplinary Team Model	Transdisciplinary Team Model
Goal 1: Jonathon will display increased language comprehension skills as evidenced by pointing to a series of pictures of familiar objects.	Goal 1: Jonathon will demonstrate increased language comprehension ability and expression in all settings.
Goal 2: Jonathon will identify body parts asked by the speech-language pathologist at a 75% level of accuracy.	
Goal 3: Jonathon will name three body parts when prompted by the examiner.	

Activities	Activities
A. The speech-language pathologist will expose Jonathon to a series of 10 pictures of familiar objects, and he will be asked to point to the desired picture.	A. The primary service provider will provide Jonathon with a variety of objects, and will encourage appropriate play behaviors with the objects while also providing the names of the objects. These will be objects that require him to stack, manipulate, and categorize.
B. Jonathon will be shown five body parts and provided with the names of each part he is shown.	B. Jonathon's family will be shown how to accurately interpret and identify Jonathon's communicative intents. They will also be shown how to take full advantage of these intents in expanding upon and encouraging his communicative attempts.
C. Jonathon will be asked to name three body parts after he demonstrates 100% comprehension of the parts he is shown.	C. Jonathon's mother will be shown how she can better use the home environment to stimulate Jonathon's overall developmental progress.

---

handicapped children], I came into the home and worked on the child's communication needs, gave the mother some activities to do until the next visit, and left. Sometimes the mothers did them; sometimes they didn't. Now, I work with the family in all areas of the child's development—not just communication. I have learned positioning, self-help skills, and all kinds of skills [from the team]. If I'm not the one going to the home, I train someone else on our staff to do what I would have done with the child. I can't speak for anyone else, but I think I give better services to families now that we use a team approach."

EARLY IDENTIFICATION OF SOCIO-COMMUNICATIVE PROBLEMS

Efforts to identify early patterns of developmental delay in social and communicative development are under way. A national study (Palfrey, Singer, Walker, & Butler, 1987) to determine the age at which developmental deficits could be identified found, in part:

1. Overall, only 4.5% of children's problems are identified at birth.
2. Only 28.7% of children's problems are identified before the age of 5 years.
3. Variation in age of identification depends on the condition (1 year for Down Syndrome and cerebral palsy versus a 6-year range for mental retardation).
4. Physicians are more likely to identify less common, more severe handicaps. Physicians identify 15 to 25% of learning disabilities, speech impairments, emotional disorders, hyperactivity, and other developmental disorders.
5. Age of identification is predicated by the complexity of the problem, the association with health and other developmental concerns, socioeconomic indicators, and whether a physician is involved in the diagnosis or not.

These results suggest that, as a whole, early identification is not well coordinated. Part of the difficulty seems to be the lack of consensus on the factors that may influence maladaptive social development and atypical communicative development. However, there is agreement that early detection of socio-communicative problems may improve the quality of later performance in all domains of development, especially prelinguistic development.

PRELINGUISTIC DEVELOPMENT AND ASSESSMENT

Socio-communicative development begins at birth. Long before children consistently vocalize or utter their first words, the foundations for socio-communicative competencies are established. Many believe that early nonverbal interchanges between the child and the parent/caregiver during the first months of life form the basis for later conversational turn-taking and language knowledge (Bruner, 1978). Consequently, interventionists must be aware of the various aspects of **prelinguistic** (preverbal) **development** which precede the emergence of first words (the linguistic period).

Prelinguistic development is related to caregiver-infant attachment and interaction, play behavior, gestural development, and the development of pragmatics. Interventionists must be familiar with the development and assessment of these factors to facilitate them, and to encourage families to facilitate them, in young children.

Infant-caregiver Attachment

A variety of researchers during several decades have elaborated on the process by which the human infant becomes attached to its primary caregiver. What has emerged from this work is a description of the critical importance of **attachment**, a unique relationship that lasts over time (Klaus & Kennell, 1976), to the survival and development of the infant.

Attachment works in both directions. Infants become attached to caregivers and caregivers become attached to infants. Generally, the mother's attachment begins during the initial planning of the pregnancy and continues to grow following the birth of the child and the undertaking of caregiving routines. The steps of attachment from the maternal perspective are outlined in Table 5–2.

Taylor and Hall (1979) have perhaps best summarized the unexpected realities that replace maternal expectations with the birth of a child who has special needs. They state that for the mother of the ill or premature infant:

1. A scrawny, underweight, high-risk infant, who is either seriously ill or likely to become so, replaces the healthy fullterm infant.
2. An unreactive or underreactive infant replaces the responsive infant with whom the parents had expected to actively interact.
3. Separation of the infant from the mother replaces the anticipated frequent and close contact.
4. An incubator in a sophisticated intensive care nursery replaces the expected bassinet beside the mother's bed.
5. Nurses, doctors, and knowledgeable strangers replace the parents as the primary caregivers.
6. The mother has failed to produce the expected baby; hence, the parents' perception of failure and its accompanying loss of self-esteem replace the expected success and increase in self-esteem.

Parents of at-risk and handicapped infants are vulnerable to difficulties in parent-child attachments and interactions. However, deficiencies in interactional style or

TABLE 5–2
Steps in attachment from the maternal perspective.

1. Pregnancy planning
2. Pregnancy confirmation
3. Acceptance of the pregnancy
4. Initial movement of the fetus
5. Mother begins to accept the fetus as an individual
6. Birth of the baby
7. Seeing and hearing the baby
8. Touching and holding the baby
9. Routine caregiving over time

Source: From *Care of the High-Risk Neonate* (p. 149) by M. Klaus & S. Fanaroff, 1979, Philadelphia: Saunders. Copyright © 1979, by W. B. Saunders. Reprinted by permission of W. B. Saunders and the authors.

attachment detected at an early age are often more amenable to intervention. If left untreated, the chances of later socio-communicative problems are greatly increased.

Assessment of infant-caregiver attachment.   Optimal parental-infant interactional patterns result only when there are sufficient levels of caregiver or maternal attachment. Attachment deficiencies may be worsened by prolonged illnesses, health issues, and stress. Fortunately, there are several strategies interventionists may use to detect patterns of attachment that may be indicative of impending deficiencies in caregiving ability.

Avant (1982) describes an assessment strategy designed to focus on maternal attachment behaviors. Using a 1-page observation checklist consisting of common attachment behaviors compiled from several sources, the Maternal-Infant Observation Scale gives information on general attachment, affectionate behavior, proximity maintaining, and caretaking. A modified score sheet for the Maternal-Infant Observation Scale is shown in Table 5–3.

This scale, and others like it, allow interventionists to structure observations so more accurate judgments regarding the development of attachment may be made. If normal attachment behaviors are observed, especially if these behaviors are observed early and persist over time, the probability that normal interaction will develop is increased. The absence of normal attachment, however, increases the risk of deficient adult-child interaction styles.

Infant-caregiver Interaction

Eye contact, crying, quieting, attention to faces and voices, and body movements are interaction cues and responses of the normal newborn. In general, infant-caregiver interactions that are considered in synchrony with the infant's signals are thought to

TABLE 5–3
Maternal-infant observation scale.

Affectionate Behavior Subscale	Proximity Maintaining Subscale
Positions infant en face	Mother holds infant
Looking at infant	Close contact with infant
Talking (singing, cooing to infant)	Encompasses infant
A-T-L (accessory/touch/love)	Infant on mother's knees
Kisses infant	
Smiles at infant	
Touches with fingertips only	
Touches with fingertips and palms	

Source: From "A Maternal Attachment Assessment Strategy" by P. Avant in *Analysis of Current Assessment Strategies in the Health Care of Young Children and Childbearing Families* (p. 172) by S. Humenick-Smith (Ed.), 1982, Norwich, CT: Appleton-Century-Crofts. Copyright © 1982, by Appleton-Century-Crofts. Adapted by permission.

have beneficial long-term effects on cognitive, social, and linguistic skills (Sparks, Clark, Oas, & Erickson, 1988). However, at times it may be more difficult to establish a responsive relationship with young children with developmental disabilities. Many factors—adjustment to the diagnosis, additional caregiving demands, financial pressures—may affect initial parent-child interactions. In other cases, children are not afforded an optimal opportunity to establish a stable relationship with their primary caregiver. Infants who spend 4 to 10 weeks in an intensive care nursery, for example, use all of their physiological energy for survival. There is little energy to spare to develop a reciprocal relationship with any caregiver.

It is generally accepted that the quality of time parents spend with their child is directly related to the quality of interactional patterns that develop. Hospitalizations may interfere with the time typically spent bonding with the infant. For example, infants between 1,501 and 2,000 g initially spend a mean of 24 days in the neonatal intensive care nursery while infants weighing less than 1,000 g spend a mean of 89 days (Committee to Study the Prevention of Low Birth Weight, 1985). Further, 40% of the infants with these birthweights are rehospitalized during the first year of life for a mean of 16 days (Committee to Study the Prevention of Low Birth Weight, 1985). In these situations, establishing optimal parent-infant interactional patterns in the early months of life with premature or sick infants clearly will be difficult, even for the most determined parents.

Interactional opportunity.   High and Gorski (1985) found that family-infant interactions in the hospital were not only limited, but any adult-infant interactions for the acutely ill premature and convalescing infant may be severely limited. These researchers quantified the interactions observed between medical personnel and infants while infants were in the intensive care nursery and then examined the opportunities for interaction. The results of their study indicate that:

1. Nurses were present for only 30% of the acute observations and 20% of the convalescent observations.
2. No caregiver of any kind was present for 63% of acute observation periods and 71% on convalescent ones. (These statistics may reflect staffing patterns that assign one nurse to several infants at a time when they no longer require critical care.)
3. Nurses spent 85 seconds for acute and 64 seconds for convalescent groups from the time of completing an intervention to the time of leaving the infant's care area.

These results dramatize the reality that less than optimal interactional opportunities and patterns are part of the normal hospital nursery routine. And yet, these patterns of interaction exist in the presence of high-quality medical care. Early physical separations caused by health crises, or emotional distances prompted by stress-related adjustments to the child's developmental disability, put the child and the child's family at risk for interaction and attachment deficits.

Assessment of infant-caregiver interaction.   In an attempt to identify deficient mother-infant interactive-communicative patterns, Klein and Briggs (1986) devised the Observation of Communicative Interaction (OCI) scale. The OCI is an informal observation guide to assist in describing the interaction strategies used by parents. The tool may be administered during any caregiver routine, and is organized around 10 interaction categories. Ratings from the OCI may help to informally identify strengths and weaknesses in caregivers' interaction patterns and provide guidance for planning individual goals to increase the match between parent and child behaviors. An adapted scoring form based on the Observation of Communicative Interaction scale is presented in Table 5–4.

Seibert and Hogan (1982) devised another means of monitoring the type and quality of interactions between parents and their children. They developed the Early Social Communication Scales (ESCS) as a measure of the degree to which the infant seeks out, responds to, and/or initiates social interaction. In the early stages of interaction, the infant establishes the tone for interactions. In fact, it has been found that helping infants with severe handicaps cry less and smile more in response to actions

TABLE 5–4
Observation of communicative interaction scoring sheet.

Item	Rarely/Never	Sometimes	Often
1. Provides appropriate tactile kinesthetic stimulation (strokes, pats, caresses, cuddles, rocks baby).	_____	_____	_____
2. Mother displays pleasure while interacting with baby.	_____	_____	_____
3. Mother responds to child's distress.	_____	_____	_____
4. Positions self and infant so eye-to-eye contact is possible (facing 7 to 12 inches away).	_____	_____	_____
5. Smiles contingently at infant.	_____	_____	_____
6. Varies prosodic features (uses higher pitch, talks slower, exaggerates intonation).	_____	_____	_____
7. Encourages conversation.	_____	_____	_____
8. Responds contingently to infant's behavior.	_____	_____	_____
9. Modifies interaction in response to negative cues from infant.	_____	_____	_____
10. Uses communication to teach language and concepts.	_____	_____	_____

Source: Adapted from *Observation of Communicative Interaction* (unpaged) by D. Klein & M. Briggs, 1986, Washington, DC: Division of Maternal and Child Health, U.S. Department of Health and Human Services. This observation scale is in the public domain.

of their parents and other adults seems to make a significant contribution to the life satisfaction of both parent and child (Rose, Calhoun, & Ladage, 1989). Consequently, the more responsive the infant is to caregivers, the richer and more complex the interactions caregivers tend to offer the child. For this reason, using direct teaching to increase positive child characteristics (e.g., smiling, initiation, soothability) to increase positive parent/caregiver-child interactions is often recommended for at-risk children and their families. The items of the Early Social Communication Scales are presented in Table 5–5.

Early interactions and attachment are precursors to later, more elaborate social and communicative patterns. Although it is accepted that responsive adult-child interactions are crucial to normal development, it is difficult to quantify the exact nature of *quality* adult-infant interactions. Despite the fact that the instruments discussed have identified certain behaviors as representative of optimal interactional patterns, it is difficult to attach weighted values to these behaviors.

Interactional styles vary across families as well as cultures. For instance, maternal age and cultural differences appear related to the amount of maternal verbalizations offered during early teaching interactions (DeCubas & Field, 1984). Although caregiver-child interactional patterns show considerable variation, certain behaviors do seem to be important for the nurturing of the young child and may be worthwhile intervention goals. Generally, it is accepted that young children need experiences that support their emotional growth. Critical areas for socio-communicative intervention seem to be related to increasing and introducing experiences that foster the following in caregiver-child interactions:

☐ attention and engagement
☐ intentional, reciprocal gestures and cues
☐ vocal/verbal turn-taking
☐ elaboration of emotional responsiveness
☐ mutually pleasurable exchanges

TABLE 5–5
Early social communication scale dimensions.

Child responds to social interaction
Child initiates social interaction
Child maintains social interaction
Child responds to joint attention
Child initiates joint attention
Child maintains joint attention
Child responds to behavior regulation
Child initiates behavior regulation
Child maintains behavior regulation

Source: Adapted from Jeffrey M. Seibert and Anne E. Hogan, "A Model for Assessing Social and Object Skills and Planning Intervention," in Dan P. McClowry, Arthur M. Guilford, and Sylvia O. Richardson (Eds.), *Infant Communication Development: Assessment and Intervention,* p. 30. Copyright © 1982 by Allyn and Bacon. Used with permission.

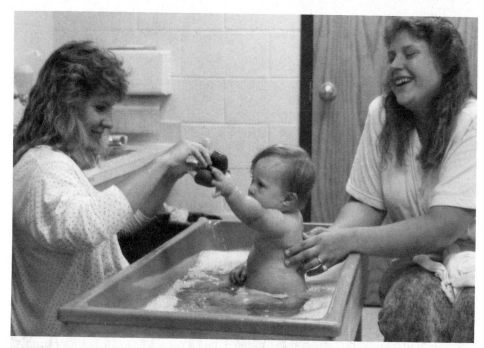

Playful, mutually rewarding interactions promote positive attachments and provide the foundation for quality socio-communicative development in infants and toddlers.

Play

Monitoring play can assist interventionists in following how the child develops representational thought. A large body of evidence relates certain cognitive skills to various features of language development. Although no one-to-one mapping of language and cognitive concepts exists, it is clear that certain behaviors reflected in the child's play express cognitive skills necessary for the development of spoken language.

Both language and pretend play require the child to mentally represent reality. Just as the child must realize that a doll is only a representation of a live baby, or that a piece of paper can serve as a blanket, the child must understand that a word is not the object but only a representation of the object. Consequently, it is important that interventionists are familiar with play and play assessments as well as how play affects language development.

A number of researchers have attempted to map this relationship. For example, The Manual for Analyzing Free Play (MAFP), proposed by McCune-Nicolich (1980), incorporates a play sequence initially suggested by Piaget (1962). The MAFP includes strategies for viewing symbolic play, relational play, and manipulative play. By categorizing the different types of play, a series of discrete judgments may be made concerning the child's play behavior. Table 5–6 presents an adapted version of one of the play levels (e.g., symbolic play) and the specific play behaviors incorporated in this tool. Manipulative and relational play are coded in a similar way.

TABLE 5–6
Categorizing symbolic play.

Level	Play Behaviors
Level 1: Pre-symbolic scheme	Child picks up comb, touches it to hair, drops it
	Child picks up phone, puts it to ear, sets it aside
	Child gives mop a swish on floor
	Child hammers
	Child rolls truck on floor
Level 2: Auto-symbolic scheme	Child simulates drinking from a toy baby bottle
	Child eats from an empty spoon
	Child closes eyes/pretends to sleep
Level 3: Single scheme symbolic games	Child feeds mother or doll
	Child grooms mother or doll
	Child pretends to read a book
	Child pretends to mop floor
Level 4.1: Single scheme combinations	Child combs own, then mother's, hair
	Child drinks from bottle, then feeds doll from bottle
	Child cleans several objects with sponge
Level 4.2: Multischeme combinations	Child holds phone to ear, then talks
	Child kisses doll, puts it to bed, puts spoon to its mouth
	Child stirs in the pot, feeds doll, pours food into dish
Levels 5.1 and 5.2: Planned symbolic sets	Child picks up bottle, says baby, then feeds the doll and covers it with cloth
	Child finds iron, sets it down, searches for cloth, then irons (5.1)
	Child puts play foods in pot, stirs, says "mommy" or "soup," then feeds mother (5.2)
	Child picks up play screwdriver, says "toothbrush," and makes the motion of toothbrush

Source: From "Beyond Sensorimotor Intelligence: Assessment of Symbolic Maturity Through Analysis of Pretend Play" by L. McCune Nicolich in *Merrill-Palmer Quarterly, 23* (April, 1977), pp. 89–99. Adapted with permission from L. McCune Nicolich, Rutgers University, New Brunswick, NJ.

Additional paradigms for charting the development of play from a Piagetian orientation are provided by Rubin, Maroni, and Hornung (1975) and Dunst (1980). Play activities are frequently arranged as a means of facilitating communicative skills in young children. Using the naturalistic teaching strategies discussed in Chapter 4, play offers opportunities for initiating and refining comprehension and expression skills in children. Westby (1980) has outlined the play activities and concurrent language skills that should be expected at various ages for young children. A sample of these concurrent play and language behaviors for symbolic play are presented in Table 5–7.

Changes in play behavior, especially symbolic play, are accompanied by concurrent changes in language function and usage (Mindes, 1982; Terrell & Schwartz, 1988). Observing the child's play skills can give interventionists an insight into the child's communicative and cognitive performance.

Gestures

Gestures are also precursors to verbal communication, and occur concurrently with other aspects of preverbal communication. The importance of gestural development on later communicative abilities has only recently been acknowledged. It is now considered important that interventionists monitor gestural development and arrange specific interventions when expected patterns do not emerge.

Several instruments have been developed for this purpose. The Assessing Prelinguistic and Early Linguistic Behaviors inventory (Olswang, Stoel-Gammons, Coggins, & Carpenter, 1987), for instance, includes a language and gesture section. This instrument represents the first comprehensive attempt to structure gestural assessment as part of a complete battery designed to assess prelinguistic and early linguistic skills. The tool organizes gestures into six distinct categories: social regulation and social games; greetings, signs of affection, and bedtime; eating and drinking; dressing, grooming, and washing; adult activities; and toys and games. A sample of the specific behaviors included in this gesture inventory is provided in Table 5–8.

In addition, the Early Language Milestone Scale (ELM) (Coplan, 1987), which was developed as a rapid means of assessing language development in children from birth to 3 years of age, can provide limited information about the child's use of gestures. Further information about gestural competence may be obtained from parents by asking questions such as, "Does your baby ever play Peek-A-Boo, Patty Cake, or wave bye-bye?" If parents respond in the affirmative, then a follow-up question about whether the child demonstrates these behaviors spontaneously or imitatively should be asked.

Two instruments that are designed specifically to assess early language skills, and which incorporate gestural items, are the Oliver (MacDonald, 1978) and the Environmental Prelanguage Battery (Horstmeier & MacDonald, 1978). The gesture items on these tools are used to compute an overall score for language ability. The Early Intervention Developmental Profile (EIDP) (Rogers et al., 1981) also incorporates gestural items as part of an overall assessment of children up to 36 months of age. The EIDP is designed to gather data on skills in the cognitive, motor, social, self-

TABLE 5–7
Symbolic play scale.

Play Activity	Language
Stage I: 9–12 months	
Aware that objects exist when not seen.	No true language. May have words associated with some actions and objects.
Does not mouth or bang all toys.	Exhibits some command and request behaviors.
Stage II: 13–17 months	
Purposefully explores toys. Discovers operation of toys through trial/error.	Single words used (context dependent).
Hands toy to adult if unable to operate on own.	Communicative functions include: request, command, protest, respond, greet, protest.
Stage III: 17–19 months	
Pretends to go to sleep or drink from a cup.	Uses words to describe own actions.
Stage IV: 19–22 months	
Symbolic play extends beyond the child's self.	Refers to objects and persons not present.
Plays with dolls. Combines two toys in play. Performs pretend activities.	Beginning of word combinations.
Stage V: 24 months	
Represents daily experiences, plays house, uses objects in a realistic manner.	Uses increased phrases and short sentences.
	Following morphological markers appear: /ing/ endings, plurals, possessives.
Stage VI: 30 months	
Represents events less frequently experienced.	Responds to what, who, whose, where?
	Asks WH questions.
Stage VII: 36 months	
Obviously sequences play activities.	Uses past tense.
Associative play.	Uses future aspects (particularly *gonna*), such as "I'm gonna wash dishes."
Re-enacts events with varying outcomes.	

Source: From "Assessment of Cognitive and Language Abilities Through Play" by C. Westby, *Language, Speech, and Hearing Services in the Schools, 3,* 1980, p. 154. Copyright © 1980 by The Council for Exceptional Children. Reprinted with permission.

TABLE 5–8

Gesture inventory behaviors.

Social regulation and social games
"Up" (reaches arms up in request to be picked up)
Shows (extends arm with object in hand)
Peek-A-Boo (covers and uncovers face)
Nods head yes
"All gone" (shrugs and puts out hands in gesture of surprise)

Greetings, signs of affection, bedtime
Waves hi/bye
Hugs (dolls, people, and/or animals)
Puts to bed (dolls, people, and/or animals)
Rocks (dolls, people, and/or animals)

Eating and drinking
Drinks (brings container to mouth)
Feeds others (puts utensil to mouth of doll)
Wipes (wipes hands or face with napkin or bib)
Pours (makes gesture of pouring from a container)

Dressing, grooming, and washing
Combs or brushes hair
Brushes teeth
Puts on hat (or tries to put on)
Diapers (takes off/puts on diapers, powders bottom)

Adult activities
Talks on telephone (puts receiver to ear)
Pushes stroller/shopping cart
Plays musical instrument (tries to play an instrument)
Writes/types

Toys and games
Throws and/or kicks ball
Rolls or pushes toy vehicles
Makes a shooting gesture
Makes a gesture of flying an airplane or helicopter in the air

Source: From *Assessing Prelinguistic and Early Linguistic Behaviors* (p. 120) by L. Olswang, C. Stoel-Gammons, T. Coggins, & R. Carpenter, 1987, Seattle: University of Washington Press. Copyright © 1987 by University of Washington Press. Adapted with permission.

care, and language domains. Because this instrument integrates multiple developmental areas, interventionists working in teams find it especially useful.

Gesture assessment instruments such as these permit early interventionists to structure observations of gestures during more traditional infant/toddler assessments. The absence of gestural behaviors may be indicative of impending language deficits. This deficit tends to become more obvious when traditional language milestones are expected, and do not develop.

Although additional research on the development of gestures is needed, there is enough information at this time to encourage the assessment of gestures as a part of comprehensive language assessments of children younger than 3 years of age. Gestural development, like other prelinguistic skill areas, appears to be related to the development of pragmatics in young children.

Pragmatics

The final area of prelinguistic language development to be discussed is pragmatic development. **Pragmatics** refers to the use of language in social contexts and includes the social rules of how language is used for communication. Pragmatics are concerned with the way language is used to communicate, rather than with the way language is structured (Owens, 1988). For the very young child, pragmatics involve the reasons for speaking, and understanding how to participate in conversations. Generally, children learn pragmatics, as well as most aspects of language, within the context of conversation.

Much of the child's language, including pragmatics, during the first 3 years concerns the here and now. For example, the 2 year old is able to respond to a conversational partner and to engage in short dialogues of a few turns on a given topic. The 2 year old may also be able to introduce a change in the topic of discussion. By age 3, the child is more aware of the social aspects of communicating, better acknowledges a partner's turn, and engages in longer conversations. By kindergarten age, the child has learned the basic rules for the social usage of language, although refinement of pragmatic learning continues for some time.

The learning of pragmatic rules is set in motion initially by the interactions between the primary caregiver and the infant. By reviewing the features of mother-infant talk, it is apparent how conducive they are to the development of pragmatic functions in children (Olswang et al., 1987):

- □ short utterance length and simple syntax
- □ object-centered, small core vocabulary
- □ topics limited to here and now
- □ heightened use of facial expressions and gestures
- □ frequent questioning and greeting
- □ infant behaviors are treated as meaningful: mother awaits infant's turn and responds even to nonturns
- □ frequent modifications of pitch and loudness
- □ frequent verbal rituals

A few instruments are available to assist interventionists in their attempt to assess and facilitate social/pragmatic uses of language in infants and toddlers. One instrument is The Social Communication-Pragmatics Screening Test (Antoniadis, Didow, Lockhart, & Moroge, 1984). Although there is no normative data, this scale may be useful for guiding intervention decisions.

Other instruments examine pragmatics in the context of other language functions. For example, The Communication and Symbolic Behavior Scales (CSBS) (Wetherby & Prizant, 1989), designed for early identification of children who have or are at risk for developing communication impairments, examine the communication, social, affective, and symbolic abilities of children functioning between a 9-month and 2-year communication age. These scales attempt to detect early communication problems. Innovative efforts such as the CSBS expand the ability of professionals to identify, monitor, and ultimately intervene in areas of communicative delay and performance that previously were too subtle for such early detection.

There is a relationship between gestural and pragmatic development. For example, children use gestures to communicate by 12 to 18 months of age; gestures plus word-like vocalizations at 12 to 18 months; conventional words or word combinations to express a range of intentions at 18 to 24 months; requests for objects or action, rejections, or protest at 18 to 24 months; and a variety of newly developed intentions (discourse functions) at 18 to 24 months (Chapman, 1981). Normally developing children incorporate many of the basic rules of conversation into their communicative repertoire as it develops.

From the previous discussion of prelinguistic development, it should be clear that early communicative and social-emotional development in early childhood overlap. To influence prelinguistic aspects of the child's socio-communicative development, interventionists must be able to assess, monitor, and encourage major preverbal skills. Because most nonprofessionals believe children learn language when they begin to speak, it is also important that interventionists communicate the importance of prelinguistic competence to families and other professionals.

LANGUAGE COMPREHENSION

The importance of prelinguistic skills to later acquisition of linguistic or verbal language has only recently been understood. A more traditional view of language development and assessment considered the process of language as primarily related to language comprehension and expression. Given the prevalence of communicative disorders, it is essential that all members of transdisciplinary teams become familiar with procedures for assessing and facilitating the broad spectrum of early speech and language abilities.

Assessment

There is a strong link between cognition, comprehension, and production in child language. Children learn language by first determining, independent of language, the meaning that a speaker intends to convey to them, and then working out the relationship between the meaning and the language. As children pass through various stages of growth in language comprehension, they tend to display behaviors reflective of this process taking place. These behaviors form the basis for what is measured as language comprehension or receptive language. **Receptive language** involves the child's ability to understand spoken language. For a more complete discussion of various aspects of language development see Owens (1988).

Many instruments and checklists have outlined a sequence of comprehension skills in children younger than the age of 3. For example, Rowan and Johnson (1988) developed a screening instrument for evaluating comprehension behaviors of children from birth through 12 months of age. The instrument lists specific behaviors and how these behaviors are observed. Observational categories include direct observation and direct testing. Table 5–9 presents a sample of comprehension items by age.

Most of the few standardized comprehension assessment instruments available use a format that attempts to measure primarily single-word vocabulary comprehension. In some cases, test items may not represent the child's comprehension reper-

TABLE 5–9
Speech and language screening comprehension items.

How Observed	PR = Parental Report O = Direct Observation DT = Direct Testing	Comprehension Item
	Birth to 3 Months	
_____		Alerting response to sound
_____		Activity diminishes/ceases when approached by sound
_____		Quieted by a familiar voice
_____		Smiles at mother's voice
_____		Often watches speaker's mouth
	3 to 6 months	
_____		Shows fear to angry voice
_____		Anticipates feeding at sight of food
_____		Recognizes and responds to name
_____		Appears to recognize words such as *up* and *bye*
_____		Responds to pleasant speech by smiling
	6 to 9 months	
_____		Moves toward or searches for family member when named
_____		Begins to show recognition of *no*
_____		Begins to anticipate visual games
_____		Shows stranger anxiety
_____		Relates sound to an object
	9 to 12 months	
_____		Action response to verbal request
_____		Shakes head yes/no
_____		Understands *hot* and *so big*
_____		Understands some action words
_____		Frowns when scolded
_____		May follow simple commands when given by gesture

Source: From *Screening and Assessment* (p. 2) by L. Rowan & C. Johnson, 1988, June. Paper presented at the Infant and Toddler Communication and Assessment Workshop, Minneapolis.

toire. One way to handle this dilemma is to interview parents prior to the assessment, and ask them to identify several items their child seems to know.

Although some reservations have been expressed regarding the use of vocabulary checklists as a valid index of child language, there is reasonable support for the claim that vocabulary checklists are valid instruments for the assessment of various aspects of child language (Reznick & Goldsmith, 1989). Performance on vocabulary checklists seems to be correlated with scores on the Bayley Scales of Infant Development and the Peabody Picture Vocabulary Test at 13 and 24 months of age (Olson, Bates, & Bayles, 1982).

Reznick (1982) used vocabulary checklists for 8-, 14-, and 20-month-old children and found a reasonable pattern of similarity between parents' assessment of child language and the child's behavior in a word comprehension procedure administered in a laboratory setting. Comprehension tasks that include items appropriate for the age and environment of the child, and that are free from cues from the individual giving the test, seem to be a valuable means to assess overall language comprehension for children younger than 3 years of age.

After the 24-month level, a number of traditional assessment instruments are available. Instruments such as the Peabody Picture Vocabulary Test (Dunn & Dunn, 1981), the Test of Auditory Comprehension of Language (Carrow, 1973), the Environmental Prelanguage Battery (Horstmeier & MacDonald, 1978), the Receptive-Expressive Emergent Language Scale (Bzoch & League, 1971), and the Miller-Yoder Test of Grammatical Comprehension (Miller & Yoder, 1982) are good examples. The Early Language Milestone Scale (Coplan, 1987) and the Assessing Prelinguistic and Early Linguistic Behaviors scale (Olswang et al., 1987) are designed for infants and toddlers and use both parent reporting and direct observation to determine language comprehension ability.

Assessing the language comprehension of children younger than 3 years of age challenges even the most experienced speech pathologist. However, by using a number of sources of information such as parent questionnaires, direct observation of behaviors during informal assessment procedures, and the administration of established language comprehension evaluation instruments, a fairly accurate assessment of the child's skills can be established. Successful assessment and intervention is always built upon the assumption that interventionists are well trained to be astute observers of spontaneous behaviors, and to use naturalistic ways to improve language comprehension. Generally, teamwork produces the best intervention plans for children.

Intervention

Language comprehension is linked to language expression. Unless the child has significant deficits with pragmatics, as in the case of some autistic children, comprehension intervention tends to be included with expressive language intervention. This is because comprehension (receptive language) tends to precede the development of expressive language (the ability to produce language). Infants understand who *mom* is long before they are able to call for her.

Comprehension can be encouraged through the use of naturalistic techniques. As stated in Chapter 4, naturalistic teaching involves using what the child is engaged in at the time to teach, reinforce, and shape desired skills. For example, to foster comprehension, the parent or interventionist would focus on objects and actions that are familiar to the child. The child would hear these objects and actions frequently labeled (e.g., "Oh, your cup!") and the child would be asked to indicate the objects or actions (e.g., "Which one is your cup?"). Nouns are taught first in this way and then verbs. Action words initially should be words that describe the child's own actions (e.g., "You drank it."). To evaluate the child's comprehension, the child could be asked to continue or discontinue the action (e.g., "Drink some more."). In the beginning, requests may need to be supported with gestural cues such as pointing or modeling as the request is given.

Chapman (1981) suggests this sequence of comprehension ability by age:

8–12 months	Understands a few single words in routine
12–18 months	Understands single words outside of routine, some contextual cues needed
18–24 months	Understands words for absent objects, some two-word combinations
24–36 months	Comprehension of three-word sentences, needs context of past experience to determine meaning

As basic comprehension is established, more difficult comprehension tasks may be attempted. The items used in previous levels may be then used as two-word units. That is, familiar nouns may be used in conjunction with familiar verbs. Later, both familiar and unfamiliar combinations of nouns and verbs may be used, as well as novel combinations. It can be assumed that if the child demonstrates appropriate performance to an utterance such as "kiss the car," appropriate comprehension is present. Other suggestions for comprehension intervention are presented in the expressive language section.

LANGUAGE EXPRESSION

Around their first birthday, most children produce their first word. This is typically an exciting time for families. However, if a child does not make this milestone, it may be a time of additional stress. Before specific activities can be planned to attempt to stimulate any child's expressive language, a description of the child's past and current expressive behaviors must be obtained.

Assessment

There are many ways to assess language expression. One method is to have parents fill out a questionnaire on their child's language usage. Table 5–10 presents a language/speech expression-oriented questionnaire. Some of the expression items in

TABLE 5–10
Speech and language screening expression items.

How Observed	PR = Parental Report	Expression Item	S = Speech Oriented
	O = Direct Observation		C = Communication Oriented
	DT = Direct Testing		

Birth to 3 months

_____	Reflexive cry
_____	Soft, throaty noises
_____	Begins differentiated cry
_____	Vocal sounds of pleasure
_____	Begins sustained laughter
_____	Vocalizes two or more different syllables

3 to 6 months

_____	Talks back in face-to-face interaction (S)
_____	Produces more vowels than consonants (S)
_____	Vocalizes to objects that move (S)
_____	Protests when objects are removed (S)
_____	Initiates simple person-oriented acts (C)

6 to 9 months

_____	Initiates conversations with toys (C)
_____	Babbles using many different phonemes (S)
_____	Inconsistently imitates noises of others (S)
_____	Shakes head *No* (C)
_____	Expresses desire by hand gesture (C)

9 to 12 months

_____	Echos speech and imitates sound (C)
_____	Copies melody pattern of familiar phrases (S)
_____	Tugs on mother for attention (C)
_____	Initiates speech games (S)
_____	Uses one to three words (S)

Source: From *Screening and Assessment* (p. 4) by L. Rowan & C. Johnson, 1988, June. Paper presented at the Infant and Toddler Communication and Assessment Workshop, Minneapolis.

the table represent speech-oriented behaviors (S), those that involve some form of verbalization; others represent communication-oriented behaviors (C), which are mostly nonverbal behaviors such as gestures.

Other methods of assessing expressive language are to conduct a parent interview and to observe the child and parents interacting in play situations. A combination of all three methods provides the most complete and useful information about the child's language expression. These activities are not intended to supplant the need for formal assessment instruments. However, instruments designed to measure language expression in children younger than 3 years of age are in an emerging state. For this reason, parent information and observed behaviors should never be overlooked or undervalued in the presence of contradictory test results.

Following a child's interests, repeating the activity often, and expanding a child's observations
during play are ways to facilitate
language skills in infants and
toddlers.

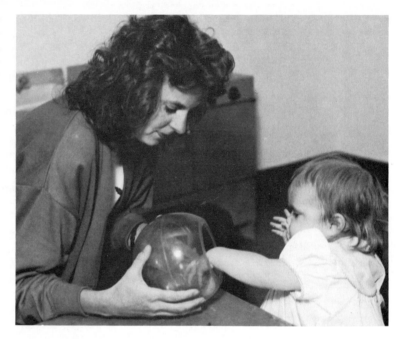

Nonstandard expressive language assessment procedures.   Still another way to
assess expressive language is to use nonstandard assessments. Nonstandard procedures are not synonymous with informal or unstructured observations. Nonstandard
procedures differ from standard procedures or tests in that they do not have a well-
established set of stimuli or instructions that must be adhered to, nor do they have
well-established standards or norms for interpretation. They do have sufficient face
validity to be used in assessing various aspects of language, and encompass both
structured tasks and unstructured observations. One of the primary assets of nonstandard procedures is that they are flexible and may be adapted to fit the needs and
characteristics of the child. Because the interventionist is not limited to a particular
method for eliciting information, the child's knowledge and abilities can be explored
by varying content, form, and presentation. Four common nonstandard assessment
procedures include nonstandard instruments, word production checklists, parent reporting, and the collection and analysis of spontaneous language samples.

First, a good example of a nonstandard assessment instrument is the Infant
Scale of Communicative Intent (ISCI) (Update Pediatrics, 1982). The ISCI is a descriptive measure developed to meet the needs of infants with developmental problems. Items on the scale are administered by observation, direct testing, or parental
reporting. Scoring is on a pass/fail basis, and both comprehension and expression
are assessed. An adapted form of the language expression portion of the ISCI is
presented in Table 5–11.

Second, word checklists may be used to obtain sample vocabulary for assessing
early language. Reznick and Goldsmith (1989) suggest that sample vocabulary is well

TABLE 5–11

Infant Scale of Communicative Intent (ISCI).

Language Expression Items

Birth to 1 Month
Some vocalizations
Nasalized vowels
Begins to cry for attention

1–2 Months
Begins differentiated cry
Gurgles in response to stimulation
Produces short vowel sounds
Cries for social stimulation

2–3 Months
Definitely coos
Makes glottal-velar consonants
Takes turns when communicating
Alerts to people

3–4 Months
Initiates babbling
Chuckles—sort of vocalized laugh
Cries for attention
Vocalizes feelings of pleasure

4–5 Months
Vocalizes laughter
Vocalizes eagerness
Cries if play disrupted
Actively engages adult interaction

5–6 Months
Vocalizes "ah-goo"
Imitates own noises
Vocalizes to interrupt others

6–7 Months
Imitates familiar sounds
Expresses anger by sounds
Initiates social contact
Tries to imitate facial expression

7–8 Months
Repeats babbling
Imitates sound sequence
Imitates gestures
Vocalizes satisfaction

8–9 Months
Shakes head "no-no"
Combines two or more consonants
Shouts for attention

9–10 Months
Intentionally communicates
Gestures with vocalizations
Uses sounds to call others

10–11 Months
Vocabulary of two words or approximation
Uses objects as tools
Laughs at own sounds
Attempts to label objects

11–12 Months
May recognize words as symbols
Uses "ma-ma" with meaning
Imitates new sounds
Imitates tones of adult

12–13 Months
Uses three to four meaningful words
Uses sounds for vocal play
Imitates animal sounds
Wakes with a "call"

13–14 Months
Has six-word vocabulary
Points to desired object
Tries to sing
Imitates other children

14–15 Months
Has up to 8-word vocabulary
Initiates give and take
Uses modifiers

15–16 Months
Starts using double syllable words
May label pictures
Pulls at wet pants/diaper
Pulls adult hand to show something

16–17 Months
Uses extended phrases for vocal play
Uses differentiated object names
Gradually increases vocabulary
May ask "what that?"

17–18 Months
Has up to 20-word vocabulary
Asks for "more"
Makes successive single word utterances.

Source: From "An Assessment Tool: The Infant Scale of Communicative Intent" by Gail Karen Sacks, M.A., CCC-SP, & Edna Carter Young, Ph.D., CCCI-SP, 1982, *Update Pediatrics*, pp. 1–4. Adapted by permission. This material is in the public domain.

correlated with other normed measures of language expression ability. In their study, they used five short lists of vocabulary items. These lists were divided into 19 semantic categories: activities, animals, body parts, clothing, food and drinks, furniture and rooms, household, outside, people, places to go, prepositions, pronouns, qualities, quantifiers, questions, time, toys, vehicles, and verbs (auxiliary). A significant correlation was found between vocabulary performance on this abbreviated task and language expression instruments of greater length and complexity.

Third, parent reporting is a valuable source of the child's overall language, for either screening or educational purposes (Dale & Bates, 1989). Despite the concerns of some interventionists, little relationship between SES and vocabulary has been noted with parent report data. Checklists with parent reports offer an easy means of initial screening for delayed language performance in children younger than 3.

Finally, language sampling is a nonstandard assessment procedure that has received widespread use for assessing language expression ability. Although the age of the child must be kept in mind when considering language sampling, this procedure may be used any time after the child begins to demonstrate some expressive competence. The first step in analyzing language production is to obtain samples of the child's language. Some have argued that when collected appropriately, language samples may constitute the most accurate picture of the child's production ability (Stickler, 1987). To be useful, language samples must be representative of the child's language. A **representative language sample** is a collection of the child's spoken words that reflects the child's optimal performance (McLean & Snyder-McLean, 1978), portrays the child's usual performance (Gallagher, 1983), and includes the child's usual productive language ability, including performance that may be somewhat below or above usual abilities (Stickler, 1987).

Language samples involve tape recording a sufficient number of examples of the child's language. Stickler (1987) suggests several guidelines for interacting with children while obtaining a language sample:

- □ begin with parallel play and parallel talk
- □ move into interactive conversation
- □ continue the topic expressed by the child
- □ limit the use of questions (one question for every four speaking turns)
- □ provide options that are expressed as alternative questions (e.g., "Should we play gas station or have a picnic?")
- □ use utterances that are slightly longer than the child's
- □ learn to be comfortable with pauses in the conversation
- □ have a variety of materials
- □ do not be afraid to be silly and have fun

Most interventionists find that the speech-language pathologists on their teams prefer to analyze language samples collected by other team members because of the use, form, and content analyses involved. However, speech pathologists who have used the analyses for team training report many practical skills are learned that may be used in a variety of ways in later interventions.

Intervention

A great deal of attention has been placed on the assessment of communication skills because clear identification of strengths and weaknesses is the groundwork for facilitating children's use of language. Quality assessment sets the stage for quality intervention.

New perspectives on language learning indicate that language acquisition is facilitated through a child-centered approach (Gable, Raver, & Sandler, 1990; Girolametto, Greenberg, & Manolson, 1986). In the child-centered approach, interventionists guide parents and other family members in learning conversational styles that are responsive to the child's utterances. Parents learn to identify their child's attempts to communicate, to follow the child's lead, to use strategies for continuing conversations (e.g., turn-taking), to use prompts to enhance the child's responses, and to use materials that may maximize comprehension and verbal expression learning.

To guide families to use these skills naturally, some interventionists use structured play situations to model the skills they would like parents to use. Some simply reinforce these skills whenever they are displayed spontaneously by parents and family members. Still others use videotaping to assist the discussion of interactive styles between the child and parents that promote socio-communicative development. Videotapes allow interventionists and families to collaboratively identify behaviors that seem to have a positive effect on the child's social and communicative abilities.

Many investigators have provided valuable suggestions for how parents can better facilitate language learning through their regular routines with their children (see Drash, Raver, Murrin, & Tudor, 1989; Hopman, 1989; Jelinek, 1975; MacDonald & Gillette, 1984; Mahoney & Powell, 1988; Raver, 1980; Raver, Cooke, & Apolloni, 1978; Rosenberg & Robinson, 1985; Simmons-Martin, 1975). One technique involves the use of **incidental language teaching**. This involves achieving expressive and receptive goals by arranging activities or focusing on ongoing activities to promote language skill informally. By talking in short sentences, repeating often, and highlighting desired language skills, children have their language stimulated throughout the day (Winitz, 1983). This type of intervention generalizes more efficiently because training closely resembles regular interaction.

The reciprocal nature of social interactions allows basic eliciting procedures for increasing expressive and receptive language to be easily incorporated into home and center-based routines. Techniques such as imitation/modeling, questions, paraphrases, language expansion, and sentence completion are useful means of distributing expressive and receptive language stimulation throughout the child's day (Raver, 1987). **Imitation/modeling** involves performing the appropriate language function and expecting the child to repeat it (e.g., "You're pushing the car. . . . (Say) 'push car.' "). **Questioning** involves asking questions that require a response from the child about the activity in which the child is currently engaged (e.g., "Where's the car now?"). **Language expansion** involves retaining the words given by the child and adding to them to make better-formed responses that match the circumstances (e.g., Child: "Car go." Interventionist/parent: "Car go down."). **Paraphrasing** involves send-

TRANSDISCIPLINARY CASES

The following case studies illustrate the transdisciplinary role of speech-language pathologists and some common circumstances professionals are likely to encounter when they work with high-risk or handicapped infants and toddlers.

THE TORRES FAMILY

José Torres was born at approximately 36 weeks gestational age. His birthweight was 1,650 g and he spent 35 days in the intensive care nursery with frequent respiratory problems (assisted ventilation was required for 4 days). José's mother, a 24-year-old homemaker, and his father, a 27-year-old factory worker, had one older child.

Initially, Mrs. Torres was reluctant to interact with her child in the nursery. However, after the speech-language pathologist answered her questions and offered practical suggestions for making the interactions more rewarding, she assumed as much of the caregiving responsibility as permitted, and visited frequently.

When José was discharged, he weighed 2,550 g (about 5 pounds, 10 ounces). He had frequent illnesses for the first 8 months. Mrs. Torres described him as very difficult to soothe and as having a weak suck. Further assessments revealed hypertonia and a heart murmur. Mrs. Torres was trained to better read José's initiations for interaction, and was rewarded eventually when José began to demonstrate reciprocal social behaviors. These early signs of social responsiveness encouraged his family to continue their work with José, even though he continued to be difficult to soothe. Follow-ups in the Torres's home at 6, 9, 12, and 18 months indicated that José's socio-communicative development reached age-appropriate levels when he was 18 months old.

THE BATES FAMILY

Kathryn Bates was born at 32 weeks gestational age, with a heart defect which required immediate surgery. She remained in the hospital for 6 weeks. During the course of the hospitalization, her parents, who were 19 and 17 years old and had no previous childrearing experience, were fearful of her condition. They visited her on three occasions.

An infant intervention team saw Kathryn for the first time in her home when she was 7 months old. At the time of the initial evaluation, Kathryn was functioning below age levels in all developmental domains. Team members conducting the assessment noted that, based on informal and formal assessments, optimal attachment did not appear to have taken place between Kathryn and her parents. Team members recorded that the family seemed to desire a distance between the team and the family.

The infant program's social worker was selected by the team as the primary service provider for the family. Intervention attempts to assist the mother in facilitating more appropriate caregiving and interactional patterns were largely unsuccessful. Using the speech-language pathologist and other team members as consultants, the social worker attempted to demonstrate to Mrs. Bates ways in which Kathryn attempted to initiate interactions. Unfortunately, these efforts were reported to be only moderately successful.

At 12 months of age better communication between mother and infant was noted; however, overall developmental scores continued to demonstrate a moderate degree of developmental delay. The main area of developmental delay was socio-communicative development. Consequently, at this point, the speech-language pathologist also began to make weekly home visits to assist the family in better understanding Kathryn's communication needs and how stimulation activities could be incorporated into daily caregiving routines. These efforts also yielded only moderate results.

By 20 months of age, Kathryn's overall language ability was delayed approximately 4 to 6 months. Home visits continued and the speech-language pathologist was made case manager and primary service provider to the Bates. By the time Kathryn was 36 months old, the only area of deficit that remained was in the area of language. Most of Kathryn's language skills were within 2 months of age-appropriate levels. She was enrolled in a center-based preschool program to enhance her overall development as well as focus on her communicative skills. The Bates continued to require a great deal of professional and personal support.

These case studies demonstrate some of the services speech-language pathologists and their team members provide. Outcomes of early intervention are never guaranteed. However, more favorable results can be expected if team intervention is begun early, if parents participate, and if intervention continues throughout the preschool years.

ing an abbreviated version of the child's message back to the child in an attempt to continue the verbal interaction (e.g., "Car fall off?"). **Sentence completion** is a non-threatening way to elicit one- or two-word responses (e.g., "You're playing with the _____ ?").

Expressive and receptive language acquisition is facilitated by adult utterances that are on the same topic as the child's utterances, and by utterances that continue and expand observations made by the child. A variety of materials and curricula are available that may be used with these eliciting techniques. For instance, the Teacher Organized Training of the Acquisition of Language (TOTAL) (Witt & Boose, 1984) offers language training embedded in traditional concept development for young children.

Other materials stress establishing an environment in which prelinguistic and linguistic language learning can take place and is expected (see Adler, 1984; Beitchman, 1985; Cole & Dale, 1986; Fitzgerald, Trabue, & Karnes, 1987; Raver, 1987; Streml-Campbell & Rowland, 1987). To maximize the child's expressive and receptive language, families must be keenly aware of which competencies the child needs to master as well as how to implement enjoyable, play-oriented, *fun* strategies to encourage the development of those skills.

SUMMARY OF PROCEDURES

There are many ways in which affective and communicative disorders and delays may be manifested in young children, and nearly as many ways to address those deficits. Some of the key procedures for facilitating age-appropriate socio-communicative development in children follow:

1. Use continuous training to share and monitor skills released by speech-language pathologists to team members.
2. When appropriate, attempt to increase opportunities for interaction in the hospital setting, matching intervention techniques to the child's state of alertness.
3. Actively monitor parent/caregiver-infant interaction and attachment patterns in the first months of life. Improve synchrony and responsiveness by modeling, feedback, and the use of videotaping, if appropriate. Attachment and interaction styles influence later cognitive, social, and language abilities.
4. Use direct teaching to increase positive child characteristics (e.g., smiling, initiations, soothability) to increase positive parent/caregiver-child interactions.
5. Assist families to arrange environments that attempt to increase attention, engagement, reciprocal gestures, vocal/verbal turn-taking, elaboration of emotional responsiveness, and mutually pleasurable interactions between the child and significant adults.
6. Use common objects and familiar actions with objects to informally assess and modify language comprehension skills in children younger than 2 years of age. After 24 months, there are a number of formal assessment instruments for this purpose.

7. Use observation, parent reporting, and nonstandard expressive language assessment procedures (e.g., language sampling) to assess expressive competence in young children.
8. Employ language eliciting techniques such as imitation/modeling, questions, paraphrases, language expansion, and sentence completion to promote spontaneous language in routine activities and interactions.

SUMMARY

The relationship between language functioning and overall developmental skill mastery is strong. Specifically, in the young child, there is overlap in early communication and social-emotional development. Consequently, deficiencies in caregiver-child attachment and interaction, and other areas of prelinguistic development, may be manifested later as deficiencies in expressive and receptive language abilities. Using the speech-language pathologist as a consultant, interventionists can work with families to collaboratively create environments that consistently and continuously promote language development.

DISCUSSION QUESTIONS

1. What is the relationship between prelinguistic and linguistic development?
2. Why are accurate language comprehension assessments difficult to make with the very young child?
3. What are the relationships between parent-child interaction and later socio-communicative development?

APPLIED ACTIVITIES/PROJECTS

1. Observe an arena assessment with a language-delayed child younger than 3 years of age. Describe behaviors observed that support the interdependence of language, cognitive, and emotional-social development.
2. Interview a speech-language pathologist working with at-risk and handicapped infants and toddlers in an interdisciplinary program and another in a transdisciplinary team arrangement. Outline how their roles differ.
3. Visit an intensive care nursery and observe the general environment. How conducive to optimal socio-communicative development is this setting?

SUGGESTED READINGS

Bromwich, R. (1981). *Working with parents and infants*. Baltimore: University Park Press.
Cole, L., & Deal, V. (Eds.). (1986). *Communication disorders in multicultural populations*. Rockville, MD: American Speech-Language-Hearing Association.
Lindemann, J. E., & Lindemann, S. J. (1988). *Growing up proud: A parent's guide to the psychological care of children with disabilities*. New York: Warner Books.
McClowry, D. P., Guilford, A. M., & Richardson, S. O. (1982). *Infant communication: Development, assessment, and intervention*. New York: Grune & Stratton.

Rossetti, L. (1986). *High-risk infants: Identification, assessment, and intervention.* Boston: College-Hill Press/Little, Brown.

Rossetti, L. (1990). *Infant-toddler assessment: An interdisciplinary approach.* Boston: College-Hill Press/Little, Brown.

Spencer, M., Brookins, G., & Allen, W. L. (1985). *Beginnings: The social and affective development of Black children.* Hillsdale, NJ: Erlbaum.

REFERENCES

Adler, S. (1984). *Lesson plans for the infant and toddler: A sequential oral communications program for clinicians and teachers.* Springfield, IL: Charles Thomas.

Antoniadis, A., Didow, S., Lockhart, S., & Moroge, P. (1984). Screening for early cognitive and communicative behaviors. *Communique, 9,* 14–19.

Avant, P. (1982). A maternal attachment assessment strategy. In S. Humenick-Smith (Ed.), *Analysis of current assessment strategies in the health care of young children and childbearing families* (pp. 171–178). Norwich, CT: Appleton-Century-Crofts.

Beitchman, J. (1985). Therapeutic considerations with language-impaired preschool children. *Journal of Psychiatry, 30,* 609–617.

Bruner, J. (1978). The role of dialogue in language acquisition. In A. Sinclair, R. Jarvella, & W. Leveit (Eds.), *The child's conception of language* (pp. 241–250). Berlin: Springer-Verlag.

Bzoch, K., & League, R. (1971). *The Receptive-Expressive Emergent Language Scale.* Austin, TX: PRO-ED.

Capute, A., Palmer, F., & Shapiro, B. (1987). Using language to track development. *Patient Care, 19,* 60–71.

Carrow, E. (1973). *Test of Auditory Comprehension of Language.* Austin, TX: Learning Concepts.

Chapman, R. (1981). Exploring children's communicative intents. In J. Miller (Ed.), *Assessing language production in children: Experimental procedures* (pp. 111–136). Baltimore: University Park Press.

Cogswell, V., & Rossetti, L. (1987). *Language and cognitive performance of children of low birthweight.* Unpublished manuscript.

Cole, K., & Dale, P. (1986). Direct language instruction and interactive language instruction with language-delayed preschool children: A comparison study. *Journal of Speech and Hearing Research, 29,* 206–217.

Committee to Study the Prevention of Low Birth Weight (1985). *Preventing low birthweight.* Washington, DC: Institute of Medicine.

Coplan, J. (1985). Evaluation of the child with delayed speech or language. *Pediatric Annals, 14,* 202–208.

Coplan, J. (1987). *The Early Language Milestone Scale.* Tulsa, OK: Modern Educational Corporation.

Dale, P., & Bates, E. (1989). *The validity of a parent report instrument of child language at 20 months.* Unpublished manuscript.

DeCubas, M., & Field, T. (1984). Teaching interactions of Black and Cuban teenage mothers and their infants. *Early Child Development and Care, 16,* 41–56.

Drash, P., Raver, S., Murrin, M., & Tudor, R. (1989). Three procedures for increasing vocal response to prompt in infants and children with Down Syndrome. *American Journal of Mental Deficiency, 94,* 64–73.

Dunn, L., & Dunn, L. (1981). *Peabody Picture Vocabulary Test* (rev. ed.). Circle Pines, MN: American Guidance Service.

Dunst, C. (1980). *A clinical and educational manual for use with the Uzgiris-Hunt Scales of Infant Psychological Development*. Austin, TX: PRO-ED.

Fitzgerald, M., Trabue, M., & Karnes, D. (1987). A parent-implemented language model for at-risk and developmentally delayed preschool children. *Topics in Language Disorders, 7*, 31–46.

Gable, R., Raver, S., & Sandler, A. (1990). Assessing developmentally disabled learners. In R. Gable (Ed.), *Annual advances in mental retardation and developmental disabilities, Vol. IV*. Greenwich, CT: JAI Press.

Gallagher, T. (1983). Pre-assessment: A procedure for accommodating language use variability. In T. Gallagher & C. Prutting (Eds.), *Pragmatic assessment and intervention issues in language* (pp. 128–151). Boston: College-Hill Press.

Girolametto, L., Greenberg, J., & Manolson, H. (1986). Developing dialogue skills: The Hanen Early Language Parent Program. *Seminars in Speech and Language, 7*, 367–382.

High, P., & Gorski, P. (1985). Recording environmental influences on infant development in the intensive care nursery. In A. Gottfried & J. Gaiter (Eds.), *Infant stress under intensive care* (pp. 131–156). Baltimore: University Park Press.

Hopman, W. (1989). Interactional approaches to parent training. *Childhood Education, 65*, 167–168.

Horstmeier, D., & MacDonald, J. (1978). *Environmental Prelanguage Battery*. New York: The Psychological Corporation.

Jacobson, C., Starnes, C., & Gasser, V. (1988). An experimental analysis of the generalization of descriptions and praises for mothers of premature infants. *Human Communication, 12*, 23–34.

Jacobson, C., & Wendler, S. (1988). Language stimulation in the neonatal intensive care unit. *Human Communication Canada, 12*, 48–51.

Jelinek, J. (1975). The role of the parent in a language development program. *Journal of Research and Development in Education, 8*, 14–23.

Klaus, M., & Fanaroff, S. (1979). *Care of the high-risk neonate*. Philadelphia: W. B. Saunders.

Klaus, M., & Kennell, J. (1976). *Maternal-infant bonding*. St. Louis: Mosby.

Klein, D., & Briggs, M. (1986). *Observation of Communicative Interaction: A model program to facilitate positive communication between caregivers and their high-risk infants*, No. MCI 06351–01–0. Washington, DC: Division of Maternal and Child Health, U.S. Department of Health and Human Services.

Largo, R., Molinari, L., Pinto, C., Weber, M., & Duc, W. (1986). Language development of term and preterm children during the first 5 years of life. *Developmental Medicine and Child Neurology, 28*, 333–350.

MacDonald, J. (1978). *Oliver*. New York: The Psychological Corporation.

MacDonald, J., & Gillette, J. (1984). Conversation engineering: A pragmatic approach to early social competence. *Seminars in Speech and Language, 5*, 171–183.

Mahoney, G., & Powell, A. (1988). Modifying parent-child interaction: Enhancing the development of handicapped children. *The Journal of Special Education, 22*, 82–96.

McCune-Nicolich, L. (1980). *A manual for analyzing free play: Experimental edition*. New Brunswick, NJ: Rutgers University.

McLean, J., & Snyder-McLean, L. (1978). *Transactional approach to early language training*. Columbus, OH: Merrill.

Miller, J., & Yoder, D. (1982). *Test of Grammatical Comprehension*. Madison: University of Wisconsin Press.

Mindes, G. (1982). Social and cognitive aspects of play in young handicapped children. *Topics in Early Childhood Special Education, 2*, 14–26.

Olson, S., Bates, J., & Bayles, K. (1982). Maternal perception of infant toddler behavior: A longitudinal construct validation study. *Infant Behavior and Development, 5,* 397–406.

Olswang, L., Stoel-Gammons, C., Coggins, T., & Carpenter, R. (1987). *Assessing Prelinguistic and Early Linguistic Behaviors.* Seattle: University of Washington Press.

Owens, R. (1988). *Language development.* Columbus, OH: Merrill.

Palfrey, L., Singer, J., Walker, D., & Butler, J. (1987). Early identification of children's special needs: A study in five metropolitan communities. *Journal of Pediatrics, 5,* 651.

Piaget, J. (1962). *Play, dreams and imitation in childhood.* New York: Norton.

Raver, S. (1980). The effect of antecedent vestibular stimulation on the receptive language learning of retarded toddlers. *Child Study Journal, 10*(2), 77–86.

Raver, S. (1987). Practical procedures for increasing spontaneous language in language-delayed preschoolers. *Journal for the Division of Early Childhood, 11*(3), 226–232.

Raver, S., Cooke, T., & Apolloni, T. (1978). Developing nonretarded toddlers as verbal models for retarded classmates. *Child Study Journal, 8*(1), 1–8.

Reznick, J. (1982). *The development of perception and lexical categories in the human infant.* Unpublished doctoral dissertation, University of Colorado, Boulder.

Reznick, J., & Goldsmith, L. (1989). Multiple form word production checklist for assessing early language. *Journal of Child Language, 16,* 91–100.

Rogers, S., Donovan, C., D'Eugenio, D., Brown, S., Lynch, E., Moersch, M., & Schafer, S. (1981). *Early Intervention Developmental Profile.* Ann Arbor: University of Michigan Press.

Rose, T., Calhoun, M., & Ladage, L. (1989). Helping young children to respond to caregivers. *Teaching Exceptional Children, 21,* 48–51.

Rosenberg, S., & Robinson, C. (1985). Enhancement of mother's interactional skills in an infant education program. *Education and Training of the Mentally Retarded, 20* (June) 163–169.

Rossetti, L. (1986). *High-risk infants: Identification, assessment, and intervention.* Boston: College-Hill Press/Little Brown.

Rossetti, L. (1989). *Infant toddler assessment: An interdisciplinary approach.* Boston: College-Hill Press/Little Brown.

Rowan, L., & Johnson, C. (1988, June). *Screening and assessment.* Paper presented at the Infant and Toddler Communication and Assessment Workshop. Minneapolis.

Rubin, K., Maroni, T., & Hornung, M. (1975). Free play behavior in middle- and lower-class preschoolers: Parten and Piaget revisited. *Child Development, 47,* 414–419.

Seibert, J., & Hogan, A. (1982). A model for assessing social and object skills and planning intervention. In D. McClowery (Ed.), *Infant communication development: Assessment and intervention* (pp. 21–54). New York: Grune & Stratton.

Simmons-Martin, A. (1975). Facilitating parent-child interactions through education of parents. *Journal of Research and Development in Education, 8,* 96–102.

Sparks, S., Clark, M., Oas, D., & Erickson, R. (1988, November). Clinical services to infants at risk for communication disorders. Paper presented at the annual convention of the American Speech-Language-Hearing Association, Boston, MA.

Stickler, K. (1987). *Guide to analysis of language transcripts.* Eau Claire, WI: Thinking Publications.

Streml-Campbell, K., & Rowland, C. (1987). Prelinguistic communication intervention: Birth to 2. *Topics in Early Childhood Special Education, 7,* 49–56.

Taylor, P., & Hall, B. (1979). Parent-infant bonding and opportunities in a perinatal center. *Seminars in Perinatology, 3,* 73–86.

Terrell, B., & Schwartz, R. (1988). Object transformation in the play of language-impaired children. *Journal of Speech and Hearing Disorders, 53,* 459–466.

Update Pediatrics. (1982). *An assessment tool: The Infant Scale of Communicative Intent*. Boston: St. Christopher's Hospital.

Westby, C. (1980). Assessment of cognitive and language abilities through play. *Language, Speech and Hearing Services in the Schools, 3,* 154–163.

Wetherby, A., & Prizant, B. (1989). *Communication and Symbolic Behavior Scales* (Experimental ed.). San Antonio, TX: Special Press.

Winitz, H. (1983). *Treating language disorders: For clinicians by clinicians*. Baltimore: University Park Press.

Witt, B., & Boose, J. (1984). *Teacher Organized Training for the Acquisition of Language (TOTAL)*. Tuscon, AZ: Communication Skill Builders.

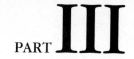

INTERVENTION STRATEGIES
FOR MEDICAL SETTINGS

6

Techniques for the Neonatal Period

Eva K. Thorp and Sharon A. Raver

OVERVIEW

This chapter discusses issues relating to premature infants and their families, including:

- medical complications frequently associated with prematurity
- characteristics and issues regarding drug-exposed infants
- issues confronting families in the course of their infants' hospitalization in neonatal intensive care nurseries
- strategies for supporting families at different stages in the hospitalization and discharge process
- assessment and developmental intervention with high-risk neonates
- discharge planning for effective transitions from the hospital to the home

Neonatal intervention has evolved from the recently acknowledged needs of premature infants hospitalized in intensive care nurseries. Research during the neonatal period suggests that developmental and emotional support may assist infants in their adaptation to the stress of a premature birth (Bennett, 1987).

Preterm infants are defined as infants who are born at less than 38 weeks gestation. Between 7 and 8% of all live births are preterm or premature (Bowden, 1988; Fletcher, 1984). The term **immature** may be used for infants born at less than 28 weeks gestational age. The infant's **corrected age** is calculated by subtracting the number of weeks of prematurity from the infant's chronologic age (the infant's age based on the time since the child's birth). Preterm and immature infants require intensive medical intervention because of their immature body systems and associated low birthweight.

As a result of medical technology and today's organization of neonatal care, more preterm and immature infants are surviving. For example, twice as many **very low birthweight (vlbw) infants**, those weighing less than 1,500 g or $3\frac{1}{2}$ pounds, are surviving now than did in the 1960s (Moore, 1988). **Low birthweight (lbw) infants** are those who weigh between 1,500 to 2,500 g or $3\frac{1}{2}$ to $5\frac{1}{2}$ pounds.

The survival of preterm infants is not without short- and long-term costs to infants and families. Some low birthweight infants die while hospitalized. The lower the infant's birthweight, the likelier the chances of death (Ahmann, 1986). Other infants require lengthy hospitalizations that may range from 2 weeks to a year and require many thousands of dollars in treatment. Once discharged, premature infants are hospitalized disproportionately more frequently than fullterm infants and are likely to experience a variety of chronic health problems. Of greatest significance for the field of early intervention is the fact that 25% or more of premature infants may experience long-term developmental problems, central nervous system disorders, and social interactive problems (Brazelton, Nugent, & Lester, 1987; Fletcher, 1984; Plunkett & Meisels, 1989).

The risks related to an infant's prematurity may be further complicated by social and economic environmental risks that initially contributed to the premature birth (Weston, Ivins, Zuckerman, Jones, & Lopez, 1989). Mothers who have not had adequate prenatal care, such as many teenage and substance-abusing mothers, are at a greater risk for premature delivery. These mothers may also have more difficulty creating a supportive environment for their fragile infants. Fortunately, as the medical field has improved its ability to save premature infants, the ability to facilitate the development of many high-risk infants has also improved.

TRENDS IN DEVELOPMENTAL INTERVENTION

Although the intensive care nursery is a life-saving environment, it can also be a hostile environment for infants (Field, 1987; Lawson, 1988). Neonatal intensive care units (NICUs) tend to have constant technical activity and, at times, a very high noise level. They may be tension-filled, because the severely ill infants in care there may have a medical crisis at any moment. There may be unpredictable times of light or darkness. The necessary patterns of caregiving, feeding, changing, and routine medical manipulations may not support infants' abilities to organize their own behavior. Caretaking routines are rarely given in response to infants' signals. Infants may be in situations of sensory overload with little or no opportunity to exert control over the NICU environment (Goldberger, 1988; Gorski, 1985; VandenBerg, 1985).

To handle neonatal intervention, a new role may be in the process of being defined. A **behavioral intervention specialist** is an infant interventionist who works in the NICU and assists the staff in identifying environmental manipulations and handling strategies that better support the developing infant (Cole & Frappier, 1983; Ensher & Clark, 1986; Gottfried, 1985; VandenBerg, 1985). Research is accumulating that demonstrates the efficacy of this type of hospital-based intervention. Increases in both infant and parental competence have been reported (Cardone & Gilkerson, 1989; Heinecke, Beckwith, & Thompson, 1988; Korner, 1987; Nugent & Brazelton, 1989).

FIGURE 6–1
Leading causes of death for infants in the United States. (Source: National Center for Health Statistics. Health, United States, 1989. Hyattsville, Maryland: Public Health Service, 1990.)

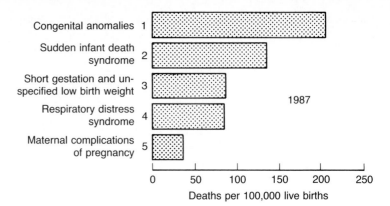

From a policy perspective, neonatal intervention is supported by Part H of P.L. 99–457 because states are encouraged to serve at-risk infants as soon as they are identified. Premature, low birthweight infants will satisfy some states' eligibility definitions for "at risk." However, extending interventionists' roles to include intensive care nurseries brings expanded responsibilities for professionals (Thorp & McCollum, 1988).

Community-based infant interventionists such as educators, occupational therapists, psychologists, and social workers are trained very differently than hospital-based neonatal nurses and other medical specialists. Because of these divergent professional perspectives, infant interventionists are learning new skills as they join medical teams in providing support to premature infants and their families. One significant new area of knowledge is the medical aspects of the neonatal period.

MEDICAL ASPECTS OF THE NEONATAL PERIOD

The risk of death during the first month of life is about 1 in 1,000 in the fullterm infant. Death may be caused by a range of conditions from congenital malformations to **sudden infant death syndrome (SIDS)** and infections (National Center for Health Statistics, 1978). The most common causes of death during the first month of life for fullterm infants in the United States are shown in Figure 6–1.

Preterm infants, on the other hand, face far greater obstacles in their first months of life. The many complications associated with prematurity are a function of

☐ the immaturity of the newborn's body systems
☐ the medical treatments needed to save the infant's life
☐ the presence of environmental factors such as infection that affect the infant's survival

Some conditions threaten the infant's initial survival, while others are associated with long-term developmental outcomes. Table 6–1 summarizes the medical complications that result from prematurity.

In general, the major medical threats to premature infants are respiratory, cardiac, neurologic, and gastro-intestinal problems; and exposure to infections. Often

TABLE 6–1
Summary of medical complications that result from prematurity.

Disorder	Possible Outcomes	Diagnostic Outcomes
Pulmonary immaturity	→ Hypoventilation and hypoxia due to insufficiently rapid synthesis of surface-active pulmonary lecithin	→ Respiratory distress syndrome
Weak sucking, swallow, gag, and cough reflexes	→ Difficulty in feeding and danger of aspiration often compounded by respiratory difficulties	→ Nutritional disturbances
Deficiency in glycogen storage and greater surface-to-body ratio	→ Decreased ability to maintain body temperature; may be compounded by pulmonary problems due to increased O_2 consumption	→ Hypothermia
Lack of or inefficient bacteria-fighting factors	→ Increased susceptibility to infection	→ Sepsis Meningitis
Liver immaturity	→ Limited ability to excrete solutes in urine	→ Hyperbilirubenemia
Immature gastrointestinal tract	→ Diminished absorption of fat and fat-soluble vitamins	→ Nutritional disturbances Hyperbilirubenemia
Presence of subependymal germinal matrix, stressful birth, and anoxia	→ Unstable intravascular pressures; ischemic injury to brain and capillaries	→ Intraventricular hemorrhage

Source: From *The development of infants born at risk* (p. 34) by D. L. Holmes, J. N. Reich, & J. F. Pasternak, 1984, Hillsdale, NJ: Erlbaum. Copyright © 1984 by Lawrence Erlbaum Associates, Inc., Publishers. Reprinted by permission.

as a result of their prematurity and treatment, premature infants are at a higher risk for hearing and visual problems. Further, drug-exposed premature infants have these medical vulnerabilities as well as special long-term developmental concerns. Each of these issues are discussed here.

Respiratory Conditions

Problems with the respiratory, or pulmonary system, occur with most neonates in the intensive care unit. **Respiratory distress syndrome (RDS)** is the primary lung disease affecting infants born before there is sufficient physical and biochemical maturation of the pulmonary system, resulting in difficult breathing after birth

(Fletcher, Brown, & Wetherby, 1987). In most cases, infants who survive the first few days of RDS will recover.

Unfortunately, the complications of RDS may have a permanent effect on the infant's growth and development. The severity (i.e., the length of the hospitalization) and the chronicity (i.e., the extent of postnatal respiratory illness) have been found to be effective predictors of cognitive and psychomotor risk in preterm infants (Meisels, Plunkett, Pasick, Stiefel, & Roloff, 1987). These variables, in addition to the presence of birth asphyxia (lack of oxygen), have been associated with delayed cognitive development in the second year of life in some preterm infants (Meisels et al., 1987).

Interventionists working with infants with RDS must avoid over-stressing the infant's respiratory system while organizing interventions to help the infant overcome developmental lags caused by this medical problem. Respiratory distress requiring more than 6 hours of mechanical ventilation may place any infant at risk because of the side effects of the treatment, such as **hypoxemia**, insufficient oxygen in the blood (Blackman, 1986).

Apnea.   In addition to respiratory distress, infants may have pulmonary insufficiency because of immature or abnormal controls of the respiratory drive. **Apnea**, the cessation of breathing, is one of the most frequent problems found in infants in NICUs. Apnea may be accompanied by **bradycardia**, or slowing of the heart rate. As the central nervous system matures, the severity and frequency of apneic episodes tend to decrease. Some episodes may respond to simple tactile stimulation (touching the child), while others may require artificial ventilation or artificial stimulation of the respiratory drive.

Seigel and colleagues (1982) found that language development was particularly affected by the severity of apnea in preterm infants. Apnea was measured by the number of days it occurred and the number of days it was treated with theophylline. However, these researchers also report that it is impossible to separate the effects of theophylline from the effects of apnea on infants' development.

Bronchopulmonary dysplasia (BPD).   The most serious complication of RDS is failure to recover normal pulmonary function. The treatment of RDS may lead to a chronic lung disease called **bronchopulmonary dysplasia (BPD)**. BPD is a description of the airways' reaction to damage from oxygen and pressure. Lungs damaged during the neonatal period by RDS, and resulting in BPD, have the potential for recovery, but infants with this condition are very likely to require rehospitalizations during their first 2 years of life due to respiratory infections.

The most severely affected infants require prolonged hospitalizations, home monitoring, home oxygen, and multiple medications. The medications required for treatment may cause gastric distress, irritability, or overstimulation. As the survival rate of infants with BPD improves, more infants are being discharged on oxygen (Cooper & Kennedy, 1989). Infants with BPD expend substantial energy in merely handling the task of breathing. Consequently, they have exceptional caloric requirements. However, they also are unable to tolerate large volumes of fluid, so they are given special formulas that cause abdominal discomfort. As Fletcher and colleagues (1987) state, this situation creates a cycle of medication and discomfort:

> To handle the fluid that goes in with the formula, they [infants with BPD] require diuretics. Then, to counteract the loss of electrolytes from the diuretics, they must take replacement salts which further upset the stomach. With their medication and chronic illness, their appetite is less than needed to assure adequate intake. Their poor nutrition occurs at a time of critical postnatal brain differentiation (p. 80).

Because infants with BPD are instrumented frequently through their mouths, oral intake of food is often resisted. Coughing and poor gag reflex may complicate circumstances, and too many calories may be used in trying to feed. Because of this, infants with BPD become candidates for alternative routes for feeding such as prolonged **oral gastric gavage feeding** (forced feeding through a tube into the stomach in which formula is either dripped or pushed so sucking is not required) and **gastrostomy feedings** (rubber tube going through a gastrostomy that has one end within the stomach and the other outside the abdominal wall, permitting feeding directly into the stomach). Infants with BPD who are able to eat enough for good rates of growth have a better prognosis than those who continue to have feeding difficulties. In general, infants with severe lung disease at the time of discharge are at the highest risk for developmental disabilities.

Tracheostomy.　A **tracheostomy**, an artificial opening through the neck into the trachea that allows air to enter and leave the lungs without going through the upper airways (nose, mouth, or voice box), enables the infant to expend less work to breathe. Blockage of the trach tube with secretions and mucus is the greatest medical complication of a tracheostomy. Infants in home care with tracheostomies are at the greatest risk of all NICU graduates for sudden death because of complications of the trach and/or underlying diseases (Fletcher et al., 1987).

Chronic lung infections.　Because of the prematurity of the immune system and the lungs, infants with RDS are especially at risk for serious infections, i.e., pneumonia. Invasive instruments such as chest tubes also increase the chances of infection. As a rule, antibiotics are administered at the first sign of infection in fragile, premature infants.

Cardiac Conditions

Congenital heart diseases encompass a wide spectrum of conditions. Generally, the later a cardiac malformation is evidenced, the less severe it is.

Patent ductus arteriosus (PDA).　This condition is frequently seen on discharge summaries of premature infants. Prior to birth, the ductus arteriosus connects the pulmonary artery and the aorta so there can be a diversion of blood flow away from the lungs. Failure of that vessel to close after birth, however, allows abnormal flow either toward or away from the lungs, which is called **patent ductus arteriosus (PDA)**. Unlike fullterm infants, premature infants appear to lack the musculature in the vessel for easy closure. A surgical closure, or **ligation**, is considered the simplest corrective surgery. Although the surgical procedure is simple, infants who require the procedure tend to be fragile and the worst surgical risks. Essentially, recovery appears dependent on the infant's accompanying medical problems. Some evidence suggests that infants with PDA have more developmental problems than infants who do not have PDA (Fletcher, 1984).

Neurologic Problems

The medical field's knowledge about body systems tends to exceed its knowledge of neonatal brain development. For this reason, it is simply not possible to predict the impact of a perinatal (around the time of birth) insult or illness on the future development of the child (Batshaw & Perret, 1981).

To measure the infant's level of development and the health of the nervous system, medical personnel use the electroencephalogram (EEG), the computerized radiographic view (CT scan), ultrasonography, and more recently, nuclear magnetic resonance imaging (NMR) routinely with premature infants. The cranial ultrasound examination can detect the position and size of ventricles in the brain and abnormal fluid collections. Physical examinations are also used regularly to evaluate neurologic function and development. For example, head circumference is monitored because it reflects brain growth (Batshaw & Perret, 1981). Excessive head growth may indicate **hydrocephalus** (abnormal accumulation of fluid within the vault containing the brain). Muscle strength is evaluated because it offers information on the infant's neurologic status.

Intraventricular hemorrhage (IVH). Bleeding in the head is known as **intracranial hemorrhage**. **Intraventricular hemorrhage (IVH)**, bleeding occurring in or around the ventricles of the brain, is the most frequently diagnosed intracranial hemorrhage. IVH is classified by location and severity. At present, there is no evidence that a specific classification of IVH may be predictive of developmental outcome. Nonetheless, IVH in premature, very low birthweight infants has been associated with poorer intellectual outcomes at 24 months of age when IVH has been accompanied by BPD or progressive hydrocephalus (Landry, Fletcher, Zarling, Chapieski, & Francis, 1984).

Seizures. Seizures occur more frequently during the neonatal period than at any other time in life (Ensher & Clark, 1986). The causes of neonatal seizures may not be determined but they tend to be associated with asphyxia, infection, intracranial hemorrhage, metabolic derangements, or brain malformations. Many of the medications used to control seizures, such as phenobarbital, have significant side effects including drowsiness.

Cerebral palsy. Brain damage that may result in cerebral palsy may occur at any time from conception to early childhood. The causes for the brain lesions that result in cerebral palsy vary, and only a few causes can be determined specifically. As indicated in Chapter 3, the incidence of cerebral palsy is not declining, in part due to the survival of the smallest premature infants. Two significant risk factors for cerebral palsy are low birthweight and birth **asphyxia**, suffocation in which there is a lack of oxygen with a build up of carbon dioxide. It is still unclear how much asphyxia may be necessary for cerebral palsy to result. Some of the high-risk factors for cerebral palsy are shown in Table 6–2.

Today, the clinical condition at birth is first established by the infant's Apgar score. In 1953, Virginia Apgar, an anesthesiologist, proposed a scoring system to examine five characteristics that are believed to correlate with recovery from intra-uterine stress:

- □ heart rate
- □ color
- □ reflex irritability
- □ respiratory effort
- □ muscle tone

TABLE 6–2

High-risk factors for cerebral palsy.

Prenatal
Hyperemesis gravidarum
Toxemia
Teratogenic drugs
Placenta previa
Placenta abruptio
Intrauterine viral or bacterial infection:
toxoplasmosis, rubella, cytomegalovirus, herpes, and syphylis
Chromosomal abnormality
Maternal malnutrition
Family history positive for cerebral palsy

Perinatal
Small for gestational age
Prematurity
Breech or face delivery
Intrauterine asphyxia
Low Apgar score at 5, 10, and 20 minutes
Seizures
Respiratory distress syndrome
Hyperbilirubenemia

Postnatal
Head trauma
Intracranial infections
Toxic encephalopathies (lead)
Cerebrovascular accident

Source: From *The Neonatal Experience* (p. 148) by M. A. Fletcher, C. Brown, & C. Wetherby, 1987, Washington, DC: The George Washington University. Copyright © 1987 by The George Washington University. Reprinted by permission.

Each variable of the Apgar score is judged 0, 1, or 2, depending on quality. A score of 0 indicates a complete absence of response, and a score of 2 indicates the best response, such as a heart rate greater than 100, regular respiratory effort, and totally pink color. Although there is much debate about the predictive value of Apgar scores (Ensher & Clark, 1986), the 5-minute Apgar score is considered to be related to **morbidity** and **mortality** rates (Drage, Kennedy, & Schwarz, 1964).

Cerebral palsy may not be manifested in early infancy. Children who develop hypertonic cerebral palsy (high resting activity or tension in the muscle), for instance, may have a latency period with initial hypotonia (low resting activity or tension in the muscle) until approximately 6 to 9 months of age when hypertonia begins to be revealed. Similarly, children with athetoid cerebral palsy may have variable tone in early infancy and not manifest a movement disorder until 1 or 2 years of age.

Gastro-intestinal Problems

Many growth and feeding problems are associated with gastro-intestinal problems. **Necrotizing enterocolitis (NEC)**, a feeding complication, and **failure to thrive**, a growth failure problem, are common difficulties seen in the neonatal period of life.

Necrotizing enterocolitis (NEC).   This problem is unique to neonates and young infants. With this condition there is a feeding intolerance with constipation, diarrhea, vomiting, abdominal distention, bloody stools, or a general appearance of **sepsis** (severe infection) (Cloherty & Stark, 1985). NEC compromises bowel circulation, which may lead to tissue death, **necrosis**, and perforation, with spillage of bowel contents into the peritoneal cavity. Bowel perforations demand immediate surgery, which tends to be high risk due to the general poor condition of the infants. When surgery is performed on the bowel, an **ostomy** (i.e., colostomy or ileostomy, depending on the site) may be performed. Recovery after surgery depends on how much bowel is left and how well it functions. Even when no surgery is performed and the child responds to medical therapy, **enteric feedings** (feeding other than by mouth) may be restarted to allow the infant's bowel to rest. Several weeks are needed for recovery.

Failure to thrive.   When growth does not follow the curves expected for age, growth failure occurs. Growth failure may be primarily in head circumference, representing poor brain growth with a poor prognosis for achievement, or it may be more limited to weight and height. Gastro-intestinal problems in infants account for the largest percentage of organic causes of failure to thrive (Gryboski & Walker, 1983). However, organic causes of failure to thrive are not the only source of growth failure. When non-organic causes of failure to thrive are identified, interventionists must focus on modifying environmental and social interactions (Haynes-Seman & Hart, 1987).

As stated earlier, children with gastro-intestinal problems tend to have feeding difficulties. Enormous amounts of effort are required for sucking. Fragile premature infants may not be able to coordinate eating and breathing at the same time. They often do not stop sucking to breathe and become apneic during feedings. Consequently, either oral or tube enteric feedings are given depending on the infant's medical problems. The following routes are choices for enteric tube feedings:

- □ **nasogastric**: tube through nose into stomach
- □ **orogastric**: tube through mouth into stomach
- □ **transpyloric**: tube crossing the **pyloric exit** of the stomach
- □ **jejunal**: nasal or oral tube ending in small intestine
- □ **gastrostomy**: tube through abdominal wall directly into stomach

Infections

The longer the infant is in the hospital, or the more equipment and personnel required for the infant's care, the more likely the infant will suffer infectious diseases. **Infection** implies that the infant's symptoms are caused by organisms that may be viral, parasitic, bacterial, or fungal (Ensher & Clark, 1986). For example, pneumonia is an infection of the lungs, and meningitis is an infection in the lining of the brain. Sepsis is a generalized infection involving the blood and more than one organ. Symptoms of sepsis are severe and life-threatening (Cloherty & Stark, 1985). Infections of specific organs may be accompanied by general sepsis as well. A common bacterial sepsis in neonates is Group B Beta Hemolytic Streptococcus (GBS). Common viral infections are cytomegalovirus (CMV), congenital cytomegalic inclusion disease (CID), herpes, and acquired immune deficiency syndrome (AIDS). AIDS is discussed in Chapter 7. Refer to Cloherty and Stark (1985) for more information about these and other conditions.

Hearing and Sight Problems

After infants are discharged from the NICU, they still are at risk for hearing and vision problems that may not be evident at the time of their discharge. The major causes of deafness in the neonatal period are familial causes such as autosomal recessive conditions and malformations, exposure to toxins, infections, defects of the head and neck, prematurity, and fullterm infants suffering encephalopathy (Fletcher, Brown, & Wetherby, 1987).

Premature infants or infants who have suffered asphyxial injury or meningitis after birth are at high risk for a variety of visual problems as well. These infants may display retinopathy of prematurity (ROP), **amblyopia** (reduction of visual acuity in the absence of any organic lesion), **strabismus** (abnormal alignment of the eye), hypermyopia (extreme nearsightedness), cortical or cerebral blindness, and visual-perceptual defects (Fletcher et al., 1987).

Retinopathy of prematurity.   The retina, the part of the eye where visible light images are turned into neurologic impulses, is one of the last structures of the eye to mature (Purohit, Ellison, Zierler, Miettinen, & Nadas, 1985). For reasons still not clearly understood, the blood vessels in the immature portion of the retina may develop abnormally when a child is born prematurely. This abnormality of maturation of the retinal vessels is called **retinopathy of prematurity (ROP)**. In 80% of the cases in which infants develop ROP, eye functioning heals itself as it matures during the first year of life. In other cases, there may be partial resolution requiring the child to seek ophthalmologic care, often in the form of glasses. In extreme cases, the retinal vessels develop so abnormally that scar tissue distorts and dislodges the retina. The smallest and most immature infants are at the highest risk of developing the most extreme forms of ROP. Infants with birthweights between 500 and 749 g have a 43% chance of ROP, while infants whose weight is between 1,500 and 1,750 g only have a 3% chance (Purohit et al., 1985).

An international classification of ROP describes the extent and location of this condition (Committee for Classification of Retinopathy of Prematurity, 1984). The degree of severity is classified by stages. Stage I indicates early, reversible changes in the blood vessels; Stage V injury results in retina detachment and blindness. Unfortunately, ROP occurs most often in infants who have already overcome the greatest odds against survival. Diagnosis seems to come after these infants appear to be over the worst, so this complication can be especially devastating to families and medical specialists alike.

Drug-exposed Infants

Medical professionals have understood the effects of nicotine on the fetus (i.e., low birthweight) and alcohol abuse during pregnancy (i.e., fetal alcohol syndrome) for some time. **Fetal alcohol syndrome** is characterized by infants who are small for gestational age, have mild to moderate mental retardation, congenital heart defects, droopy eyelids, microcephaly (small cranium), and joint abnormalities (Batshaw & Perret, 1981). The immediate and long-term effects of exposure to other drugs such as cocaine, crack, and heroin on the developing fetus and infant are just beginning to be understood.

Although most infants exposed to drugs in utero are referred to as addicted infants (Jones & Lopez, 1988), some drugs (such as cocaine) are addictive while others (such as marijuana) are toxic (Weston et al., 1989). The THC in marijuana retards placental development, which reduces blood flow to the fetus. Both addictive and toxic drugs can cause the newborn to be sick, small for gestational age, low birthweight, and/or premature. Whatever the specific drug, infants exposed to drugs in utero tend to be irritable, have hypertonicity or hypotonicity, and may be less responsive and rewarding than even difficult healthy infants (Weston et al., 1989). Their ability to communicate their needs through smiles, frowns, cries, and eye contact tends to be compromised.

Cocaine-addicted infants tend to manifest poor body-state regulation, tremors, chronic irritability, and poor visual orientation. Crack-addicted infants may have strokes, seizures, small heads, and various malformations. In reality, drug-abusing mothers tend to mix alcohol, cigarettes, and illicit drugs, so their infants are actually the products of polydrug exposure (Zuckerman, Amaro, Bauchner, & Cabral, 1989).

In addition to the immediate effects of prenatal drug exposure, drug-exposed infants may have compromised developmental functioning, in part related to the impact of living in a family that abuses substances (Howard, in press). Developmental deficits may persist into early childhood. For example, follow-up data suggests that affective-communicative deficits are commonplace with drug-exposed, school-aged children (Howard, Beckwith, Rodning, & Kropenske, 1989).

Because both drug-dependent mothers and their drug-exposed infants have difficulty coping with even moderate levels of frustration and tension, comprehensive services are necessary to promote the infant's health and development (Green, Silverman, Suffett, Taleporos, & Turkel, 1979; Tittle & Claire, 1989). Unfortunately, there are few specialized services for either mothers or their children. Most of the hospitals responding to a 1988 survey indicated that they have no place to refer drug-abusing pregnant women for treatment (Miller, 1989). Consequently, interventionists may have to actively solicit long-term, comprehensive intervention for substance-abusing mothers and drug-exposed infants to reduce the effects of drug exposure on the infant's future health and development. Interestingly, the problem of substance abuse during pregnancy does not seem to be confined to urban settings, nor is it limited to low-income women (Weston et al., 1989).

Though no cost studies specific to drug-exposed infants have been conducted, Miller (1989) found the hospitals he surveyed acknowledged the high cost of care for low birthweight and sick infants, and the increasing number of these infants who have been exposed to drugs. A Los Angeles hospital estimates the average cost of a drug-exposed newborn in the ICN as approximately $750 a day for a mildly drug-exposed infant and $1,800 a day for a severely affected newborn.

The number of drug-exposed infants is increasing so rapidly that some suggest that the medical community may have to define a new, organic brain syndrome based on the damage to fetal brains by drug-abusing mothers (Greer, 1990). Drug-exposed infants have the same medical vulnerabilities as other low birthweight, premature infants, as well as additional problems imposed by their exposure to drugs and their multi-risk home environment in which substance abuse may continue. In spite of this, there is limited clinical evidence that some of the effects of cocaine exposure in utero, for example, may be modified by intensive developmental interventions (Schneider, Griffith, & Chasnoff, 1989).

In summary, the medical complications of prematurity may be extensive and lasting. Low birthweight premature infants are usually not suited for independent extrauterine life. Because they were denied the benefits of full gestation, they require significant medical and environmental supports. To increase their chances of survival and handle complications encountered in therapy, they require lengthy hospitalizations.

Nonetheless, some children do not develop the major problems their risk conditions may predict (Bennett, 1987). Although neonatal care units keep infants alive who weigh as little as 500 g, these infants are at significant risk for developmental problems (Frohock, 1986; Klein, 1988; Seigel et al., 1982). Infants between 1,500 and 2,500 g are less likely to experience complications but still require monitoring. The medical needs of preterm infants place significant stress on families. Refer to the Glossary for definitions of other conditions interventionists will encounter with premature and medically fragile infants and toddlers.

IMPLICATIONS FOR FAMILY-CENTERED CARE

In order to offer family-centered intervention and care, interventionists must understand the family crisis that begins with the premature birth of the child and continues through long, often repeated, hospitalizations.

Weathering the Crisis of the Birth

The birth of a preterm at-risk infant is an extremely stressful event for families. Parents often feel anxious and guilty, and wonder if they did something, or did not do something, that may have prompted the premature delivery (Porter, 1983a). The premature at-risk infant is small, fragile, undeveloped, and may appear less attractive than the fullterm infant. It is not surprising that parents grieve for the anticipated perfect baby. Parents may feel let down by one another or by their at-risk infant, and may blame one another for their disappointments (Lowenthal, 1989). During this initial period, families need to be supported as they recall and resolve the pain of the delivery.

There are many practical ways to alleviate stress in families during the crisis of the premature birth. To mediate the stress of separation, research suggests that mothers see their infants before they are transferred from community hospitals to hospitals better equipped to care for high-risk infants, and that parents should be offered a picture of their infant before the transfer occurs (Garrand, Sherman, Rentchler, & Jung, 1978). A call to the mother after the infant makes a safe arrival also provides vital assurance to the family (Fleischman, 1986). Further, pamphlets describing the NICU and books about the infant's conditions are other concrete supports that may help to reduce the initial stress (Flynn & McCollum, 1989).

Sharing Information

There are many ways for interventionists to assist parents in working through grief, building attachments, and reducing the stress associated with parenting the premature at-risk infant. Information regarding prognosis and the potential treatment course should be given to parents honestly, in amounts they appear able to manage. Parents report that an honest, gentle, and supportive discussion of their child's condition, with compassion shown for the family's most immediate needs, is the best way to be told of their child's special needs. Because of stress and exhaustion, information may have to be given frequently to parents. Murdoch (1983) found that most parents expressed a need to talk to someone who understood their problems, and to gain more information about future prospects for their child. Some evidence suggests that the earlier diagnostic information is provided to families, the better parents' adjustment may be (Weber & Parker, 1981).

In the initial period of the infant's hospitalization, parents must deal daily with the potential life and death of their child. Often decisions must be made that require exploration of values and ethical dilemmas (Bowden, 1988; Churchill, 1985; Kohrman, 1988; Murray, 1985). This requires professionals to be sensitive to family issues and to have a structure for ongoing communication. Unfortunately, one of the least met needs of families is the need for a good listener (Fortier & Wanlass, 1984).

When interacting with families, it is best, as Lowenthal (1989) has noted, to avoid false rescuing behaviors. Statements such as, "It will be OK—these babies always make it. You'll see," do not alleviate grief and pain, and they may be untrue. Usually emotional support and active listening are the best tools in helping parents manage stress.

It may also be unwise to make assumptions about what may be best for parents or a family. Each family is unique, so what may be helpful for one family may be completely inappropriate for another. Flexibility and empathy are the most useful qualities for early interventionists, especially in high-risk nurseries.

Although the trend is to support families in making decisions about their child's care, this as well must be approached with delicacy. As Frohock (1986) says,

> It is a mistake to think that parents are the equal partners of doctors in assessing their children's condition and choosing therapy. . . . When parents are influenced by community values far removed from, and even antagonistic to, the guiding principles of medicine, parents and doctors may disagree sharply. (p. 161)

The challenge for interventionists is to respect and support the family's need to be empowered, while at the same time to recognize that certain practices may need to be followed in order to prevent or ameliorate risk conditions.

Managing Long-term Hospitalizations

After the infant's medical condition has stabilized, parents are usually able to take on more of their child's caretaking needs. The philosophy of family-centered care suggests that fostering family well-being promotes the child's well-being. Consequently, during the hospitalization, interventionists may focus on

- ☐ encouraging parent-infant interactions
- ☐ increasing parents' control in the neonatal high-risk nursery
- ☐ increasing parents' pride in their child
- ☐ supporting parents so they are able to recognize their own strengths (Lowenthal, 1989)

Establishing Communication Procedures

Open communication between all professionals involved with the premature infant's care is essential. Interventionists must be careful to avoid power struggles among themselves, the family, and medical personnel when dealing with the child who has complex health needs (Thomas, 1988). Parents often complain about the lack of control they experience in the neonatal unit. Regular consultations between parents and medical personnel during visiting and feeding times may increase feelings of control and reduce stress in parents (Kaiser, 1989).

Exhaustion is the most common state for parents as they attempt to handle new stresses, visit their child, take care of the rest of the family, and deal with an apparently endless string of unpredictable crises. Parents may respond to these stresses with hypersensitivity, hostility, or with decreased decision-making skills (Lowenthal, 1989).

Preparing for Discharge

Discharge commonly occurs around the time of the originally expected birth date, even when there are complications. In preparation for discharge, parents tend to be asked to increase their caregiving responsibilities (Ahmann, 1986). However, many parents report that they feel inadequately prepared for their infant's technical care-taking (Thorp, 1987). Others, because they have been deprived of the normal sequences of parenting with their child, fear that attachment may be more difficult. Formal and informal community supports are particularly critical for the family in ensuring a successful transition to the home (Thorp & Brown, 1987).

PROGRAMMING IN THE INTENSIVE CARE NURSERY

Effective intervention in the intensive care nursery requires interventionists to acknowledge and balance the infant's need for medical stability and a responsive environment, as well as the family's need for support.

The Central Role of Medical Stability

The purpose of the neonatal intensive care unit is to establish medical stability. Medical efforts are aimed at treating complications associated with the immaturity of the preterm infant's organs. Medical interventions also attempt to promote temperature regulation, stabilized respiration, heart rate, elimination, and feeding. A primary goal of the NICU is to promote growth by attempting to prevent medical crises, such as the occurrence of sepsis, that may compromise growth. Although some believe that infant-caregiver social interaction in some neonatal units may not facilitate infant development (Bennett, 1987), the first objective of neonatal nurseries is to promote the survival of unprepared, fragile infants.

Developmental Intervention

The central task in implementing developmental intervention in the intensive care nursery is establishing procedures for systematic observation of infants. Due to the fragile and changing nature of these infants, intervention often bears little resemblance to the hands-on intervention employed with older, healthy infants with developmental disabilities. In fact, for infants weighing less than 1,500 g, stimulation must be minimized because they do not have the developmental maturity to tolerate simultaneous tactile, auditory, or visual stimulation (Cooper & Kennedy, 1989).

Similarly, cocaine-exposed infants tend to be hypersensitive and irritable, crying inconsolably at the slightest provocation (Cloherty & Stark, 1985). A sudden noise, talking, or even looking at the infant may trigger prolonged crying. Other cocaine-exposed infants may escape stimulation by sleeping for extended periods of time. In such cases, observation and minimal handling are the backbone of developmental intervention in hospital settings. Generally, intervention involves attempts to structure the hospital environment so that it is supportive and contingently responsive to the medical and developmental needs of the growing premature infant.

Observational systems may be informal, such as a simple record of behavior kept by the infant's isolette. Or, observations may be formal such as using instruments as the Brazelton Neonatal Behavioral Assessment Scale (Brazelton, 1984), the Feeding Interaction Scales and Teaching Interaction Scales (Barnard & Eyers, 1979), and the Assessment of Preterm Infant Behavior (Als, Lester, Tronick, & Brazelton, 1982). Structured observations lead to an understanding of the infant's unique behavioral style, the infant's response to environmental stress, and the infant's ability to recover from environmental stress. Observations also provide parents with a means of obtaining feedback from their infants that can lead to greater competence and confidence in their caregiving abilities (Flynn & McCollum, 1989).

Data from structured observations are useful guides in establishing caregiving routines. Ideally, procedures that minimize stress to the infant and promote the infant's ability to recover can then be encouraged. Caregivers who understand the infant's pattern of responsiveness can identify when the child may be most able to participate in social interactions. Parent-child interactions that do not overload the infant's sensory system allow parents to perform normal parenting roles and allay anxieties about the child and their own caretaking abilities (Als et al., 1982). For example, to lengthen the duration of the infant's gaze toward parents, parents can imitate or mirror the child's gestures and movements (Field, 1975; Winnicott, 1971).

Any handling of the premature infant requires attention to the infant's signals of overstimulation. Common indicators of overstimulation include changes in skin color, extension of limbs, flaring of fingers and toes, and arching of the back, as well as apnea and bradycardia. Early signs of an over-loaded nervous system in the drug-exposed infant include hiccoughs, yawns, sneezes, grimaces, jerky movements, flushed skin, averted or closed eyes, and crying (Cloherty & Stark, 1985).

Bennett (1987) summarized 12 studies that offered auditory, tactile, vestibular, and multimodal stimulation to neonates. The results are mixed, and at times, they contradict one another, with some reporting benefits of weight gain, mental development, or motor development and others reporting opposite results. Although the nature of neonatal intervention, the role of parents, and the characteristics of the child undoubtedly influence the results of neonatal intervention, most professionals consider developmental intervention useful for the child and the child's family. Developmental intervention should be individualized and is best when it promotes recovery, supports the infant's emerging competence, embraces optimal interaction with caregivers, and promotes optimal growth and development following the hospital stay.

Family Support

The goal of family support in the intensive care nursery is to assist families in managing the immediate crisis of giving birth to a medically fragile infant and to prepare them for caring for that infant at home. The amount and type of support given will vary according to individual family needs and will depend on whether the infant is newly admitted, is facing long-term hospitalization, or is being prepared for discharge (Bendell, Goldberg, Urbano, Urbano, & Bauer, 1987; Brown, 1987; Porter, 1983b).

As stated, initially parents must deal with the crisis of birth while also beginning to develop an understanding of their infant's condition. Some parents find support groups with other parents of high-risk infants beneficial because they are able to share their feelings and fears with others experiencing the same crisis.

During long-term hospitalizations, parents, as well as extended family members, continue to need access to information about the infant's medical status. As the recovery process begins, families may need to be prepared to take on caretaking routines. At this point, new information is required that will assist families in reading and understanding the infant's behavioral cues. Other means of support may include matching "veteran parents" with new parents of the NICU, and "Family Evenings" following discharge so families may participate in an evening of activities and support that focuses on their entire family (Kaiser, 1989).

Klaus and Kennell (1981) explored the effects of rooming in with mothers of preterm high-risk infants. Mothers lived in a room adjoining the premature nursery and fed their infants. They ate with other mothers so support and experiences could be easily shared. These researchers also arranged for premature infants to be brought to the mothers' rooms. Because of this arrangement, parents had an opportunity to become acquainted with their newborns under more natural circumstances. Infants who weighed between 1,500 and 2,000 g were monitored by the primary care nurse for any signs of distress while they were in their mothers' rooms. The mothers in this study reported increased feelings of control over their lives and their infants' lives as a result of this arrangement.

Although a critical goal of neonatal intervention is family adaptation, there are many ways in which interventionists may facilitate this process. Because family characteristics and circumstances vary so greatly, there is never only one way to support families and their infants. Some forms of support may be better suited to individual families than others.

PLANNING FOR DISCHARGE AND FOLLOW-UP

As families begin to prepare for the infant's discharge, it is important again to establish procedures for support and communication. Families may miss the security of the nursery's procedures and be fearful about their ability to provide the same care as highly skilled medical professionals. Some parents may need help in making connections with community support services, including early intervention programs; other families may require only periodic monitoring by the neonatal follow-up clinic. It is especially important that families are provided contact with other parents of high-risk infants through individual parent-to-parent connections or formal parent support groups.

Anticipatory Guidance

During the discharge period interventionists become more reliant on the use of **anticipatory guidance**. They try to anticipate difficulties the child and family may encounter and take steps to either prevent or minimize those difficulties. For example, parent-child interactions and bonding are areas of concern at the discharge phase and following hospitalization. Because of long separations, parents may need a good deal of reassurance that their parenting skills are satisfactory for their child. Additionally, after their child's medical stability is achieved, interventionists begin teaching parents/caregivers to read and respond to the infant's behavioral cues.

Infants with sleep and feeding problems and those unable to give positive feedback through smiling or cooing, such as some drug-exposed infants, may be especially trying for caregivers. The stresses from the responsibilities of apnea monitoring, administering medications around the clock, and feeding complications may simply overwhelm the otherwise competent, but emotionally and physically exhausted, parent. Parents must be alerted to these potential problems and work toward identifying ways to reduce their own stress (e.g., child care relief) before significant problems arise.

Coordination with Community Programs

One goal in the discharge process is to avoid gaps in services and supports during the hospital to community transition. There are several practical, activity-oriented books available to guide families in better understanding their infant's cues and facilitating the child's development. For instance, books such as *Handling Your Young Premature Baby at Home* (Valvano & Givens, 1986), *Understanding My Special Signals* (Hussey-Gardner, 1989), and *Home Care for the High-Risk Infant* (Ahmann, 1986) are useful for interventionists and families alike.

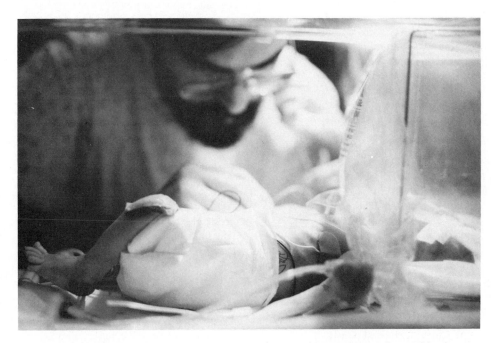

For some children, the medical complications of prematurity are extensive and lasting.

TRANSDISCIPLINARY CASES

The following two case studies demonstrate the variability in the course and range of complications associated with premature birth. They also represent the range of interventions necessary to meet families' needs. Despite the fact that both infants were born at similar gestational ages and had similar birthweights, one is expected to have long-term, widespread developmental delays; the other will probably function in mainstreamed settings. Both families required intensive crisis support while their infants were in the hospital and also were assisted in long-term planning issues.

THE JONES FAMILY

Joel Jones was born at 26 weeks gestation weighing 989 g. He is now 2 years old and experiencing general developmental delay. His intervention continues to require collaboration between medical and educational professionals. He was hospitalized for more than 3 months and continued to require medical management after discharge. In the intensive care nursery, Joel developed hydrocephalus secondary to severe intraventricular hemorrhage. This required the placement of a shunt that is still in place. He had seizures throughout his nursery stay and continues to take medication for seizure control. Joel appears to have experienced central nervous system damage resulting in significant motor impairment.

Joel was primarily tube fed for the first 2 months of his life. However, bottle feedings were increased and at discharge he was able to be entirely bottle fed. Joel was on a ventilator for more than 2 months. Although he was eventually weaned from the ventilator, he still required supplemental oxygen at discharge. As a result of his early respiratory complications, Joel has bronchopulmonary dysplasia. He experiences frequent upper-respiratory infections and has a wheezing cough. In addition, Joel had patent ductus arteriosus that required surgical correction when he was 2 weeks old. He has had no further cardiac complications.

Family-centered Intervention Issues

Joel is the family's third child. His siblings, both brothers, were 15 and 17 years old at the time of his birth. Mr. and Mrs. Jones are both 42. Mr. Jones is a government statistician; Mrs. Jones was not employed outside the home at the time of Joel's birth. His parents are now divorced; they separated during the pregnancy. Joel's mother reported that despite problems for years, they finally separated because her husband did not want a third child. Mr. Jones's whereabouts are now unknown, and he provides no child support.

All three children now live with Mrs. Jones. Both older brothers are employed part-time and attending a local junior college. Mrs. Jones is working as an instructional aide in Joel's preschool program.

During Joel's hospitalization, interventionists had to consider the status of the family prior to his birth as well as the added crisis of his hospitalization. It was clear that Mrs. Jones was committed to caring for Joel. Despite her sadness at the loss of her marriage and Joel's premature birth, she showed no signs of initial rejection. She identified the following resource needs:

1. Knowledge about community resources to assist her in finding affordable housing that was adequate for Joel's care needs and to assist her in finding employment that would also allow her to be primary caretaker for Joel.
2. Knowledge about Joel's condition and about his special care needs after discharge.
3. Emotional support in dealing with the shock of her losses and re-establishing herself and her family. She had no family nearby, and many of her friends were unsure how to help.
4. Information and support for Joel's siblings.

Based on Mrs. Jones' identified needs and Joel's condition, the following goals guided family intervention:

1. Assist Mrs. Jones in establishing home routines that enable her to visit Joel while in hospital.
2. Connect Mrs. Jones with appropriate community resources to assist her in re-establishing her household. These included a

housing assistance program and a job placement program.

3. Assist Mrs. Jones in identifying and accessing sources of emotional support, including a local parent-to-parent program as well as Parents Without Partners.
4. Provide information necessary to involve Mrs. Jones in Joel's care including handling techniques and supporting her natural ability to read his cues.
5. Assist Joel's siblings in understanding his condition and provide them with opportunities to visit him in the nursery and to handle him as his condition improved.
6. Prepare the family for bringing Joel home, for providing medications and other care needs, as well as for dealing with his medically fragile status and his probable developmental delays.

Developmental Intervention Issues

Joel was an irritable infant. All of his body systems were stressed by even the most non-invasive caretaking procedures. Once stressed, he was very difficult to calm. His body posture was primarily extended, and he had increased muscle tone. Developmental intervention goals were as follows:

1. Minimize handling.
2. Minimize noise and light in the nursery by establishing regular patterns of lights out and reduced noise and limiting noise and light levels at all other times.
3. Following any handling, staff were encouraged to stay with Joel and use careful touching and a calm voice to ensure that he was stable.
4. Use blanket rolls for containment to facilitate a flexible position for Joel and to minimize his excessive movements.

Hospital to Home Transition

In preparation for Joel's transition home, hospital staff did the following:

1. They provided Mrs. Jones and Joel's siblings with CPR training and training necessary to care for Joel's oxygen equipment and monitors.
2. They gave Mrs. Jones the opportunity to take over Joel's care for a full day prior to discharge.
3. They referred Mrs. Jones to a local early intervention program in order to assure coordinated therapy and support, given Joel's probable delays.
4. They scheduled a meeting attended by hospital discharge staff, Mrs. Jones and her sons, and staff of the early intervention program to establish transition goals.
5. They established a schedule for routine follow-up assessment of Joel's medical and developmental status in the intensive care nursery follow-up clinic.

Follow-up

Joel continues to be seen twice weekly, once by a home visitor and once in a center-based program attended by other parents and their infants. He receives physical, occupational, and speech therapy, and educational intervention through his home visitor. He has continued to be reasonably healthy, except for frequent respiratory infections. He was completely off oxygen support by 1 year of age. According to recent assessments, he has mild cognitive delays. His motor delays are more severe, and he has been diagnosed as having cerebral palsy. His early intervention program has referred him to a preschool special education program that he will enter at age 3.

THE MITFORD FAMILY

Sarah Mitford was born at 27 weeks weighing 900 g. She is the first child for her mother, who is 23, and her father, who is 27. She was delivered by emergency Caesarean.

Sarah experienced severe respiratory distress and required a ventilator for nearly 6 weeks. After being weaned from the ventilator, she required supplemental oxygen for an additional 6 weeks. She was discharged home requiring no additional oxygen support.

continued

Prior to discharge, Sarah was also diagnosed as having retinopathy of prematurity. This has resulted in a visual impairment; however, corrective lenses have proved adequate. When Sarah was 4 weeks old, she also developed an infection. Although she became very ill and unresponsive at the time, she was treated with antibiotics and appears to have no long-term complications. Finally, Sarah had patent ductus arteriosus, which complicated her respiratory status, but was treated with medication and did not require surgery. Sarah was discharged after a 4-month hospitalization.

Family-centered Intervention

The first task in providing family-centered intervention was to assist Sarah's mother in adjusting to the disappointment of her premature labor and delivery. Ms. Mitford repeatedly expressed her shock and grief at the abruptness and pain associated with Sarah's birth. She stated that she had no desire to see Sarah in the intensive care nursery because she was certain Sarah would die. Sarah's mother received counseling support by the hospital social worker. At her request, she was also referred to another mother who had a similar experience and whose child was now at home. Sarah's father visited her regularly.

As Sarah's condition began to stabilize, her mother took more interest in visiting her. However, any medical setback, such as the infection, was a major crisis for Ms. Mitford. It was nearly a month before she visited regularly and began to take active interest in Sarah's care. At that time, Ms. Mitford's primary intervention need was to receive as much information as possible. It became critical that hospital staff, accustomed to supporting her emotional needs, be equally supportive of her information needs. It was especially critical that they establish a collaborative relationship with her and avoid impatience with her constant questions. During this time, intervention consisted of careful explanation and providing printed materials.

As the hospital began to prepare for Sarah's discharge, her mother was encouraged to take on more of Sarah's caretaking. At first Ms. Mitford enjoyed this, but as she became more responsible, her earlier fear of Sarah's death re-emerged, as did her feelings of anger about her delivery. Efforts to provide emotional support were increased. At the same time, her caretaking efforts were reinforced as much as possible to assist her in developing a strong sense of parental competence.

Both parents were trained to handle Sarah's routine care, and assisted in anticipating the re-emergence of their fears and sadness over Sarah's birth. Also, they were referred to a community parent support group. Mr. Mitford expressed willingness to come back to talk with other fathers in similar circumstances.

Developmental Intervention Issues

While in the NICU, Sarah was often fussy and difficult to calm. Initially, interventions were aimed at preventing her from becoming overly fussy when handled. Hospital staff and parents were encouraged to minimize stimulation, to provide visual or auditory input, but not both at once. They were encouraged to talk to her quietly before handling and to ensure that she was calm before they left her.

She began to respond without fussing to quiet voices and, prior to discharge, was alerting differentially to the voices of caregivers. She continued to be less organized in response to visual input. Special care was taken to avoid overwhelming her with bright lights or too many visually stimulating objects at once.

Transition from Hospital to Home

At the time of discharge, Sarah was already performing as though she had no central nervous system damage. She also appeared to be functioning appropriately for her gestational age. However, given her low birthweight and her uneven hospital course, she was referred to a community early intervention program for a weekly center-based parent-infant group and monthly home visits. She was also referred to the hospital's infant follow-up clinic for monitoring of medical and developmental status.

At age 2, Sarah is functioning within normal limits in all areas except language, in which she appears to have some expressive delay. She has been diagnosed as having bronchopulmonary dysplasia resulting from treatment of respiratory complications in the newborn period. She has a chronic cough and asthma. She will enter a nursery school program for normally developing preschoolers and receive supplemental speech therapy. Sarah's parents report that they believe Sarah would not have done as well without the early intervention program that enabled them to work with her at home and to better understand her behavior.

Interventionists who deal with neonates are being challenged to learn medical terminology and develop a working knowledge of medical complications and their implications for child development. At the same time, it is incumbent upon hospital personnel to address the emotional as well as immediate and ongoing medical needs of high-risk infants and their families. Clearly, medical and educational professionals have different styles of handling problems and interacting with children and families. Flynn and McCollum (1989) state that the union of education, social services, and medicine has the capacity to rectify some of the obvious weaknesses in professional-parent interactions experienced by families of high-risk, premature infants. As Ensher and Clark (1986) remark:

> Ultimately, to bridge the gap from profession to service we must forgo our academic preciousness and learn new skills in translating areas of specialization into practice. ... Such changes should contribute to a new concept of role that diminishes misunderstanding and rivalry, enhances the personalization with which service is delivered, and helps to focus on the family as the responsible agent in the growth and progress of the child. (p. 277)

SUMMARY OF PROCEDURES

Neonatal intervention is unique in that it requires simultaneous attention to the health and developmental status of the infant while also assisting the family's adjustment during a period of crisis. Some of the key strategies discussed in this chapter to accomplish these goals follow:

1. Provide concrete supports for families during the crisis of the premature delivery. For example, offering photos of the infant, calling the family when the infant arrives at the high-risk care hospital, providing pamphlets about the NICU, and sharing books about the infant's condition may work to mediate the family's stress.
2. Provide individualized intervention for both the premature, high-risk infant and all the infant's caregivers. Intervention is best when it promotes recovery, supports the infant's emerging competence, enhances optimal interaction with caregivers, and promotes optimal growth and development following discharge.
3. Solicit long-term, comprehensive intervention for both the substance-abusing mother and the drug-exposed premature infant to reduce the effects of drug exposure on the infant's health and development.
4. In collaboration with the medical care team, establish an observation system for infants in the intensive care nursery that generates data to be used in developing an environment that is supportive, and to the extent possible, responsive to the infant. Observational systems are also helpful in identifying when infants may be most responsive to social interaction as their medical conditions stabilize.
5. Provide active supports for families to assist them in managing the crisis of the medically fragile infant and to prepare them for successfully caring for that infant at home. Active supports include identifying and building support

systems within the family, involving extended family members, and when appropriate, arranging interactions with other families in similar circumstances.

6. As medical stability is achieved, assist parents/caregivers to read and respond to the infant's behavioral cues in the intensive care setting and later in the infant's home.

7. Involve all professionals and family members in identifying the infant's signals of overstimulation and to adjust interactions accordingly. Common signs of overstimulation include changes in skin color, extension of limbs, flaring of fingers and toes, and arching of the back, as well as apnea and bradycardia.

8. Avoid making assumptions about what may be best for parents by using rescue behaviors. Emotional and instrumental support, and active listening are the most appropriate means of individualizing supports for families.

9. Involve parents and medical caregivers, in some way, in all phases of intervention. Increasing parental pride in their infant and assisting parents in identifying their own strengths and resources encourages coping mechanisms for stress management and helps parents to feel more competent.

SUMMARY

Infants are surviving at younger ages and with lower birthweights. Although many infants may recover from this initial insult, others will have long-term developmental disabilities with varying degrees of severity. Most of these infants will require a long hospitalization and a minimum of short-term specialized interventions to assist them in their recovery.

The families of hospitalized newborns will likewise need either short- or long-term supports. These supports may be provided by the medical care team in conjunction with a developmental specialist in the intensive care nursery. This interventionist promotes handling and interactive strategies that facilitate the growing infant's development. This professional assists parents and caregivers in better interpreting their infant's behavior and in assuming caretaking that is responsive to the infant's unique behavioral style. The specialist may also take a significant role in organizing the discharge from hospital to home and connecting the family with community-based early intervention programs when appropriate.

The earliest possible intervention and prevention efforts take place in the neonatal intensive care nursery. The quality of services in the NICU are critical for infant survival and may be linked to family adaptation. Equally important, in the intensive care nursery effective partnerships are forged that set the stage for future positive, collaborative parent-professional interactions.

--- **DISCUSSION QUESTIONS** ---------------

1. What are the most common medical complications related to prematurity and what are some of the developmental implications of each?
2. What preparations are programs making to meet the needs of substance-abusing mothers and drug-exposed infants in light of the fact that the number of these at-risk infants and families is projected to increase dramatically in the next 10 years?
3. Reread the two transdisciplinary case studies. What were the medical complications of each of the children? How may the medical complications of the newborn period have led to later developmental problems?
4. What issues were unique to each family in the case studies? How did the needs of the families change from initial hospitalization to discharge? What specific strategies may be used to involve parents and other medical staff in the infant's developmental intervention program in the nursery?

--- **APPLIED ACTIVITIES/PROJECTS** -------------

1. Arrange an observation in a neonatal intensive care nursery, and consider the following:
   □ Why are particular beds used with particular infants?
   □ What are the functions of the different types of equipment?
   □ What are the medical conditions of the infants? Choose one of the medical complications found in this nursery and research its causes and potential long-term complications.
   □ Which family members are permitted on the unit?
   □ To what degree are families involved in the caregiving of their child? In what ways are they encouraged to become involved in caregiving?
   □ What services are available for parents, for siblings, for grandparents?
   □ What is different about family involvement in the evenings or on weekends?
2. In the NICU, observe one infant who is stable for at least 15 minutes.
   □ What are the predominant states? What is the range of states observed? How do states change with handling and other forms of environmental stimulation? How easily does the infant move from one state to another?
   □ What movement efforts does the infant make? How do the movements affect the child?
   □ What are the influences of caregiving procedures on temperature, respiration, and heart rate?
3. Interview two members of the intensive care nursery staff. What are their roles? What specialized training was required for their positions? What do they see as their special contribution to the nursery team? What is stressful about their jobs? What do they like about their jobs? What do they consider to be their role with the families of infants who are in the nursery?
4. Arrange to observe a prenatal behavioral assessment of a premature infant and a drug-exposed infant. What did you learn about each infant that you had not observed in the nursery? What does this information suggest for later intervention with each child?
5. What issues/strategies are critical for effective parent-professional communication in the hospital setting?
6. Interview a family whose child was in an intensive care nursery and discuss the following:
   □ What has been your experience?
   □ What was most stressful?

- ☐ In what ways did the nursery staff and environment support your involvement with your infant?
- ☐ What forms of support would you have liked?
- ☐ How were you prepared to take your infant home?
- ☐ What has been difficult/easy since your child has been home?
- ☐ How do you think your experience has been different from families who have a fullterm, healthy infant?

7. Develop a parent resource booklet. What post-discharge support resources, print materials, and community services are available to parents of high-risk infants in your community?

SUGGESTED READINGS

Ahmann, E. (1986). *Home care for the high-risk infant*. Rockville, MD: Aspen.

Cloherty, J., & Stark, A. (Eds.). (1985). *Manual of neonatal care*. Boston, MA: Little, Brown.

Cole, J., & Frappier, P. (1983). *Developmental intervention in a special care nursery: A new approach to providing care for the preterm infant*. Boston, MA: Wheelock College, Center for Parenting Studies.

Ensher, G. L., & Clark, D. A. (1986). *Newborns at risk: Medical care and psychoeducational intervention*. Frederick, MD: Aspen.

Fletcher, M. A., Brown, C., & Wetherby, C. (1987). *The neonatal experience* (training manual) Washington, DC: The George Washington University.

Harrison, H., & Kositsky, A. (1983). *The premature baby book*. New York: St. Martin's Press.

Porter, S. (1983). *Organizing support programs for parents of premature infants*. Boston, MA Wheelock College, Center for Parenting Studies.

Stinson, R., & Stinson, P. (1983). *The long dying of baby Andrew*. Boston: Little, Brown.

Thorp, E. & Brown, C. (1987). *The family experience* (training manual). Washington, DC: The George Washington University.

REFERENCES

Ahmann, E. (1986). *Home care for the high-risk infant*. Rockville, MD: Aspen.

Als, H., Lester, B., Tronick, E., & Brazelton, T. B. (1982). Toward a research instrument for the assessment of preterm infants' behavior (APIB). In H. Fitzgerald, B. M. Lester, & M. W. Yogman (Eds.), *Theory and research in behavioral pediatrics, Vol. 1* (pp. 35–132). New York: Plenum.

Apgar, V. A. (1953). A proposal for a new method of evaluation of the newborn infant. *Anesthesia and Analgesia, 32,* 260–267.

Barnard, K. E., & Eyers, S. J. (1979). *Child health assessment, Part 2: The first year of life*. (DHEW Pub. No. HRA 79–25). Hyattsville, MD: U. S. Department of Health, Education and Welfare.

Batshaw, M. L., & Perret, Y. (1981). *Children with handicaps: A medical primer*. Baltimore: Paul H. Brookes.

Bendell, D., Goldberg, M. S., Urbano, M. T., Urbano, R., & Bauer, C. (1987). Differential impact of parenting sick infants. *Infant Mental Health Journal, 8,* 28–36.

Bennett, F. C. (1987). The effectiveness of early intervention for infants at increased biological risk. In M. J. Guralnick & F. C. Bennett (Eds.), *The effectiveness of early invention for at-risk and handicapped children* (pp. 96–103). Orlando, FL: Academic Press.

Blackman, J. (1986). *Basic criteria for tracking at-risk infants and toddlers*. Washington, DC: National Center for Clinical Infant Programs.

Bowden, V. (1988). Selective nontreatment of handicapped newborns: How do we decide? *Children's Health Care, 17,* 12–18.

Brazelton, T. B. (1984). *Neonatal Behavioral Assessment Scale*. Philadelphia: Lippincott.

Brazelton, T. B., Nugent, J. K., & Lester, B. M. (1987). Neonatal behavioral assessment scale. In J. D. Osofsky (Ed.), *Handbook of infant development* (pp. 780–817). New York: Wiley.

Brown, C. (1987). *The community experience*. Washington, DC: The George Washington University.

Cardone, I., & Gilkerson, L. (1989). *Family administered neonatal activities: A first step in the integration of parental perceptions and newborn behavior*. Unpublished manuscript.

Churchill, L. R. (1985). Which infants should live? On the usefulness and limitations of Robert Weir's selective nontreatment of handicapped newborns. *Social Science and Medicine, 20,* 1097–1102.

Cloherty, J., & Stark, A. (Eds.). (1985). *Manual of neonatal care*. Boston, MA: Little, Brown.

Cole, J., & Frappier, P. (1983). *Developmental intervention in a special care nursery: A new approach to providing care for the preterm infant*. Boston, MA: Wheelock College, Center for Parenting Studies.

Committee for Classification of Retinopathy of Prematurity. (1984). An international classification of retinopathy of prematurity. *Archives of Ophthalmology, 102,* 1130–1134.

Cooper, C. S., & Kennedy, R. D. (1989). An update for professionals working with neonates at risk. *Topics in Early Childhood Special Education, 9*(3), 32–50.

Drage, J., Kennedy, C., & Schwarz, R. (1964). The Apgar score as an index of neonatal mortality. *Obstetrics & Gynecology, 24,* 222–230.

Ensher, G. L., & Clark, D. A. (1986). *Newborns at risk: Medical care and psychoeducational intervention*. Rockville, MD: Aspen.

Field, T. M. (1975). *Infants born at risk: Behavior and development*. New York: SP Medical & Scientific Books.

Field, T. M. (1987). Alleviating stress in ICU neonates. In N. Gunzenhauser (Ed.), *Infant stimulation: For whom, what kind, when, and how much?* (pp. 121–128). Skillman, NJ: Johnson & Johnson.

Fleischman, A. (1986). The immediate impact of the birth of a low birthweight infant on the family. *Zero to Three, 6,* 1–5.

Fletcher, M. A. (1984). Prematurity. In J. J. Sciarra (Ed.), *Gynecology and obstetrics* (Vol. 3), (pp. 1–16). Philadelphia: Harper & Row.

Fletcher, M. A., Brown, C., & Wetherby, C. (1987). *The neonatal experience*. Washington, DC: The George Washington University.

Flynn, L., & McCollum, J. (1989). Support systems: Strategies and implications for hospitalized newborns and families. *Journal of Early Intervention, 13*(2), 173–182.

Fortier, L., & Wanlass, R. (1984). Family crisis following the diagnosis of a handicapped child. *Family Relations, 33,* 13–24.

Frohock, F. M. (1986). *Special care: Medical decisions in the first year of life*. Chicago: University of Chicago Press.

Garrand, S., Sherman, N., Rentchler, D., & Jung, A. (1978). A parent-to-parent program. *Family and Community Health, 1,* 103–113.

Goldberger, J. (1988). Infants and toddlers in hospitals. *Zero to Three, 8,* 1–6.

Gorski, P. (1985). Examining the NICU: Its environment, functions, and purposes. In Contemporary Forums, *Developmental interventions in neonatal care* (pp. 1–3). Danville, CA: Author.

Gottfried, A. (1985). Environmental neonatology: Consequences for the neonate under stress in the NICU. In P. Gorski (Ed.), *Contemporary forums, Developmental interventions in neonatal care* (pp. 4–17). Danville, CA: Author.

Green, M., Silverman, I., Suffett, F., Taleporos, E., & Turkel, W. (1979). Outcomes of pregnancy for addicts receiving comprehensive care. *American Journal of Drug and Alcohol Abuse, 6,* 413–429.

Greer, J. (1990). The drug babies. *Exceptional Children, 56,* 382–387.

Gryboski, J., & Walker, W. (1983). *Gastrointestinal problems in the infant.* Philadelphia: Saunders.

Haynes-Seman, C., & Hart, J. (1987). Doll play and failure to thrive toddlers: Clues to infant experience. *Zero to Three, 7,* 10–13.

Heinecke, C. M., Beckwith, L., & Thompson, A. (1988). Early intervention in the family system: A framework and review. *Infant Mental Health Journal, 9,* 111–141.

Howard, J. (in press). A prevention/intervention model for chemically dependent parents and their offspring. In S. Goldston, C. Heinecke, R. Pynoos, & J. Yager, *Preventing mental health disturbances in childhood.* Washington, DC: American Psychiatric Press.

Howard, J., Beckwith, L., Rodning, C., Kropenske, V. (1989). The development of young children of substance-abusing parents: Insights from 7 years of intervention and research. *Zero to Three, 9*(5), 8–12.

Hussey-Gardner, B. (1989). *Understanding my special signals.* Palo Alto, CA: VORT.

Jones, C., & Lopez, R. (1988). *Direct and indirect effects on the infant of maternal drug abuse.* Washington, DC: U. S. Department of Health and Human Services, National Institutes of Health.

Kaiser, C. (1989). Earlier family support through a NICU IFSP. *DEC Communicator, 16*(1), 4.

Klaus, M., & Kennell, J. (1981). *Parent-infant bonding.* St. Louis: Mosby.

Klein, N. (1988). Children who were very low birthweight: Cognitive abilities and classroom behavior at 5 years of age. *The Journal of Special Education, 22*(1), 41–54.

Kohrman, A. F. (1988). Selective nontreatment of handicapped newborns: A critical essay. *Social Science and Medicine, 20,* 1091–1095.

Korner, A. (1987). Preventive intervention with high-risk newborns: Theoretical, conceptual, and methodological perspectives. In J. D. Osofsky (Ed.), *Handbook of infant development* (pp. 1006–1036). New York: Wiley.

Landry, S., Fletcher, J., Zarling, C., Chapieski, L., & Francis, D. (1984). Differential outcomes associated with early medical complications in premature infants. *Journal of Pediatric Psychology, 9,* 385–401.

Lawson, J. (1988). Standards of practice and the pain of premature infants. *Zero to Three, 9,* 1–5.

Lowenthal, B. (1989). Alleviating stress in parents of high-risk preterm infants. *Teaching Exceptional Children, 3*(3), 32–33.

Meisels, S., Plunkett, J., Pasick, P., Stiefel, G., & Roloff, D. (1987). Effects of severity and chronicity of respiratory illness on the cognitive development of preterm infants. *Journal of Pediatric Psychology, 12*(1), 117–132.

Miller, G. (1989). Addicted infants and their mothers. *Zero to Three, 9*(5), 20–23.

Moore, J. A. (1988). Medical costs associated with children with disabilities or chronic illness. *Topics in Early Childhood Special Education, 8,* 98–105.

Murdoch, J. (1983). Immediate postnatal management of the mothers of Down Syndrome and spina bifida children in Scotland, 1971–1981. *Journal of Mental Deficiencies Research, 28,* 67–72.

Murray, T. H. (1985). Why solutions continue to elude us. *Social Science and Medicine, 20,* 1103–1107.

National Center for Health Statistics. (1978). *Hospital handbook on birth registration and fetal death reports.* Hyattsville, MD: U.S. Department of Health, Education and Welfare.

Nugent, J. K., & Brazelton, T. B. (1989). Preventive intervention with infants and families: The NBAS model. *Infant Mental Health Journal, 10,* 84–99.

Plunkett, J. W., & Meisels, S. (1989). Socioemotional adaptation of preterm infants at 3 years. *Infant Mental Health Journal, 10,* 117–131.

Porter, S. (1983a). *The early years: A guide for parents of premature infants.* Boston, MA: Wheelock College, Center for Parenting Studies.

Porter, S. (1983b). *Organizing support programs for parents of premature infants.* Boston, MA: Wheelock College, Center for Parenting Studies.

Purohit, D. E., Ellison, R., Zierler, S., Miettinen, O., & Nadas, A. (1985). Risk factors for retrolental fibroplasia: Experiences with 3,025 premature infants. *Pediatrics, 76,* 339–344.

Schneider, J., Griffith, D., & Chasnoff, I. (1989). Infants exposed to cocaine in utero: Implications for developmental assessment and intervention. *Infants and Young Children, 2*(1), 25–36.

Seigel, L., Saigal, S., Rosenbaum, P., Morton, R., Young, A., Berenbaum, S., & Stoskopf, B. (1982). Predictors of development in preterm and fullterm infants: A model for detecting the at-risk child. *Journal of Pediatric Psychology, 7,* 135–148.

Thomas, R. B. (1988). The struggle for control between families and health care providers when a child has complex health care needs. *Zero to Three, 8,* 15–18.

Thorp, E. (1987). *Mothers coping with home care of severe chronic respiratory disabled children requiring medical technology assistance* (No. 8715646). Ann Arbor, MI: University Microfilms International.

Thorp, E., & Brown, C. (1987). *The family experience.* Washington, DC: The George Washington University.

Thorp, E., & McCollum, J. A. (1988). Defining the infancy specialization in early childhood special education. In J. B. Jordan, J. J. Gallagher, P. L. Hutinger, & M. B. Karnes (Eds.), *Early childhood special education: Birth to three* (pp. 147–162). Reston, VA: The Council for Exceptional Children.

Tittle, B., & Claire, N. (1989). Promoting the health and development of drug-exposed infants through a comprehensive clinic model. *Zero to Three, 9*(5), 18–20.

Valvano, J., & Givens, R. R. (1986). *Handling your young premature baby at home.* Alexandria, VA: R. R. Givens.

VandenBerg, K. (1985). Infant stimulation versus developmental intervention: Practical suggestions for what really works. In K. VandenBerg (Ed.), *Contemporary forums, Developmental interventions in neonatal care* (pp. 87–92). Danville, CA: Author.

Weber, G., & Parker, T. (1981). A study of family and professional views of the factors affecting family adaptation to a disabled child. In N. Stinnett, J. DeFrain, & K. King (Eds.), *Family strengths 3: Roots of well-being* (pp. 379–395). Omaha: University of Nebraska Press.

Weston, D., Ivins, B., Zuckerman, B., Jones, C., & Lopez, R. (1989). Drug-exposed babies: Research and clinical issues. *Zero to Three, 9*(5), 1–7.

Winnicott, D. W. (1971). *Playing and reality.* London: Travislock.

Zuckerman, B., Amaro, H., Bauchner, H., & Cabral, H. (1989). Depressive symptoms during pregnancy: Relationship to poor health behaviors. *American Journal of Obstetrics and Gynecology, 160,* 1107–1111.

7

Coordinating Services for Medically Fragile/Complex Infants and Toddlers

Cordelia Robinson and Barbara Jackson

OVERVIEW

This chapter discusses issues relating to intervention with chronically ill and medically fragile infants and toddlers, and the roles of health care professionals on the transdisciplinary team, including:

- □ issues and concerns relating to coordination of care for medically fragile/complex infants and their families
- □ effects of complex medical conditions on infants' health and development
- □ effects of chronic/complex medical conditions on families
- □ appropriate assessment procedures for seriously ill infants
- □ coordination of health care and other professionals serving medically fragile and/or complex infants and their families

The health, developmental, and therapeutic care of medically fragile infants is an area of growing concern. Advances in medical technology, a growing understanding of newborn physiology, and organ transplantations have enabled children to survive who even 10 years ago would not have done so. The number of chronically ill/medically complex children who are limited in activity nearly doubled between the 1960s and the 1980s (Butler, Budetti, McManus, Stenmark, & Newacheck, 1985). These changes in the medical field have coincided with philosophical changes in the care of people with disabilities. For infants who are medically fragile or who have complex medical problems, the current emphasis on community-based coordinated care has increased the chances that these children will return to their families, specialized foster care, or extended care units. Care that was once thought to be so technical that only skilled professionals in hospitals could execute it is now being taught to parents, child care workers, and other professionals.

Traditionally, health care professionals have provided medical services with little attention to coordinating their efforts with the educational services the child may have received. However, for some infants that practice seems to be changing. Today, more health care professionals recognize the value of working in teams with professionals from other disciplines, and dialogue between medical and educational settings is becoming an expected occurrence.

ROLES OF HEALTH CARE PROFESSIONALS

Many different disciplines are involved in the health and habilitative care of medically fragile/complex infants. A congenital condition of liver disease, for example, can require the combined expertise of several medical specialties, specialty and general pediatric care nurses, nutritionists, and physical and occupational therapists. If complications occur after surgery, such as the need for a tracheostomy, the speech pathologist is likely to become involved in the child's care. The health team may request psychological or developmental evaluations of the child's functioning prior to surgical interventions that may involve still more professionals. Interestingly, the special education/infant interventionist is a relative newcomer to the health care team.

Children with complex medical problems are likely to make multiple transitions between hospital and home care. Such changes in care demand special coordination so families are not overwhelmed with professionals, or caught without adequate health care services. Krammer (1987) describes her family as having substantial contact with more than 100 different professionals in a 6-month period in her twin sons' lives. One son has spina bifida and the other has hemiparesis, a weakening of muscle strength but not complete paralysis, on one side of the body. Krammer's experience makes the need for coordination and collaboration between health care professionals and other disciplines very apparent. Unfortunately, this is not always the case in practice. Smooth coordination may be hampered by the large number of professionals who may be involved in the child's care. The professionals most likely to be involved in the child's care in the hospital are the nurse, the child life specialist, and other related professionals.

Hospital Nurse

Nursing is the "diagnosis and treatment of human responses to actual or potential health problems" (American Nurses' Association, 1980, p. 9). Nurses consider physical, emotional, psychological, and social development when writing their plans of care. Nurses are not simply concerned with the person's physical response to a health problem, but are also sensitive to how the person and that person's family responds in all areas.

Each of the disciplines that are part of the health care team for medically fragile/complex infants has a unique role. Disciplines have specific assessment or treatment techniques that they use to develop their plans of care. Although there is some overlap among the disciplines, each tends to have a particular focus or area of the individual's functioning. For example, the speech pathologist is acknowledged as the specialist in the development of communication. The developmental therapist (physical or occupational) is particularly concerned with the development and maintenance of motor functioning. Members of these disciplines frequently discuss the importance of a holistic approach to care and propose integration of developmental domains. Nursing assumes this integrated perspective. Nurses develop a **Nursing Care Plan** that involves assessment of functioning; and identification of needs in all domains of development, areas affected by the presenting health problems, and any additional problems that may be secondary to the original problem.

The 24-hours-a-day responsibility for care that nurses assume requires them to develop uniform procedures for their work with the child (e.g., standard physical treatments, standard diets, standard administration of medications). Such routines help establish conventions for physical care in much the same way that psychologists use test manuals for standardized testing procedures. These conventions of care, however, do not prescribe ways to handle the individual's responses to care routines.

To meet the need for consistency in individualized aspects of care, most pediatric care settings now use the concept of primary nursing in their staffing patterns. **Primary nursing** means that one member of the hospital unit staff is assigned as the principal nurse for a given child. Although that person is not available on a round-the-clock basis, assigning the role of primary nurse facilitates consistency because the primary nurse develops the child's Nursing Care Plan. The main objective of primary nursing is to provide optimal care and services to patients and their families by focusing on patients' individual and unique needs. The primary nurse is responsible and accountable for providing comprehensive and continuous patient-centered care during hospitalization, as well as planning for the patient's discharge. Coordinating and communicating all aspects of care to families, other staff members, and physicians are integral components of this model of nursing care delivery (Marram, Schlegel, & Bevis, 1974). Generally, the primary nurse's role follows these parameters, whether the nurse is in general or intensive care unit settings.

Child Life Specialist

The **child life specialist** may be encountered in some hospital settings, and is probably the closest counterpart to early intervention educators in the hospital. The child life specialist is sometimes referred to as the Play Lady. The child life specialist typically has at least a bachelor's degree, with an extensive background in child development. This professional's role often includes direct intervention with both the child and the family, as well as consultative support to other team members. The child life specialist is frequently instrumental in setting up parent support groups and sibling support activities. This individual is a primary resource to nursing staff regarding the effects of disease and hospitalization on development. *Children's Health Care,* a journal of the American Association for the Care of Children's Health, an interdisciplinary national organization, provides additional information about the role of child life specialists in the care of medically fragile infants and toddlers. Basically, child life specialists make efforts to coordinate the child's physical and emotional needs.

Related Team Members

Many other specialists make up the hospital care team including social workers; physical, occupational, and communication therapists; nutritionists; and numerous medical specialists. The therapists' roles are discussed in other chapters, so they are not discussed here. These specialists are likely to be involved in both direct and consultative care. After the child returns to the home, the community health nurse and the pediatrician may assume more responsibility.

Community Health Nurse

The philosophy and responsibility of the **community health nurse** are basically the same as that of the primary care nurse in the hospital or extended care setting. The community health nurse develops a comprehensive plan of care that includes coordination of goals and strategies for implementing goals in the home or alternate care setting with all other care providers, including staff in the hospital setting. Because of an increase in the number of drug-exposed infants and infants with AIDS, the relationship between community health nurses and infant intervention service personnel will continue to grow.

Primary Care Physician

The role of the pediatrician in the care of medically fragile/complex infants involves responsibility for the overall general health care of the child as well as the coordination of health-related services. Medical specialists providing care to hospitalized children generally view it as their responsibility to communicate regularly with the pediatrician and/or the family practitioner. This **primary care physician** generally wishes to be involved with the family when alternatives in procedure and treatment are available. Although the primary care physician frequently turns over the day-to-day care of a medically fragile/complex infant to medical specialists during periods of hospitalization, involvement in the infant's care is frequently critical for comprehensive and well-coordinated care.

After the child is home, responsibility for initiating care conferences is often assumed by the primary care physician. A major role of the pediatric primary care physician and nurse is that of anticipatory guidance. These professionals address current health problems, but also anticipate potential areas of concern. When health issues are handled in a timely manner, problems consequent to the condition or treatments may be prevented; if prevention is not possible, the deleterious impact of illness may be minimized.

Any of these medical professionals discussed may serve as members of an early intervention team. When this occurs, the opportunity to share and learn across disciplines is greatly enhanced. Although basic nursing curricula include information on normal growth and developmental landmarks, primary care nurses working with medically fragile children in a hospital setting may need to increase their skills in assessing developmental functioning and implementing appropriate developmental interventions. Further, because the children in care come from a number of communities, the nurse must translate information onto several different forms depending on the support available in the child's home community. These tasks facilitate direct communication between hospital and community staff, and ultimately may lead to better coordinated transitions for children and families. The differences in the primary care nurse's role in the interdisciplinary and transdisciplinary team models are illustrated in Table 7–1.

ISSUES IN CHRONIC HEALTH CARE

The inclusion of the hospital in educational early intervention with children with disabilities is a new arrangement. The issues health care professionals encounter in such collaborations are similar to issues educational interventionists may face. The concerns health professionals have for disabled infants and toddlers are similar to the concerns they hold for all sick children in their care: the importance of continuity of care, and the importance of family in the child's recovery.

Importance of Continuity of Care

Children with complex medical problems critically need continuity in their health care. Medically fragile infants experience repeated changes in routines by virtue of the multiple transitions they make between hospital and home. Because of their medical conditions, many different adults may implement their care plans. Efforts are typically made to find out how the family or caregivers approach daily care routines, so that the nursing personnel may provide some continuity for the child and vice versa, but it can be difficult to communicate such information to all members of the care team. Additionally, medications (with accompanying side effects) and medical procedures may change often with chronically ill children. In some cases, the individuals who train parents/caregivers in care procedures may not be the ones who conduct follow-up sessions to evaluate the accuracy of their implementation.

Some groups of medically complex children present more challenges to providing continuity of care than others. For example, children with AIDS often present unique challenges because the medical and educational care of the child and the care of the infected parent may have to be considered. **Acquired Immune Deficiency Syndrome** (AIDS) reduces the body's ability to fight special types of infection and cancers, and is caused by the **Human Immunodeficiency Virus (HIV)**. After the child's immune system has been impaired, the child easily develops one or more specific opportunistic infections or rare cancers that become life threatening. The HIV virus is transmitted to infants by direct exposure to infected blood or blood products, or by an infected mother (Halleron, Pisaneschi, & Trapani, 1989).

Perinatal transmission of **pediatric AIDS**, clinical AIDS in children younger than 13 years of age, occurs through the placenta before the infant is born, during the birth process itself, or soon after birth through breast milk (Rennert, Parry, & Horowitz, 1988). It is now estimated that there is a 50% chance that an infected mother will pass the virus to her child. The risk of perinatal transmission is believed to be higher if the mother is, or becomes, seriously ill during her pregnancy (Rennert et al., 1988). Children with AIDS often have multiple caregivers (frequently foster care parents who require training), and multiple or sustained illnesses, all of which add complexity to efforts to provide continuity in medical care.

However, several model programs have been recently developed to assist professionals in devising systems to increase continuity of medical care. Project Continuity, for example, a program at the Nebraska Medical Center Hospital and Meyer

TABLE 7–1
Comparison of the primary care nurse's role in the interdisciplinary and transdisciplinary team models.

Child: Mark, a 29 month old, has AIDS. He is about to be discharged from the hospital after his third bout of pneumonia. He had the same primary care nurse for his last two hopitalizations.

Interdisciplinary Team Model	**Transdisciplinary Team Model**
Goal 1: Write discharge plan, identify means to control for further infections.	Goal 1: Mark will continue health care plan in all settings.
Goal 2: Refer to nutritionist to plan for discharge.	Goal 2: Members of Mark's family will be offered support services to assist them in dealing with his medical issues and eventual death.
Goal 3: Refer to Child Life Specialist to discuss hospital's programs for bereavement, family support, and sibling issues. Involve hospital social worker if family requests.	
Goal 4: Develop discharge nursing care plan for home care. Refer to list of private care nurses.	

Activities	**Activities**
1. Primary care nurse will meet with the family to discuss discharge plan and list of private nurses.	1. Primary care nurse will meet with Mark's family, the early intervention program staff members, and key medical personnel to devise a coordinated plan of service for the family.
2. Primary care nurse will make referrals.	2. Primary care nurse will train early intervention staff and family in care maintenance skills and make recommendations for nursing care in the home, as needed.
	3. Family will be given a list of services/supports available to them and will develop a list of services they would like to participate in, with appropriate timelines.
	4. The primary care physician will serve as the central information source for medical specialists.
	5. As appropriate, the primary care nurse will encourage developmentally appropriate experiences for Mark during hospitalizations.

Children's Rehabilitation Institute in Omaha has approached the need for continuity in care for medically fragile infants by implementing standards for care planning and family education. Examples of the ways in which these standards are put into practice are illustrated in the case studies.

Importance of the Family

Families with children with complex medical problems report that incorporating their child's care routines into their home life significantly alters the family's privacy and ability to live according to their own lifestyle preferences. Technology-dependent children, for example, require extensive medical support equipment that can restrict the family's mobility. Chronically ill infants, such as those with cystic fibrosis, may require frequent and specialized therapies that can leave little discretionary time in the family's day. Expenses not covered under medical plans may require choices between a piece of medical equipment for one child and a desired toy, such as a bicycle, for another child in the family. Some families become excessively stressed by their child's care needs. Medical personnel tend to recognize that the family's ability to perform and follow through with medical procedures will directly affect the child's recovery. Consequently, more medical settings are making efforts to either provide services to families or assist families in identifying community support programs and services.

EFFECTS OF CHILD'S CHRONIC AND COMPLEX MEDICAL PROBLEMS

When compared to the total number of births, children with chronic and complex medical problems are relatively few in number. Nonetheless, the resources required for their survival and well-being are tremendous. In general, it is difficult to predict the developmental future of children younger than 3 years of age (McCall, 1982). The manner in which health and development are affected is related to the child's disease or condition, the availability of treatment, the timing of diagnosis and treatment, as well as the family's ability to cope with the child's condition and care. Children who are medically fragile/complex face prolonged hospitalizations, limitations in experience secondary to the condition itself or restrictions in experience due to the demands of the medical interventions, separations from their families, and frequently, complications related to their conditions or treatments.

As a rule, medical problems that do not affect the central nervous system, such as congenital heart defects, liver disease, and congenital anomalies of organs (e.g., kidneys), do not, in and of themselves, have major effects on overall developmental potential. However, when complications occur following a medical intervention (such as the occurrence of a stroke) a whole new set of potential effects and limitations can occur. The potential for limited development is greater for the smallest birthweight premature children because all their systems (gastro-intestinal, cardiac, respiratory, and central nervous systems) are immature and unprepared for extra-uterine life.

Families with children with complex medical needs report that incorporating their child's routine care into their home life significantly alters the family's privacy and ability to live according to their lifestyle preferences.

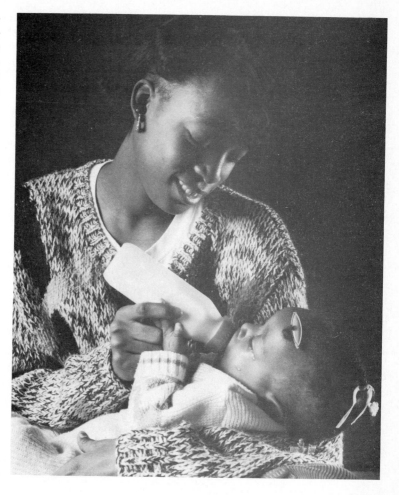

Systematic follow-up information regarding developmental functioning of medically fragile/complex infants tends to be limited and restricted to graduates of the most technologically advanced neonatal intensive care units. From these follow-up studies, it is clear that grade III and IV intracranial hemorrhages produce the most serious motoric **sequelae** (any lesion or infection following or caused by disease). However, because of the limitations in motor functioning observed in these children, the implications on cognition are difficult to immediately determine (Robinson & Fieber, 1988).

With some technology-dependent infants who have reached school age, there are indications of a higher incidence of more subtle developmental problems such as learning disabilities. Nevertheless, it is not possible at present to sort out whether these are primary or secondary conditions.

Family circumstances into which the child is born also affect the developmental outcome of medically fragile children. Developmental theory emphasizes an interactional position that looks on development as influenced by the interaction of biological potential and the ongoing biological integrity of the child, and the physical and social environments experienced by the child. Sick children of drug-addicted, teenage, or emotionally disturbed parents, for instance, face greater risk. The timing and the circumstances of an event, consequently, will mediate the overall impact of the event.

Further, substantially compromised nutrition during the first 6 months limits brain size. The lack of adequate nutrition later in development will affect growth and overall development, but will not limit potential in the same way that early severe malnutrition will. Chronic medical conditions may affect the child's physical growth, eating experiences, developmental experiences, and require the child to experience multiple hospitalizations.

Physical Growth

It has long been noted that, in general, children with cerebral palsy are small. This small size is now a cause for concern. Paban and Piper (1987) found that among a number of motor, neurological, and physical variables obtained in the first year, the child's weight at 3 months for both preterm and term at-risk infants was the best, and earliest, predictor of infant neurological status at 1 year.

The origins of growth failure in children with cerebral palsy have been attributed both to the lack of adequate nutritional intake and/or higher calorie expenditures due to the cerebral palsy. Recent studies conducted with severely retarded children with quadriplegic cerebral palsy demonstrate that ensuring nutritional intake through gastrostomy feedings results in increased physical growth when children are compared to children who received oral feedings by skilled caretakers (Shapiro, Green, Krich, Als, & Capute, 1986). Campbell, Wilhelm, and Slaton (1989) also note the high potential for inadequate nutritional intake in young children with cerebral palsy. They stress that interventionists should track the child's physical growth and initiate prompt referral to nutritionists if problems are observed.

Although poor physical growth among children with cerebral palsy has been reported for decades (Sterling, 1960; Tobis, Saturen, Larios, & Posniak, 1961), consistent monitoring of physical growth, particularly after the first year of life, is rarely done. Accurate recordkeeping regarding growth status and nutritional intake is frequently overlooked with other conditions as well. Yet, careful recordkeeping could mitigate the effects of serious illness on some children's development as may attention to children's eating experiences.

Eating Experiences

A critical issue in the care of medically fragile/complex infants is the need for normalization of eating experiences. Many fragile infants use some form of tube feedings. When this is the case, continuous consultation is necessary with the speech pathologist and occupational therapist or nutritionist. Interventions should provide substitute oral-motor stimulation necessary for the development of oral-motor musculature, vocal production, and dentition. Fletcher, Wetherby, & Brown (1986) cite case studies that illustrate strategies for moving children from tube to independent feeding.

Normalizing social experiences during mealtimes is equally important. Interventionists must be concerned with the nutritional adequacy of the child's diet as well as the need for arranging developmentally appropriate experiences. Nurses report that young patients can tell them the sequences of steps to a dressing change but do not have any idea what a tea party is with dolls or teddy bears. The use of pacifiers and the arrangement of more typical eating circumstances during tube feedings will assist the child in the transition to more typical means of eating, when or if such a transition occurs.

Impact on Developmental Experiences

Most healthy children experience some consistency in both their physical and social environments. Consistency has been related to appropriate emotional and cognitive development in children (Lamb, 1981; Wachs, 1984; Yarrow, 1979). In addition, consistency is important for language and social development. Most healthy children form a close relationship with a limited number of caregivers. Consistency in caregivers occurs infrequently for severely handicapped children, especially for those who are repeatedly hospitalized. Although continuity of circumstances and interpersonal consistency are the foundations for appropriate development, these situations simply may not exist for infants with extensive medical problems.

As indicated earlier, primary care nurses make efforts to offer some sense of continuity and consistency to their young patients. To the extent the child's medical condition permits, and with support from community intervention team members, some primary care nurses make attempts to offer developmentally appropriate experiences to children. Interventionists advise nurses to periodically alternate or change the infant's toys so experiential variety is provided. Also, they advise that too many toys or mobiles can be overstimulating and ineffective. Essentially, the infant's environmental space should be regularly monitored for the amount as well as the variety of materials or toys (Yarrow, Rubenstein, & Pederson, 1975).

Hospitalizations

Healthy children live with their families and learn to adjust to the families' goals, priorities, and patterns. Many medically fragile children have this adjustment interrupted by illness and repeated hospitalizations. The effects of hospitalization on these children are difficult to assess, as they depend on the child's age and the length of the hospitalizations.

Physical illnesses can be stressful for infants and toddlers. The additive effects of separation, particularly from 7 to 12 months of age, may intensify the impact of illness on the child (Lewis, 1982). In a long-term follow-up study of the impacts of hospitalization, Quinton and Rutter (1976) found that a single separation due to hospitalization rarely had long-term consequences. However, repeated hospitalizations, especially for children from low-income homes, had a higher relationship with later psychiatric problems.

In summary, survival through the preschool years and into middle childhood for medically fragile/complex children is a recent accomplishment. Consequently, little definitive information is available on the influence of severe medical conditions and treatment upon children's development. Because of many compounding factors, even less can be said with any assurance about the impact of fragile health on the future developmental functioning of children younger than 3 years of age.

IMPLICATIONS FOR THE FAMILY

The provisions of P.L. 99–457, Part H, recognize the importance of the child's family to the quality of life the child will experience. Families with infants and toddlers with chronic health needs have the same needs as other families with handicapped children. Additionally, these families have unique needs that arise from their efforts to maintain some stability under unpredictable circumstances and vacillating prognoses that often accompany serious illnesses and diseases.

In the Hospital

When a child is born with medical complications that require extended hospitalization, stresses for the family tend to stem from the

- extraordinary needs of the child
- grief and intrafamilial strains associated with the failure to produce a normal child
- economic burdens resulting from the care of an ill infant
- interruption in forming mutually rewarding interactions between family members and the child (Robinson, Rosenberg, Hartley, & Jackson, 1986)

The adverse effects of separation are evident in studies of mother-child interactions following the infant's dismissal from the hospital. Mothers who had been separated from their infants held their babies differently, changed position less often, burped their infants less, and were not as skillful in feeding as were mothers who were not separated from their infants (Klaus & Kennell, 1970). Others have found that early mother-infant separation may erode maternal self-confidence (Seashore, Leifer, Barnett, & Leiderman, 1973). The difficulties in forming an emotional attachment with an infant who is fussy, who has physical anomalies, and/or who is separated from the parents during the neonatal period may place the child at risk for neglect or abuse (Klein & Stein, 1971).

In addition to separations, other conditions interfere with the parent-infant relationship. Frequently, hospital staff form strong attachments to the infants in their care. The staff may become possessive of the infants, and in fact, assume the parental role, which may make it more difficult for parents to assert themselves in providing care. Staff may feel that the parents are not capable of caring for the infant at home, and thus a cycle of lack of confidence and undermining of responsibility may occur (Thomas, 1988).

The physical care of medically fragile infants is usually a matter of great concern for professionals and family members. Incidents in other families that might represent a small problem may represent a serious stressor for the family of the medically fragile infant. For example, a toddler may continue to require feeding every 3 hours through the day and night. If there is no relief for the caregiver, the sleep and feeding patterns of both the infant and the parent will be disrupted. A father of a 2-year-old chronically ill son put it this way: "We think we are holding up pretty well and something small will happen—like my older son's teacher calling me at work because my son's homework wasn't turned in—and I go crazy. The poor lady didn't know why I lost it; I didn't even bother to explain it. It was just one more pressure that I couldn't hold in anymore. . . . If I could only get some sleep."

After Discharge

Other stresses are also associated with the infant's care after discharge (Jeffcoate, Humphrey, & Lloyd, 1979). The frequent demands of the infant coupled with delays in reciprocal affection may cause some parents to experience feelings of inadequacy. Fathers of preterm infants report that they assumed more household and child care responsibilities than they had anticipated, and as a consequence, their work performance suffered. Parents of premature infants are more likely to divorce within the first 12 months after birth than parents of fullterm infants (Leifer, Leiderman, Barnett, & Williams, 1974).

When discharged from health care facilities, medically fragile infants often come home with intimidating life support devices (Richards, 1979). The use of such equipment causes stress to families in dealing with the infant's care and the use of technology. In other cases, the discharge may mean that the family or caregivers must begin actively coping with the child's terminal prognosis. For instance, only 20% of individuals with diagnosed AIDS are alive after 3 years (Rennert et al., 1988). For families in which there are other children and, perhaps, the need for the mother to return to work outside of the home, these demands can be extremely stressful.

Fortunately, children with medically complex conditions are receiving home care through funding waiver programs with increasing frequency. One problem in this option, however, is the lack of preparation of community health nurses to undertake highly technical care. Many times the parents must train the nurses. Unskilled respite care providers frequently are not useful to families under such circumstances. At times, out of desperation, children are rehospitalized, especially on weekends when no other alternative to meet the family's needs is available.

The outcomes for families living with these circumstances vary greatly. Some families experience problems with their other children, the break-up of marriages due to the neglect of personal needs, and/or the stress of living in a fishbowl with the ever-present health care providers. Further, parents may suffer from exhaustion, resulting in errors in care and maladaptive emotional responses that may take the form of resisting professional assistance.

Perrin (1989) cites a rule of thumb that has become conventional wisdom in the field of chronic illness. That rule is that 85% of the client's needs are based upon the chronicity of the person's condition and 15% on the needs specific to the condition. This appears to be a useful principle to keep in mind when considering the needs of both the medically fragile/complex infant and the infant's family. Theories of family functioning may also be useful in considering families' needs.

Family Theories

Family Systems Theory (Turnbull & Turnbull, 1990), Hill's ABCX Model (1949) regarding the impact of events, and the Family Life Cycle Model (Turnbull, Summers, & Brotherson, 1986) are prominent theories used to understand how families adapt to the handicapped child, and to identify the best ways to support families. When considering families with medically fragile/complex young children, none of these theories alone is adequate. However, when elements of each are combined, a better framework for supporting families can be developed.

The Family System Model reminds professionals that while families have individual members, those members do not behave in isolation. Each person's behavior affects all the others, either directly or indirectly.

The ABCX Model provides a framework for understanding the individual's or the family's response to atypical events. When this framework is applied to the event of a disabling or chronic illness in the child, it reminds professionals that individuals and individual families respond differently, depending on their own characteristics and circumstances. In this framework, a response to a stressful event will be the outcome of an interaction between the family's resources (A) and the family's definition of the event (B), which will determine the extent to which the event becomes a crisis for the family (C). This framework is supported in more recent literature. The family's perception of social support affects the extent to which the family reports increased stress following the birth of a handicapped child (Beckman, Pokorni, Maza, & Balzer-Martin, 1986; Bristol, 1979; Crnic, Friedrich, & Greenberg, 1983). Figure 7–1 represents an adaptation of the ABCX model.

The framework that is currently influencing thinking regarding families' needs is the Family Life Cycle Model (Duvall, 1957; Merderer & Hill, 1983; Turnbull et al.,

FIGURE 7–1
Families' responses to stressful events may result from an interaction between families' resources and the event. This interaction shapes the degree to which the event becomes a crisis for families.

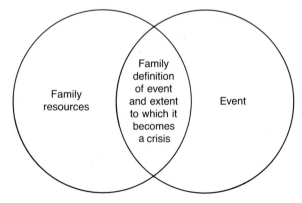

1986). The point of this conceptual framework is that family structure, priorities, interests, and needs change over time primarily in relation to the age of the child. The stages of the life cycle have implications for intervention with the family because the presence of the disabled chronically ill child may compound the difficulties of some transitions or may put families out of synchrony between ages and stages (Turnbull et al., 1986).

Although these theoretical models are helpful for interventionists in understanding family functioning, none were specifically formulated as a way to understand the issues faced by families with handicapped or medically fragile/complex infants. Rosenberg (1977) developed a model based upon small group research that seems to provide guidance in identifying factors that affect family functioning, and seems to have specific implications for intervention strategies with families with medically fragile children (Robinson, Rosenberg, & Beckman, 1988). The key variables considered in this framework are resources, expectancies, and consensus.

Effects of resources.   Resources include personal resources, such as coping strategies; emotional resources, such as family support; and material resources. In 1975, Bronfenbrenner argued for an ecological approach in considering the needs of families. He pointed out that inadequate nutrition and health care, poor housing, lack of education, limited income, and the necessity for long hours all constitute components of an environment that can sap parents of time and energy. Additional data for this position are found in the work of Patterson, Cobb, and Ray (1973) who observed that mothers lacking financial and people resources had difficulty learning child management techniques.

Families with chronically ill children are affected by the personal and social resources available to them. Parental depression (McLean, 1976), chronic illness, limited intellectual abilities (Kaminer, Jedrysek, & Soles, 1981; Rosenberg & McTate, 1982), and adverse family relationships are characteristics that can limit parental management of the child with serious medical needs. Exhaustion, a hazard of keeping the disabled child at home (Holt, 1958), is associated with families with severely handicapped children, as are increases in tension, illness, and/or incapacity to work (Lonsdale, 1978). It appears that any support that reduces parental distress may have a positive effect on the child. For example, children have been found to have an improved rate of recovery from surgery when efforts are made to reduce the anxiety of their mothers (Skipper & Leonard, 1968).

Long-term hospitalizations affect every aspect of the family's daily life and each family member in some way. Whether parents share time at the hospital or one parent takes the responsibility while the other maintains the home, normal routines are lost and there is minimal time together. If there are other children in the family, they may understand the needs of their sibling and still feel left out emotionally.

Families with severely handicapped children or children with complex medical problems often require substantial caregiving assistance, financial resources, and individualized medical services. Gaps in services and coordination problems are reported when the child's needs fall outside the traditional boundaries of health care, education, or social service systems (Moore & McLaughlin, 1988). This occurs more frequently with medically complex children. Wolfensberger (1969) first argued that families should be eligible for housekeeping assistance, child care, and income subsidy so that they could continue to maintain their children in their homes. Now, many states have subsidy and waiver programs that provide some assistance to families (Moore & McLaughlin, 1988).

Effects of expectancies and goals.   Caregivers' expectancies and goals for children affect their involvement with the children (Rosenberg, 1977). The expectations of caregivers of drug-exposed infants and infants with AIDS may be complicated by societal and legal restrictions (Rennert, Parry, & Horowitz, 1988). Additionally, public misinformation may contribute to social isolation that may further depress expectations. Parents who can value their children regardless of their developmental attainments will have an easier time becoming invested in the education and development of their children than parents who are highly concerned with the physical care and with the social status of their family and their children. Rosenberg (1977) found that mothers of handicapped infants who placed greater emphasis on economic goals and social status were judged to be less involved in their child's educational program.

Effects of consensus.   Family members must reach some agreements among themselves about the nature of their goals, the allocation of tasks, and the coordination of activities, including child care and therapy. Lack of consensus regarding the execution of household and therapeutic activities, or disagreement between parents and professionals over home program goals, will lead to inconsistent treatment for the child. Parents who disagree on child care issues, for example, will be unable to agree on activities related to their child's program. Patterson, Cobb, and Ray (1973) observed that marital discord is associated with failure to learn childrearing skills.

When there is a lack of consensus between spouses, and the father is unfamiliar with the rationale for the procedures his wife uses, Radin (1972) suggests that fathers be involved in ways that are consistent with their role in the family. She found that involved fathers are more likely to reach agreement with project staff and their wives on goals and procedures than are fathers who remain uninvolved. Beyond this, parents' skills in resolving differences can be enhanced by teaching them ways to negotiate and seek compromise solutions (Weiss, Hops, & Patterson, 1973). Strategies for negotiation, recommended for professionals but also appropriate for parents, are discussed in Chapter 13.

If parents are reluctant to become involved in their child's care and learning, the use of **time-limited contracting** can be useful for interventionists. These short-term agreements (e.g., days, weeks, months) reduce parental anxiety and change perspectives from long-term commitments, which some parents may view as overwhelming. These agreements allow parents to control their involvement and permits them a trial period in which to familiarize themselves with program and caregiving responsibilities.

It is impossible to delineate the exact way terminal or chronic illness affects families because each individual, and each family, approaches crisis, stress, responsibility, and conflict in a unique way. However, the family of the medically high-risk child requires efficient coordination of services, access to resources, and flexible case management that anticipates their changing needs throughout the course of their child's illnesses and/or care.

ASSESSMENT

There are several areas of assessment that are especially pertinent to the development of comprehensive, coordinated family-centered intervention plans for mentally fragile/complex infants. These assessment areas are the child's health and development, parent-child interactions, and the family's strengths and needs in relation to the care needs of the child.

Health and Developmental Status

Generally, in the hospital an interdisciplinary team that includes physical, occupational and communication therapists, a child life specialist or educator, a pediatric psychologist, and a primary care nurse provides input for the developmental assessment of the child. Ideally, this team shares data sources so each professional does not find it necessary to individually assess the child. The primary concern of developmental assessments of the medically fragile/complex infant is to identify the child's current level of functioning, and any developmental atypicalities, so appropriate interventions can be planned and implemented. If the child feels well physically, standard assessment tools such as the Bayley Scales of Infant Development (1969) may be administered. However, frequently these children do not feel well physically or they have physical or secondary impairments that make administration of standardized assessment inappropriate (Robinson & Fieber, 1988; Rosenberg & Robinson, in press).

Significant adaptations may need to be made with complex children. It is essential that assessment is adapted to the child's health condition, the environment, and the characteristics of the individual child. Rather than using a standard set of materials, interventionists may use materials familiar to the child and observe the child's behavior in relationship to behavioral landmarks associated with each stage of development. Such a tool, the Sensorimotor Profile (Project Continuity, 1985), an adaptation of the Uzgiris-Hunt Scales (1975), is shown in Table 7–2.

This tool and the Developmental Intervention for Care Planning and Family Education (Project Continuity, 1989) are examples of tools that permit developmental and care interventions to be simultaneously planned for children. Information gathered from these types of assessments may then be translated by team members into

- □ instrumental plans for parents (e.g., training in equipment sterilization)
- □ bedside developmental care suggestions (e.g., feeding procedures)
- □ developmental interventions with the child (e.g., environmental modifications to promote developmental functioning, such as tying a responsive toy to the side of the crib).

Sample items of the Developmental Intervention for Care Planning and Family Education tool are shown in Table 7–3, pp. 186–189.

TABLE 7–2

Sensorimotor Profile (pp. 182–185).

Substages	Age	Visual Pursuit and Object Permanence	Means-End	Causality	Schemes for Relating Objects
I. **Reflexive:** Modification of reflexes **Communication:** Shift from internal to external elicitors of affective responses; intrinsic elicitors and regulators of infant and maternal behavior	Birth– 2 months	(Momentary fixation) (Eye tracking partial arcs) Visual fixation/ tracking	(Grasp reflex) (Activity change to presented obj.) (Approach to contact— patterned stimulus) (Mouths hand)	(Grasp reflex) (Activity change to presented obj.) (Approach to contact— patterned stimulus) (Mouths hand)	(Sucks: nutritive/ non-nutritive) (Brings hand to obj. in mouth)
II. **Primary circular reactions:** Initial adaptation and beginning coordination of schemes **Communication:** Pre-intentional/ Idiosyncratic/ Perlocutionary	2–5 months	Brief gaze at point of disappearance	Hand watching (Sustained obj. grasp) Repetition of movement producing spectacle Reach/grasp obj., obj./hand in view Reach/grasp obj. in view	Hand watching Repeats movement producing spectacle Use of procedure to request repetition of event caused by adult	Incidental use/ mouthing Attention to obj.: hold/look Simple schemes, e.g. shake, bang
III. **Secondary circular reactions:** Schemes- systematic practice of schemes **Communication:** Pre-intentional/ Idiosyncratic/ Perlocutionary	5–8 months	(Searching at point of disappearance) Look/reach— partially covered obj. Anticipation— disappearing obj. (Remembers contacted obj. when covered with cloth)	Purposeful release—grasp new obj. Attached tool—pulls support	Idiosyncratic actions to request repetition of events, e.g. hand on object	Examine: visual, manual, oral Investigate object properties Differentiate simple schemes by object property (e.g. shake bell)
IV. **Coordination of secondary circular reactions:** Intentional combination of schemes **Communication:** Pre-intentional/ Conventional/ Illocutionary	8–12 months	Visible displacement (V. Dpl.)—1 screen V. Dpl.—2 or more screens	Locomotes to get obj. Differentiate spatial relationship of tool Attached tool—long string	(Signals expanded and have greater clarity) (Replication of toy's action to reproduce spectacle)	Complex schemes derived from obj. properties New complex schemes, e.g. slide, stretch, drop Brief recognitory use of functional objects (Combines functionally related objects, e.g. stir in cup)

Scoring Codes: F = Failed; E = Emerging; A = Achieved; G = Generalized; M = Motor Impairment Interferes; N/A = Not Applicable

Source: Sensorimotor Profile: Adapted from Uzgiris-Hunt Ordinal Scales of Psychological Development by C. Robinson, K. Bataillon, N. Fieber, B. Jackson, J. Rasmussen, & J. Rose, 1985, Media Resource Center, Meyer Rehabilitation Institute, University of Nebraska Medical Center, 444 South 44th St., Omaha, NE 68131–3795. Copyright © 1985, Meyer Rehabilitation Institute, University of Nebraska Medical Center. Reprinted by permission.

Spatial Relations	Gestural Imitation	Verbal Imitation	Communication
(Coordinates face/voice in view) (Visual preference/paired stimuli)	(Synchronous movements in response to adult) (Pseudo-imitation)	(Alerts to auditory stimuli) Vocalizes without distress Positive response to own sounds made by adult	(Displays regulators of interaction) (Smiles to external, social stimuli) (Responsive vocalizations) (Preferential responsiveness to caregiver)
Slow alternating (alt.) glance—2 objs. Rapid alt. glance—2 objs. Visually localizes lateral sound Accurate grasp—stable obj.	(Adult imitates child's movement, child attends) Adult imitates child's movement, child makes motor response	Adult imitates child, child repeats single sounds (Adult initiates child's sound, child repeats, e.g. cooing)	(Turn-taking, [looks, vocal, motor]) (Child initiates/terminates interaction) (Differentiated cry) (Anticipates familiar events) (Affect is content mediated, e.g. smiles with assimilation)
Looks where obj. falls in view Searches for obj. fallen from view Reorients reversed obj.	Following adult imitating child, adult initiates another familiar movement, child repeats Adult initiates child's movements, child repeats Imitation—expansion of familiar schemes	(Adult imitates child, child repeats, e.g. babbling) (Adult initiates child's sounds, child repeats a sound, e.g. babbling) (Adult initiates child's sounds, child repeats same, e.g. babbling)	(Recognizes, participates in games) (Consonant—vowel syllables, beginning repetition) (Emotions: negation, joy, anger, surprise) (Generalization of neg./pos. categories in social responses)
(Takes objs. out of container) Places single obj. in/out	(Partial imitation—visible novel movement [VNM]) Imitates—VNM, gradual approx. Imitates—VNM, directly	Adult initiates novel sound, child repeats a sound, e.g. babble Adult intitiates novel sound, child repeats same sound, e.g. babble	(Recognizes words—ritual, context) (Initiates familiar games—familiar others, strangers) (Gives obj.—turn-taking rituals) (Emotions: laughter/fear—violation expectancy) (Variety babbling, proto-words, intonation)

TABLE 7–2
(continued)

	Substages	Age	Visual Pursuit and Object Permanence	Means-End	Causality	Schemes for Relating Objects
V.	**Tertiary circular reactions:** Trial and error problem solving **Communication:** Intentional/ Conventional/ Illocutionary	12–18 months	Sequential V. Dpl.—two or more screens V. Dpl.— superimposed screens Invisible displacement (Inv. Dpl.)—1 screen Inv. Dpl.—2 or more screens Sequential Inv. Dpl.—two or more screens	Attached tool use— obj. out of view Unattached tool use (Trial and error strategies)	Combines obj. and person schemes to cause event Imitative attempt to activate toy	Functional use play—self (Functional use play—other/doll) Refers to obj. in shared interaction
VI.	**Invention of new means through mental combinations:** Representational/ foresightful problem solving **Communication:** Intentional/ Conventional/ Locutionary	18–24 months	Systematic search—sequential Inv. Dpl.—3 screens	Foresightful problem solving	Explores to activate toy (Combines steps to activate toy)	Representational play: combined schemes (Planned schemes in play, e.g. doll to bed and looks for blanket)

Parent-child Interactions

Each discipline that observes parents interacting with their child is likely to make some observations regarding the parents' degree of comfort in caregiving and the degree of warmth and affection displayed (Rosenberg & Robinson, 1988). Parent-child interactions are the foundation from which the child acquires social, cognitive, and language development. Because separations can have deleterious effects upon development of parent-infant attachment, assessment of parent-child interactions is particularly relevant for families of medically fragile infants.

The Teaching Skills Inventory (TSI) discussed in Rosenberg and Robinson's work (1988) offers a basis for the assessment of parent-child interactions and the development of teaching goals for parents and all others delivering bedside care to

Spatial Relations	Gestural Imitation	Verbal Imitation	Communication
Sequences objs. in/out Dumps objs. out Stacks objs. Experiments with gravity Moves to get obj. visible behind barrier Moves to get obj. invisible behind barrier	Imitates invisible movement, e.g. pat head Partial imitation—invisible facial gesture Imitates—familiar invisible facial gesture	Imitates novel sounds, gradual approx. (Imitates some familiar words) Imitates novel sounds directly Imitates most simple new words	(Proto/imperative—reach/request, give) (Proto/declarative—give/point to share) (Recep. vocab. 10-50 words) (Jargon, proto-words, single words, gestures) (Expands intents—comments, greetings) (Emotions: shame, defiance)
Remembers whereabouts/recognizes absence of familiar people/objs. (Nests 3 cups—trial/error)	Imitates—novel invisible facial gestures	(Imitates more complex new words/short phrases.)	(Recep. vocab. several hundred words) (Expresses variety of communicative intents) (Same words—varied intonations—diff. meanings) (Begin conventional yes/no forms for wants) (Begin 2 word phrases)

the child. The basic assumptions underlying the TSI include

□ the necessity of a developmental match between the child's skills and the requests made of the child

□ consideration of the child's interest as the basis for selection of content and materials used in play, and

□ the necessity for the child's active participation in developmental activities.

Tools such as this and others discussed in previous chapters allow interventionists to select objectives and strategies for child and family interventions with the family's collaboration. However, with medically fragile young children, the child's strength and general state of health dictate the intensity and quality of interactional efforts.

TABLE 7-3
Developmental Intervention for Care Planning and Family Education (pp. 186–189).

Developmental Characteristics	Suggested Care Plan Interventions
Age: 0–4 Months	
Motor:	
□ Lifts head when placed at shoulder or when placed on his/her stomach	Provide the child opportunities to improve head control by laying the infant on your shoulder or supported sitting
□ Holds head steady	
□ Moves arms and legs in play	
□ Swats, reaches or grasps objects	
Social/Emotional/Communication:	
□ Vocalizes, smiles and reaches toward familiar people	Provide opportunities for face-to-face interactions that encourage smiles and vocalizations
	Utilize safety mirrors in crib and during play time
□ Communicates needs using differentiated cries	
Cognitive:	
□ Visually tracks moving objects	
□ Alternates visual attention between objects	
□ Turns to source of sound	
□ Utilizes banging, shaking, mouthing, looking in play with toys	Give the infant safe, hand-held toys that are easily manipulated
	Position toys within the child's reach

Appropriate Play Materials & Equipment: Music box, tapes with soothing music or parents' voices, black/white mobiles, bright-colored objects, small rattles, cradle gym, slinky, mirrors, bells, infant seat, infant hammock.

Developmental Characteristics	Suggested Care Plan Interventions
Age: 5–8 Months	
Motor:	
□ Sits with little support progressing to independent sitting	Provide the infant opportunities for supportive sitting and rolling
□ Rolls in both directions	
□ Stands firmly when held	
□ Transfers objects from one hand to another	Give the infant safe, hand-held toys that are easily manipulated
□ Grasps with whole hand	
Social/Emotional:	
□ Pats and smiles at images in mirror	Utilize safety mirror in crib and during play-time
□ Recognizes familiar people and discriminates strangers	Provide a balance of quiet and stimulating interactions
Cognitive:	
□ Examines and explores toys	Utilize a variety of toys that promote examination
□ Imitates familiar action	

Communication:
□ Vocalizes using syllables, e.g., ba, ma, with repetition
  - Imitate child's vocalizations/gestures, pause and wait for the child to respond
□ Communicates wants, e.g., touches toy for more or vocalizes/ smiles for more in a game situation
  - Establish routine games with the infant, pausing and allowing time for the infant to respond

Self-Help:
□ Eats food from a spoon with assistance
□ Holds, sucks, or bites cookie

Appropriate Play Materials & Equipment: Slinky, squeak toys, toys that can be poked and examined, e.g., helicopter rattle, toys with moving parts, radios, musical toys, mirrors, happy apples, hard-paged books, mat, crib gym, infant chair.

Age: 9–12 Months

Motor:
□ Moves in and out of sitting position
□ Crawls
□ Pulls to standing
□ Uses pincer grasp to pick up small objects
□ Hits two objects together at midline
  - Provide opportunities to practice crawling and standing skills
  - Provide opportunities to grasp small food items, e.g., Cheerios or raisins, if within prescribed diet

Social/Emotional:
□ Shows interest in other adults' or children's activities
□ Exhibits difficulty separating from familiar people and displays stranger anxiety
□ Displays full range of emotion, e.g., laughter, fear, anxiety and anger
  - Provide continuity of care givers to minimize separation anxiety

Cognitive:
□ Places objects in and out of containers
□ Searches for object that is covered
□ Uses a variety of actions with toys, e.g., stretch, slide, drop, squeeze
  - Provide a variety of toys with which the infant can discover new actions

Communication:
□ Communicates wants, e.g., repeats action of a game to signal for more or reaches to make wants known
  - Collaborate with family in interpreting and responding to child's indication of wants
  - Introduce games such as Peek-a-Boo, Row-row-row your boat, allowing the child to communicate his desire to continue or discontinue the game
□ Recognizes words that are familiar to them
□ Uses expressive jabbering (vocalizes with intonation using most vowel and consonant sounds)
□ Imitates unfamiliar vocalizations
  - Refer to toys and actions consistently using simple language
  - Respond to infant jabbering by mimicking the child or by verbally interpreting the message

TABLE 7–3
(continued)

Developmental Characteristics	Suggested Care Plan Interventions
Age: 9–12 Months (continued)	
Self-Help:	Introduce cup and spoon to promote eating skills
□ Drinks from a cup with assistance	
Appropriate Play Materials & Equipment: Books, busy boxes, See 'N' Say, balls, squeak toys, blocks, music, containers, pull toys.	
Age: 13–18 Months	
Motor:	Provide assistance in walking
□ Walks independently	
□ Crawls up and down steps	
□ Walks up and down steps with assistance	
□ Stacks 2-3 blocks	
□ Dumps objects from containers	
Cognitive:	Provide child with familiar household or medical items, e.g., comb, stethoscope
□ Demonstrates functional use of objects in play, e.g., gives doll a bite, combs hair	Schedule reading time with simple, realistic picture books
□ Identifies pictures in books	Provide materials for sequencing, e.g., pegboards, shape boxes, stacking poles
□ Sequences objects into containers	
Communication:	Expand toddler's single words by using them in short sentences, *Toddler: "Ball." —Adult: "You want the ball?"*
□ Uses up to 20 words	Maintain conversation with toddler during daily care
□ Follows simple directions	Refers to body parts during typical care routines.
□ Begins to point to body parts when named	
Self-Help:	
□ Removes some articles of clothing	
□ Drinks and eats with assistance	

Appropriate Play Materials & Equipment: Books, peg boards, shape boxes, household items, balls, ride toy, bristol blocks, Fisher Price little people play sets, big mouth singers, wind-up toys, wagon.

Age: 19–24 Months

Motor:
- ☐ Climbs on & off furniture and play equipment
- ☐ Kicks a ball
- ☐ Runs
- ☐ Marks with drawing materials

Social/Emotional:
- ☐ Begins negativism
- ☐ Increases interactions with other children through parallel play

Cognitive:
- ☐ Completes simple puzzles
- ☐ Begins to engage in pretend play
- ☐ Activates mechanical toys

- ☐ Imitates actions in simple finger plays

Communication:
- ☐ Understands more words than can express
- ☐ Begins expressing two-word phrases
- ☐ Listens to short stories

Self Help:
- ☐ Eats & drinks independently
- ☐ Indicates wet or soiled diapers

Assist child in opportunities to engage in climbing activities

Provide art experiences including coloring, painting, etc.

Provide toddler with a sense of control by offering choices
When appropriate, allow play in proximity of other children

Provide puzzles with large, non-interlocking pieces
Identify familiar routines and engage child in pretend play
Offer a variety of mechanical toys (See 'N' Say, tape recorder, jack-in-box, Pop-n-Pals)
Introduce simple, short finger plays (e.g., itsy bitsy spider, wheels on the bus)

Communicate in a clear & simple manner when interacting with child
Avoid pressuring child by requesting child words to be said
Utilize books with short, simple story lines

Promote independence with meal time skills

Appropriate Play Materials & Equipment: Pretend play materials, e.g., kitchen set, blocks, dolls, books, Pop-n-Pals, See 'N' Say, large Legos, vehicle sets, colors, paints, bubbles, balls, tape recorder, puzzles, shape boxes, non-pedal riding toys.

Recommended Referrals: ____ Child Life ____ Psychology ____ Physical Therapy ____ Occupational Therapy
____ Speech Therapy ____ Social Work Other: _____

Primary Nurse: _____   Date: ___/___/___
                        Signature

Source: Developmental Intervention for Care Planning and Family Education by Project Continuity, 1989, Media Resource Center, University of Nebraska Medical Center, 444 South 44th St., Omaha, NE 68131-3795. Copyright © 1989, Meyer Rehabilitation Institute, University of Nebraska Medical Center. Reprinted by permission.

Intervention with medically frag-
ile/complex young children centers around efforts to make all
experiences as normal as possible while remaining sensitive to
the child's energy level for interaction.

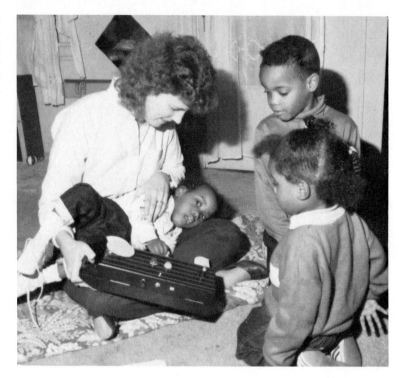

Family Strengths and Needs

Considerable concern has been expressed about the potentially invasive nature of
family needs assessments. For this reason, it is recommended that only information
that will be used productively should be collected. The types of information needed
may include

- □ the material and emotional resources available to the family
- □ the family's expectations and goals for intervention
- □ the degree of consensus between parents regarding their child and family
  goals
- □ the extent and nature of resources outside the family needed for the family
  to accomplish its goals (Rosenberg, 1977)

By using this framework to collect information, the intervention team, which
includes the parents and any family members and advocates the family chooses, has
a basis for developing an Individualized Family Service Plan that builds upon the
family's strengths and gives the family control over the areas in which they desire

assistance. Refer to Chapters 12 and 13 for detailed discussion of IFSP development and family collaboration.

SUMMARY OF PROCEDURES

Infants with chronic medical conditions require an array of services. These services must be tailored to the resources and needs of the child's family. Some of the key strategies for assisting these children and their families discussed in this chapter follow:

1. Organize support groups for family and extended family members to assist home care procedures, and encourage continuity and consistency of care-giving routines. Emotional support is particularly critical in the first year of life for families with medically fragile children because of the high rate of family conflict and divorce during this year.
2. Coordinate medical and educational services so families are not over-whelmed by professionals. Families of medically high-risk children require efficient coordination of services, access to resources, and flexible case management that anticipates needs throughout the course of the child's care and/or illness.
3. Track physical growth and nutritional intake in medically fragile children to the age of 3 years. Adequate weight gain is particularly important for development in the first year of life.
4. Use time-limited contracts to increase involvement with families who express feelings of inadequacy and/or are intimidated by the technology necessary for their child's developmental and health care needs.
5. Monitor the home and hospital environments for the amount and variety of developmentally appropriate toys and experiences.
6. Provide additional child and family support for families whose children are hospitalized between 7 and 12 months of age. Although separations caused by hospitalizations may always be difficult for the child, infants seem to be especially vulnerable during this period.
7. Coordinate activities and developmental assessments in the hospital setting so each professional on the child's health care and educational team does not find it necessary to individually assess the child.

SUMMARY

The numbers of chronically ill children are increasing. Figures gathered by the National Center for Health Statistics indicate that the number of children who are limited in activity nearly doubled between 1967 and 1979 (Butler et al., 1985). Advances in

TRANSDISCIPLINARY CASES

The first case illustrates some of the effects of a terminal illness on a toddler's development, and the effects of this situation on the child's family. The second case focuses on the demands of caring for a chronically ill child. Though there are many similarities, the situations also have poignant differences.

THE GRIFFIN FAMILY

At birth, Susan Griffin was diagnosed with Down Syndrome. Susan was the youngest child of a two-parent family. When she was 2 years old, she received a diagnosis of granulocytic sarcoma. Following the second diagnosis, Susan was hospitalized on a regular basis for chemotherapy treatment. When she was at home, Susan participated in an early intervention program for special needs children within her local school district. However, school participation was interrupted frequently by her rehospitalizations.

A primary goal of the hospital staff was to provide consistency in Susan's care while she was in the hospital, to minimize the effects of the hospitalizations. Input from a variety of disciplines including the child life specialist, the early intervention educator, and the physical and speech therapists was sought so the goals established by her early intervention program could be continued in the hospital. However, developmental interventions in the hospital were hindered by Susan's chemotherapy, which left her feeling so badly that she did not have the energy to interact with hospital staff. Susan was frequently isolated to control infection, which further complicated and limited her experiences in the hospital.

Nonetheless, the hospital's primary care nurse made efforts to provide consistent daily schedules and routines for Susan to promote her development. Attempts were made to create experiences that were similar to those Susan would have experienced in her home or in her school program.

Support to the Griffins was an integral component of Susan's intervention plan. The family identified several major needs, including financial support for the family's bills for travel and housing when they were away from their community and at the hospital, support in talking with Susan's siblings about her developmental problems and to prepare them for her death, and general emotional support for the parents. (One emotional support for the family involved a videotape of Susan that was made by the hospital staff while she was in the unit).

Many professionals provided support to the family at various times during Susan's treatment, including the nurses, the child life specialist, and the social worker. The child life specialist was instrumental in assisting the family with the siblings' issues by loaning pamphlets and books which helped to explain Susan's medical condition and dealt with issues related to dying and death. Financial resources were obtained to assist the family with travel and housing costs. Emotional support was provided by health and educational professionals as needed. However, much of the support came from the primary care health staff who spent the most time with the family during Susan's lengthy treatments.

Identifying the family's needs was an ongoing process. As new family needs developed, they were supported collaboratively by all professionals involved. Hospital staff encouraged the Griffins to participate in a bereavement program established at the hospital to support families who have had a member of their family die. The case manager and the primary care nurse continued support to the family following Susan's death, and conducted a 1-

year follow-up. The videotape of Susan was found to be an especially valuable source of comfort for Susan's parents and siblings after her death.

THE SMITH FAMILY

Jennifer Smith is 12 months old, and has a medical diagnosis of **biliary atresia**. She received a liver transplant at the age of 6 months. Jennifer experienced multiple complications following her transplant including viral infections and respiratory distress. As a result of these complications she had a tracheostomy and required **C-pap ventilation** (continuous positive airway pressure; provides supplemental oxygen and enough pressure to keep the lungs expanded so they do not collapse). She received her nutrition primarily through nasogastro feedings and hyperalimentation. Jennifer spent 5 months in the pediatric intensive care unit.

When Jennifer was admitted for her liver transplant, she was extremely ill and no developmental testing had been conducted. Following the transplant, her medical condition continued to be guarded. In the first 3 months following transplantation, it was difficult to find times when Jennifer was in an alert quiet state optimal for interaction. As a result, developmental intervention was provided only when her medical condition allowed, and varied from day to day. When Jennifer was 11 months of age, she was transferred from the Pediatric Intensive Care Unit to the Infant/Toddler Unit. At that time, developmental intervention was more consistently implemented because her health condition had stabilized.

Jennifer's mother and her primary care nurse were instructed, using group meetings and consultations, in the most appropriate ways to play with and stimulate Jennifer during her routines in the hospital by the child life specialist, developmental therapists, the infant interventionist, and other parents. The current goal is to encourage Ms. Smith and the primary care nurse to incorporate developmental strategies into as many care routines and play activities with Jennifer as possible.

The stress of Jennifer's hospitalizations and fragile health has overwhelmed her family at times. Ms. Smith is a single parent and has chosen to stay with Jennifer during her hospitalizations even though the hospital is approximately 400 miles from her family. During those times, Jennifer's three siblings stayed with their aunt. Because of Jennifer's prolonged illness, Jennifer's mother took a leave of absence from her job. These circumstances have placed financial constraints on the family and caused them to use Medicaid funds during the past year. Due to limited funds, few visits have been possible for other family members.

The Smiths live in a small rural community in a midwestern state. The nearest early intervention program and respite program are an hour from the Smiths' hometown. Further, Ms. Smith needs child care for Jennifer when she returns to work. Jennifer needs skilled nursing care providers, who are scarce.

Having a child with Jennifer's medical history has resulted in multiple stresses for Ms. Smith. The hospital in which Jennifer is treated is a liver transplant center. As a result, many children having transplants are hospitalized at one time. Not only has Jennifer's mother had to deal with her daughter's unpredictable medical course, but she also has watched many other children follow similar courses or die. This has added to her already nearly unmanageable stress. Ms. Smith reports that one of the most helpful supports for her has been her participation in a weekly transplant support group offered by the hospital.

surgical procedures for congenital conditions of the heart and gastrointestinal systems, and advances in technology for the survival of very low birthweight and premature infants have affected the numbers of infants with chronic and complex medical problems, as well as the way in which treatments are conducted.

Parents of medically fragile/complex children are extremely stressed, and may routinely make significant sacrifices such as giving up jobs, altering career plans, and/ or maintaining public assistance in order to care for their medically compromised child (Moore et al., 1988). Consequently, the family's needs are paramount for serving the child. The best care of medically fragile children involves consideration of the child's emotional, psychosocial, physical, and developmental needs. To accomplish this, health care and educational professionals must have open communication and smooth coordination of their services. Fortunately, today more health care professionals desire collaboration with non-medical professionals. As with all populations of at-risk and handicapped infants and toddlers, services for medically complex infants and their families are most helpful when they are individualized to the family's needs and complement the family's goals and values regarding their child's upbringing.

DISCUSSION QUESTIONS

1. What are the advantages of coordinated, family-centered health-educational services for families? What are some of the disadvantages?
2. What are the effects of hospitalizations on child development and parent-child interactions?
3. What is the value of continuity of care for medically fragile/complex infants and their families? How can interventionists insure that continuity is provided?

APPLIED ACTIVITIES/PROJECTS

1. You are the director of an early intervention program. A 6-month-old child has been referred to your program. The child's nutrition is handled by nasogastric tube feedings using soy formula. The primary care nurse has indicated that it is appropriate for the child to begin weaning from tube to oral feeding. What staff would you need? What skills would staff members need, and who should train them? How would you insure coordination and collaboration of services?
2. A middle-class family of a child in your infant program has just been told that their child has a terminal illness. The family is devastated. Describe 10 ways you might offer social and material support for the family. Additionally, the family has a limitation in their insurance that will leave them unprotected in the later stages of their child's illness. What financial resources can you uncover for the family? Find out all you can about governmental programs, private foundations, and insurance claim restrictions.
3. Attend one session of a bereavement support group. Identify four strategies you observed that were used for supporting families as they deal with the finality of a loved one's death. How could these strategies be used in different settings with less severe circumstances?

SUGGESTED READINGS

Appelbaum, S. H., & Rohrs, W. F. (1981). *Time management for health care professionals.* Frederick, MD: Aspen.

Batshaw, M., & Perret, Y. (1981). *Children with handicaps: A medical primer.* Baltimore, MD: Paul H. Brookes.

Blackman, J. A. (1989). *Medical aspects of developmental disabilities in children: Birth to 3.* Frederick, MD: Aspen.

Children with AIDS. (Newsletter published six times annually by the Foundation for Children with AIDS, Inc., 77B Warrent Street, Brighton, MA 02135).

Goldfarb, L. A., Brotherson, M., Summers, J., & Turnbull, A. (1986). *Meeting the challenge of disability or chronic illness: A family guide.* Baltimore: Paul H. Brookes.

Katz, K., Pokorni, J., & Long, T. (1989). *Chronically ill and at-risk infants: Family-centered intervention from hospital to home.* Palo Alto, CA: VORT.

Orque, M., Bloch, B., & Monnrroy, L. (1983). *Ethnic nursing care: A multicultural approach.* St. Louis: Mosby.

Powell, T., & Ogle, P. A. (1985). *Brothers and sisters: A special part of exceptional families.* Baltimore: Paul H. Brookes.

Rennert, S., Parry, J., & Horowitz, R. (1988). *AIDS and persons with developmental disabilities: The legal perspective.* Washington, DC: American Bar Association.

U. S. Department of Agriculture/Department of Health and Human Services Nutrition Education Committee for Maternal and Child Nutrition. (1986). *Cross-cultural counseling: A guide for nutrition and health counselors.* Washington, DC: Food and Nutrition Service, U. S. Department of Agriculture. (Available from National Maternal and Child Health Clearinghouse, Washington, DC).

Vogel, S., & Manhoff, D. (1989). *Emergency medical treatment: Infants.* Wilmette, IL: National Safety Council.

REFERENCES

American Nurses' Association (1980). *Nursing: A social policy statement.* Kansas City, MO: Author.

Bayley, N. (1969). *Manual for Bayley Scales of Infant Development.* New York: Psychological Corporation.

Beckman, P. J., Pokorni, J. L., Maza, E. A., & Balzer-Martin, L. (1986). A longitudinal study of stress and support in families of preterm and fullterm infants. *Journal of the Division for Early Childhood, 11*(1), 2–9.

Bristol, M. M. (1979). *Maternal coping with autistic children: Adequacy of interpersonal support and effect of child characteristics.* Unpublished doctoral dissertation, University of North Carolina.

Bronfenbrenner, U. (1975). Is early intervention effective? In B. A. Friedlander, G. M. Sterrit, & G. E. Kirk (Eds.), *Exceptional infant: Assessment and intervention* (Vol. 3), (pp. 449–475). New York: Brunner/Mazel.

Butler, J., Budetti, P., McManus, M., Stenmark, S., & Newacheck, P. (1985). Health care expenditures for children with chronic illness. In N. Hobbs & J. Perrin (Eds.), *Issues in the care of children with chronic illness* (pp. 827–863). San Francisco: Jossey-Bass.

Campbell, S. K., Wilhelm, I. J., & Slaton, D. S. (1989). Anthropometric characteristics of young children with cerebral palsy. *Pediatric Physical Therapy, 1,* 105–108.

Crnic, K. A., Friedrich, W. N., & Greenberg, M. T. (1983). Adaptation of families with mentally retarded children: A model of stress, coping, and family ecology. *American Journal of Mental Deficiency, 88,* 125–138.

Duvall, F. M. (1957). *Family development.* Philadelphia: Lippincott.

Fletcher, M., Wetherby, C., & Brown, C. (1986). *The neonatal experience.* Washington, DC: The George Washington University.

Halleron, T., Pisaneschi, J., & Trapani, M. (Eds.). (1989). *Learning AIDS.* New York: American Foundation for AIDS Research (AmFAR).

Hill, R. (1949). *Families under stress.* New York: Harper & Row.

Holt, D. S. (1958).The home life of severely retarded children. *Pediatrics, 22,* 744–755.

Jeffcoate, J. A., Humphrey, M. E., & Lloyd, J. K. (1979). Role perception and response to stress in fathers and mothers following pre-term delivery. *Social Science and Medicine, 13,* 139–145.

Kaminer, R., Jedrysek, E., & Soles, B. (1981). Intellectually limited parents. *Developmental and Behavioral Pediatrics, 2*(2), 39–43.

Klaus, C., & Kennell, J. (1970). *Maternal-infant bonding.* St. Louis: Mosby.

Klein, M., & Stein, L. (1971). Low birthweight and the battered child syndrome. *American Journal of Diseases in Children, 122,* 14–17.

Krammer, S. (1987). Personal report.

Lamb, M. E. (1981). The development of social expectations in the first year of life. In M. E. Lamb & L. R. Sherrod (Eds.), *Infant social cognition: Empirical and theoretical considerations* (pp. 155–175). Hillsdale, NJ: Erlbaum.

Leifer, A. D., Leiderman, P. H., Barnett, C. R., & Williams, J. A. (1974). Effects of mother-child separation on maternal attachment behavior. *Child Development, 43,* 1203–1218.

Lewis, M. (1982). *Clinical aspects of child development.* Philadelphia: Lea & Febiger.

Lonsdale, G. (1978). Family life with a handicapped child. *Child Care, Health and Development, 4,* 49–120.

Marram, G. D., Schlegel, M. W., & Bevis, E. O. (1974). *Primary nursing: A model for individualized care.* St. Louis: Mosby.

McCall, R. (1982). The process of early mental development: Implications for prediction and intervention. In N. J. Anatasiow, W. K. Frankenberg, & A. W. Landal (Eds.), *Identifying the developmentally delayed child* (pp. 3–11). Baltimore: University Park Press.

McLean, P. D. (1976). Parental depression: Incompatible with effective parenting. In E. J. Marsh, L. C. Handy, & L. A. Hammerlynck (Eds.), *Behavior modification approaches to parenting* (pp. 209–220). New York: Brunner/Mazel.

Merderer, H., & Hill, R. (1983). Critical transitions over the family life span: Theory and research. In H. McCubbin, M. Sussman, & J. Patterson (Eds.), *Social stresses and the family: Advances and developments in family stress theory and research* (pp. 39–60). New York: The Haworth Press.

Moore, J., & McLaughlin, J. (1988). Medical costs associated with children with disabilities or chronic illness. *Topics in Early Childhood Special Education, 8*(3), 98–103.

Paban, M., & Piper, M. C. (1987). Early predictors of 1 year neurodevelopmental outcome for "at risk" infants. *Physical and Occupational Therapy Pediatrics, 7*(3), 17–34.

Patterson, G. R., Cobb, J. A., & Ray, R. S. (1973). A social and engineering technology for the retaining of aggressive boys. In H. Adams & L. Unikel (Eds.), *Issues and trends in behavior therapy* (pp. 139–210). Springfield, IL: Thomas.

Perrin, J. (1989, June). *Childhood chronic illness: Coordination, technology, and care.* Presentation at the UAPDD Tenth Annual Conference on Coordination of Interdisciplinary Care for Persons with Developmental Handicaps and Chronic Illness, Rochester, NY.

Project Continuity. (1985). *Sensorimotor Profile*. Omaha: Meyer Children's Rehabilitation Institute, University of Nebraska Medical Center.

Project Continuity. (1989). *Developmental intervention for care planning and family education*. Omaha, NE: Meyer Children's Rehabilitation Institute, University of Nebraska Medical Center.

Quinton, D., & Rutter, M. (1976). Early hospital admissions and later disturbances of behavior: An attempted replication of Douglas' findings. *Developmental Medicine and Child Neurology, 18,* 447–459.

Radin, N. (1972). Three degrees of maternal involvement in the preschool program: Impact on mothers and children. *Child Development, 43,* 1355–1364.

Rennert, S., Parry, J., & Horowitz, R. (1988). *AIDS and persons with developmental disabilities: The legal perspective*. Washington, DC: American Bar Association.

Richards, M. P. (1979). Effects of development of medical interventions and the separation of newborns from their parents. In D. Shaffer & J. Dunn (Eds.), *The first year of life* (pp. 37–54). New York: Wiley.

Robinson, C., & Fieber, N. (1988). Cognitive assessment with motorically impaired infants and preschoolers. In T. Wachs & R. Sheehan (Eds.), *Assessment of developmentally disabled children* (pp. 127–159). New York: Plenum.

Robinson, C., Rosenberg, S., & Beckman, P. J. (1988). Parent involvement in early childhood special education. In J. B. Jordan, J. J. Gallagher, P. L. Hutinger, & M. B. Karnes (Eds.), *Early childhood special education, birth to 3* (pp. 109–128). Reston, VA: The Council for Exceptional Children.

Robinson, C., Rosenberg, S., Hartley, R., & Jackson, B. (1986). Early Referral and Follow-Up Project: Individualizing family and child interventions for chronically ill disabled children. In J. Hurth, E. Lynch, & J. Olson (Eds.), *Individualizing family services: Monograph four of the family support network series* (pp. 22–36). Moscow, ID: Warren Center on Human Development.

Rosenberg, S. A. (1977). Family and parent variables affecting outcomes of a parent-mediated intervention. Unpublished doctoral dissertation, George Peabody College for Teachers, Nashville, TN.

Rosenberg, S., & McTate, G. (1982). Intellectually handicapped mothers: Problems and prospects. *Children Today, 11,* 14–26.

Rosenberg, S. A., & Robinson, C. (1988). Interactions of parents with their young handicapped children. In S. Odom & M. Karnes (Eds.), *Early intervention for infants and children with handicaps: An empirical base* (pp. 159–177). Baltimore: Paul H. Brookes.

Rosenberg, S. A., & Robinson, C. (in press). Assessment of the infant with multiple handicaps. In E. Gibbs & D. Teti (Eds.), *Interdisciplinary assessment of infants: A guide for early intervention professionals*. Baltimore: Paul H. Brookes.

Seashore, M. J., Leifer, A. D., Barnett, C. R., & Leiderman, P. H. (1973). The effects of denial on participation in an early mother-infant education program. *Education and Training of the Mentally Retarded, 8,* 163–169.

Shapiro, B., Green, P., Krich, J., Als, D., & Capute, A. (1986). Growth of severely impaired children: Neurological versus nutritional factors. *Developmental Medicine and Child Neurology, 28,* 729–733.

Skipper, J. K., & Leonard, R. C. (1968). Children, stress, and hospitalization: A field experiment. *Journal of Health and Social Behavior, 9,* 275–287.

Sterling, H. M. (1960). Height and weight of children with cerebral palsy and acquired brain damage. *Archives of Physical Medicine and Rehabilitation, 41,* 365–369.

Thomas, R. B. (1988). The struggle for control between families and health care providers when a child has complex health care needs. *Zero to Three, 8*(1), 15–18.

Tobis, J. S., Saturen, P., Larios, G., & Posniak, A. (1961). Studies of growth patterns in cerebral palsy. *Archives of Physical Medicine and Rehabilitation, 42,* 475–481.

Turnbull, A., & Turnbull, H. (1990). *Families, professionals, and exceptionality: A special relationship* (2nd ed.). Columbus, OH: Merrill.

Turnbull, A. P., Summers, J. A., & Brotherson, M. J. (1986). Family life cycle: Theoretical and empirical implications and future directions for families with mentally retarded members. In J. Gallagher & P. Vietze (Eds.), *Families of handicapped persons: Current research, treatment, and policy issues* (pp. 45–66). Baltimore: Paul H. Brookes.

Uzgiris, I., & Hunt, J. (1975). *Assessment in Infancy: Ordinal scales of psychological development*. Urbana: University of Illinois Press.

Wachs, T. D. (1984). Proximal experience and early cognitive-intellectual development: The social environment. In A. W. Gottfried (Ed.), *Home environment and early cognitive development* (pp. 273–328). Orlando, FL: Academic Press.

Weiss, R. L., Hops, H., & Patterson, G. R. (1973). A framework for conceptualizing marital conflict. In L. A. Hammerlynck, L. C. Handy, & E. J. Marsh (Eds.), *Behavior change: Methodology, concepts, and practice. The Fourth Banff Conference on behavior modification* (pp. 309–342). Champaign, IL: Research Press.

Wolfensberger, W. (1969). A new approach to decision making in human management services. In R. B. Kugel & W. Wolfensberger (Eds.), *Changing patterns in residential services for the mentally retarded* (pp. 367–381). Washington, DC: President's Committee on Mental Retardation Monograph.

Yarrow, L. (1979). Historical perspectives and future directions in infant development. In J. Osofsky (Ed.), *Handbook of Infant Development* (pp. 897–913). New York: Wiley.

Yarrow, L. J., Rubenstein, J. L., & Pederson, F. A. (1975). *Infant and environment: Early cognitive and motivational development*. New York: Wiley.

PART IV

INTERVENTION STRATEGIES FOR SPECIFIC POPULATIONS

8

Techniques for Infants and Toddlers At-Risk

Doris Bergen and Sharon A. Raver

OVERVIEW

This chapter describes the broad range of influences that may result in infants being at risk for developmental problems, including:

☐ characteristics of infants who may be considered at risk
☐ practices for identification and assessment of at-risk infants
☐ prevention of conditions leading to risk conditions
☐ monitoring and intervention strategies for at-risk infants and their families

One of the landmark features of P.L. 99–457, Part H, is that services may not only be provided for infants with specifically identified handicaps and delays, but also for infants who may eventually evidence developmental problems. Conditions that are biological, medical, or environmental and that are likely to lead to health problems, developmental delays, or maladaptive behavioral patterns fall into the broad at-risk category defined in this law.

However, not all children who may be at risk for developmental delays will receive the services they need. This is because P.L. 99–457 gives individual states the responsibility of defining the scope of their early intervention services. Consequently, the manner in which each state defines *developmental delay* and *at risk* determines the way each state identifies the populations to be served, and dictates the extent and quality of delivery systems.

As of 1988, about half of the states had defined *high risk*. According to Graham and Scott (1988) the states' definitions are extremely varied and "many of the definitions lack conceptual clarity and indicate widespread misunderstanding of the concept" (p. 23). It appears that definitions of *at risk* have been shaped by political and bureaucratic influences as much as by best practices (Dickin, McKim, & Kirkland, 1983). Using the parameters outlined by each state, interventionists identify, monitor, and program for at-risk children, relying on their professional judgment and knowledge of characteristics of children who tend to be considered at risk.

CHARACTERISTICS OF AT-RISK CONDITIONS

Because there is debate about which child characteristics and which family characteristics should be included in the definition of at risk, governmental policymakers and early intervention advocates have differed in how they define the characteristics of at-risk conditions in their attempts to interpret the broad definitions outlined in P.L. 99–457. A wide range of problems can fall under at-risk categories, and infants may have more than one risk-inducing problem. Categories of risk may include both biological and environmental conditions, or they may be more narrowly described. In this chapter, the characteristics of the child included in the definition of at risk will be organized using adaptations of Tjossem's definitions (1976) of established, biological, and environmental risks.

Established Risk Characteristics

Established risk conditions include the presence of a diagnosed physical or medical condition that is likely to lead to developmental delay. Established risk disabilities include both physical or mental abnormalities present at birth that predict early developmental problems as well as diagnosed conditions that are biological, but may not contribute to developmental delay until later in life. Such potential risk conditions include neurological disorders, genetic disorders/syndromes, orthopedic abnormalities, mental retardation, and sensory impairments (Blackman, 1986).

Neurological disorders include conditions such as spina bifida, **microcephaly** (retarded brain growth), **anencephaly** (absence of brain), hydrocephaly, and **neoplasms**/tumors. Although some of these conditions, such as hydrocephaly, may be treated by medical and surgical procedures, they are still likely to result in developmental delay. Other conditions that will influence developmental progress include cerebral palsy, **muscular dystrophy** and similar degenerative neurological disorders, **aphasia** (brain-associated symbolic communication impairment), and other neurological abnormalities that may lead to learning disabilities. Depending on the severity, these problems may be apparent at birth or may become evident during the first months or years of life.

There is also a group of genetic disorders/syndromes that make developmental delays likely. For example, children with **cleft lip or palate** (and/or tongue abnormalities due to Pierre Rosin Syndrome) may have difficulty eating and speaking. Children with chromosome abnormalities (e.g., **Cri du Chat Syndrome, Turner's Syndrome**, Trisomy 21) will exhibit mental retardation and physical deformities. Children with congenital cardiovascular problems, **osteogenesis imperfecta** (brittle bones), **arthrogryposis** (limb defects), or **Von Recklinghaus Disease** (skin lesions) will have severe physical developmental problems that can affect their development.

Orthopedic problems affecting developmental progress include **clubfoot, scoliosis** (spine curvature), **kyphosis** (spine flexion), **torticollis** (spasmodic contractions), **metatarsus adductus** (foot deformity), hip dislocation, **abnormal tibial torsion** (twisting of shin bone), and other congenital limb deficiencies. Although some of these disorders may be corrected eventually by medical procedures, developmental delays may occur before or during the time corrective procedures are implemented. Other orthopedic problems may require children to learn alternate styles of interaction with their world. If educational support is not provided for this learning, development may be affected.

In addition to mental retardation that is related to syndromes/genetic disorders, mental deficiencies of unspecified etiology may result in developmental delay. Because mental retardation may range from mild to severe, the extent of the delay may be initially difficult to predict. Early intervention during the infant and preschool period may make delays less pronounced.

Sensory impairments, especially visual and auditory impairments, can greatly affect the rate and nature of the infant's development. Visual problems include **strabismus** (lack of eye parallelism), **hemianopsia** (loss of part of the visual field), other **visual field** defects, **anophthalmia** (absence of eye tissue), and retinopathy (inflammatory degenerative disease believed to be influenced by oxygen treatments on premature infants). Severe visual impairment is usually apparent in the first few weeks of life when infants fail to demonstrate eye contact or visual tracking. Other visual impairments may not be obvious until later in early childhood.

Auditory problems include **conductive hearing loss, sensorineural hearing loss,** and hearing distortion impairments. The ability to detect auditory problems also varies with severity and type. For example, failure to progress past the babbling stage of language development may be an indication of major hearing impairment, but lower-grade hearing distortions may not be suspected until toddlers exhibit hyperactivity and low frustration tolerance.

Any of these established risk conditions may result in developmental delay and all warrant close monitoring by early interventionists. Strategies for dealing with problems resulting from established risk factors are described in Chapters 7, 9, 10, and 11.

Biological Risk Characteristics

Biological insults to the nervous system in children during the **prenatal** (before birth), **perinatal** (during birth), and **neonatal** (following birth), or early infancy period that make normal development problematic are considered **biological risks**. The majority of children who fall into at-risk categories have no specifically identified handicapping condition or syndrome that is known to affect development negatively. Biological risk factors may be further categorized as pregnancy conditions affecting fetal health or birth processes, and trauma experienced at birth or in the neonatal period. Infants often experience more than one type of biological risk and often the risk is compounded by environmental factors. Major biological risk characteristics are described by Bennett (1987), Blackman (1986), and Frohock (1986).

Pregnancy conditions affecting fetal health or birth processes.   Complications include **toxoplasmosis** (parasitic infection), **phenylketonuria** (deficiency of amino acids), exposure to radiation, **cytomegalic** (cell enlargement), AIDS, sexually transmitted diseases such as syphilis and herpes, diabetes, rubella (measles), and intrauterine growth retardation.

Substance abuse (e.g., cocaine, heroin, alcohol) by mothers causes physical deformities and neurological disorders in their infants and can negatively affect the quality of the nurturing environment provided by the parent after the infant's birth. Use of therapeutic drugs such as anticonvulsants or anticoagulants can cause birth defects or central nervous system abnormalities.

Infants whose birthweights are two standard deviations below the mean for their gestational age, indicating intrauterine growth retardation, may have been subjected to maternal infection, genetic disorder, or substance abuse.

One major cause of infant risk is premature delivery, which results in low birthweight and complications due to the immaturity of the infant's systems. As discussed in Chapter 6, birthweight of less than 1,500 g is problematic, and infants who weigh less than 1,000 g are particularly at risk for developmental problems (Blackman, 1986). Nonetheless, larger premature infants have a good potential for normal development if they survive the first few months of life.

Prematurity and other infant developmental problems are associated with maternal age at the time of pregnancy. In a review of the literature, Landerholm (1982) outlines the correlates of teenage pregnancy as low socioeconomic status, inadequate health care and nutrition, low educational achievement, and poor interaction skills. She reports that one of every five births is to teenage mothers, 94% of whom keep their infants. Teenage mothers have 20% more medical problems during pregnancy than older mothers. Although early and continuing prenatal care appears to ameliorate some problems, teenage mothers are less likely to seek prenatal care.

Trauma experienced at birth or in the neonatal period.   As discussed in Chapter 6, a number of traumatic events can occur at the time of birth that place infants at risk. A few common problems are fetal **anoxia** (absence of oxygen), premature rupture of membranes, brain contusions/hemorrhages, fractures, central nervous insult, respiratory distress, and **Erbs Palsy** (paralysis due to birth injury). Severe asphyxia at birth, intracranial hemorrhage, seizures, and respiratory distress can greatly impair the infant's potential for normal development. Bacterial and viral infections of the central nervous system can result in permanent central nervous system injury.

Some problems that occur in the neonatal period may be diagnosed only later in childhood. For example, attention deficits, autistic-like behaviors, metabolic disorders, and chronic health impairments (e.g., **sickle cell anemia, hemophilia, asthma, cystic fibrosis**) may put young children at risk for developmental delay.

Strategies for improving the developmental functioning of biologically at-risk infants include prenatal health care to prevent conditions that could be injurious to the infant, and intensive interventions by neonatal specialists during the first weeks of life to prevent risk conditions from leading to permanent disabilities. Depending on the severity of the infant's biological risk at the time of discharge from the hospital, some infants will need immediate interagency intervention while others will need to be referred to a monitoring or tracking system that will activate interventions only if developmental delays become evident.

Environmental Risk Conditions

Environmental risk is the presence of factors in the family, community, social, or economic system that predict early life experiences that may result in developmental delay. This category may be narrowly or broadly defined. That is, environmental risks can be restricted only to those environmental conditions that focus on specific parental behaviors (e.g., child abuse, teenage pregnancy, mental illness) or they may include family, socioeconomic, and health factors that put infants who have the potential for normal development at risk for achieving their optimum potential. These risks are often intertwined with biological risk factors. The definition of environmental risk shapes both the cost and the coverage of early intervention services.

Environmental risk factors can be described using Bronfenbrenner's (1979) ecological model that includes microsystems, mesosystems, exosystems, and macrosystems. That is, environmental risks may include:

- parental behaviors and capabilities (microsystem)
- family system characteristics and level of infant-parent support (microsystem, mesosystem)
- health care, social/mental health services, and education availability and quality (mesosystem)
- community social and economic conditions (mesosystem, exosystem)
- policy and cultural value conditions (macrosystem)

An understanding of each of these systems may assist interventionists in their attempts to assist families in prioritizing the multiple factors that may place young children at environmental risk.

Parental behaviors and capabilities. Bronfenbrenner (1979) defines **microsystem** as the "pattern of activities, roles, and interpersonal relations experienced by the developing person in a given setting with particular physical and material characteristics" (p. 22). Numerous research studies show that developmentally appropriate parental behaviors and interaction patterns are essential for the growth of cognitive, language, and social/emotional abilities (Beckwith, 1985; Bruner & Sherwood, 1976; Field, 1979; Frodi & Lamb, 1980; Stern, 1977). In fact, Beckwith (1984) found that medical factors did not predict preterm infants who would have later problems in mental development, whereas the nature of the environment in which they were being reared did.

Problems with interactional patterns may occur for many reasons related to parent personality, maturity, disabilities, health practices, values, expectations of child behavior, and/or economic problems. The stress of having a high-risk infant can also disrupt the development of positive interactions between parents and their children (Hutinger, 1988).

Limited or dysfunctional parent-infant interactions place the child at risk for developmental delay (Rogers & Puchalski, 1984). For example, the parent who spends little time holding or touching the infant, gives too much or too little stimulation, and rarely talks to or faces the child does not provide an appropriate interactive environment. Placing severe limits on the child's physical movement, sudden and unpredictable intrusive control, harsh physical punishment, lack of play with the child, lack of consolation and comfort of child distress, inconsistent feeding patterns, and generally erratic expressions of emotions inappropriate for the situation may lead to developmental problems for the child. Children who are identified as failure to thrive often have experienced these conditions (Haynes-Seman & Hart, 1987).

Maternal age of less than 15 years seems to be associated with many of these maladaptive social behaviors (Cappleman, Thompson, DeRemer-Sullivan, King, & Sturm, 1982). Mothers facing their own adolescent developmental crises may have difficulty understanding and meeting the developmental needs of their infants, if infant needs are in conflict with their own needs (Helm, 1988). Adolescents need to develop an independent identity, so young mothers may perform relatively well during the first year of their child's life because the dependent infant adds to the mother's feelings of being an adult. However, the adolescent parent may have trouble dealing well with the autonomy needs of toddlers, which directly conflict with the mother's own developmental needs for control and independence (Helm, 1988; White, 1975). In most cases, the father of the child provides no parenting support or exhibits immature behaviors similar to those of the young mother, making it difficult for the infant to get the parenting care needed from either parent. Increasing efforts to reduce teenage pregnancy through in-school and/or out-of-school clinics that provide birth control, health information, and intensive follow-up services may prevent such high-risk births (Helm, 1988).

Individual differences in infants also contribute to problems in parenting (Murphy, Heider, & Small, 1986). At-risk infants often have behavior patterns that make it more difficult for their parents to feel successful, such as special feeding problems, lack of eye contact, low responsiveness, and/or irritability. Parents may either reduce attempts to interact or become over-intrusive in attempts to interact with their infant (Bailey & Slee, 1984; Klein & Briggs, 1987).

Parental disabilities and/or maladjustment problems also can place infants at risk. For parents with sensory impairments, such as visual or auditory handicaps, the care, stimulation, and communication interactions required by the infant may be difficult to maintain effectively (Rogers & Puchalski, 1984). Developmental delay may occur unless these parents learn to monitor and interact appropriately with their children. Parents with physical disabilities must also have assistance in adapting their environment to be able to care appropriately for an infant (Kirshbaum, 1988). Because of genetic or environmental factors, mental retardation in the parent may lead to mental retardation in the infant. However, with guidance mentally retarded parents can learn to provide appropriate stimulation and nurturing for their infants (Garber, 1988).

Maladjustments and/or psychiatric disorders in parents, such as schizophrenia or severe depression, often result in developmental delays or maladjustments in young children because the parents are not capable of providing a nurturing environment. Similar developmental problems tend to occur in infants whose parents have personality disorders or other types of psychological stress that distort their parenting skills. Infants in these situations may not be adequately protected from injury; may not experience stable, warm, and trust-inducing interaction patterns; and may not learn to communicate ideas or feelings or to initiate autonomous actions (Shapiro, 1983; Silber, 1989).

Additionally, ecological factors may trigger dysfunctional or disorganized parental behaviors. These factors may include stress from interpersonal situations such as imminent separation or divorce, financial crises, family illness or death, or family violence (Crnic, Greenberg, Robinson, & Ragozin, 1984).

Family system characteristics and level of infant-parent support. The extended family of the infant may be living in the same environment (microsystem) or may not live in the home but be part of the interactional system (mesosystem). Bronfenbrenner (1979) defines **mesosystems** as the "interrelations among two or more settings in which the developing person actively participates" (p. 25). The presence of an extended family system that provides support for the parent can be helpful in caring for infants with developmental delays, or this arrangement may contribute to the infant's problems.

For example, other persons in the family may be substance abusers or contribute to an atmosphere of family violence. The family may have a pattern of teenage pregnancy or a history of psychological problems, physical or sexual abuse, or other dysfunctional interaction patterns. Infants born into such family systems may fail to thrive even when they are without specific disabilities.

One of the difficulties that may be encountered in working with parents to improve their interactions with their infants is that other members of the family may not be supportive of changing interactional patterns. Family systems theory predicts that, because systems are biased toward preserving stability and established roles, other family members may inadvertently or deliberately undermine changes in parenting behavior that the caregiver is being encouraged to exhibit (Barnard & Corrales, 1979). A parent who begins to take more control of self and infant may change family roles and balance of power, which may be seen as a threat to older family members.

Primarily due to overlapping economic, cultural, and health issues, a number of at-risk infants may be found in minority or diverse ethnic groups. However, this should not suggest that all culturally diverse families have children who may be at risk. Situational and environmental conditions such as poverty, homelessness, lack of formal education, and other factors that place children and families at risk are *not* cultural attributes, but conditions that cut across all cultural groups (Anderson & Fenichel, 1989).

The family systems of culturally diverse families may affect the types of early intervention that will be successful. If the infant's principal caregiver, for example, is the grandmother or another adult in the extended family, a program training parents in caregiving skills may not have much impact on the child (Ortiz, 1981). Further, if interventionists do not understand and respect the language, values, and customs of culturally diverse families, the effects of intervention will be undermined.

Health care, social/mental health service, and education availability and quality. Mesosystem factors such as health care, social/mental health care, and educational services may be denied to infants and families at risk due to high costs, poor transportation, or lack of information. The inability to access such services may increase the likelihood that infants experience conditions that cause poor health and/or developmental delay.

Lack of health care during the prenatal period, for example, has been closely linked to a variety of risks for both mother and child. Poor prenatal care may result in infants who are biologically at risk or have established risks. A national study indicated that 6% of infants had birthweights less than 2,500 g when mothers started care in the first trimester of pregnancy but that 9% had low birthweights when their

mothers' care did not begin until the third trimester (Blackman, 1986). More difficulties during pregnancy, labor, and delivery also occur in mothers who have had
little prenatal care. Poor nutrition and substance abuse are linked to lack of prenatal
care. Consequently, access to prenatal health care is critical in preventing many at-
risk conditions.

The availability of quality health care during the first few years of the infant's
life is also crucial to the prevention of developmental delays. Nutritional deficits in
the first year of life have especially severe consequences because much of the growth
of the brain and central nervous system occurs during that period (Kagan & Segal,
1988). If access to medical services is limited, at-risk infants may not receive routine
immunizations that can prevent childhood illnesses or periodic medical check-ups
that can identify potential developmental or health problems.

Lack of access to social and mental health services may lead to developmental
delay, especially if the infant-parent interaction system or the family system is dysfunctional, as in the case of a drug-addicted parent. The ability of the various agencies
in the mesosystem to work collaboratively to track potential at-risk infants and families
and to provide services can be a key to the prevention of developmental delay. Lack
of child access to early educational experiences can also lead to delays in development. One of the consistent findings of early intervention research is that out-of-
home group experiences reduce the declines in developmental progress that usually
occur when children have high-risk home environments (Bryant & Ramey, 1987).

Community social and economic conditions.   In most environmentally at-risk situations, there are co-occurring problems in the **exosystem**, which Bronfenbrenner
(1979) describes as "settings that do not involve the developing person as an active
participant, but in which events occur that affect, or are affected by, what happens in
the setting containing the developing person" (p. 25). At-risk conditions include low
socioeconomic situations where unemployment is high. In addition to nutritional and
health care problems, unsafe or inadequate housing conditions and poor sanitation
facilities accompany poverty.

Underfunded schools, high crime rates, drug abuse, poor transportation, and
lack of safe play areas are factors from the broader economic community that may
make children's developmental opportunities less than optimal. Parental communication of high goals to their children and positive expectations for their children's
future have been related to positive long-term outcomes of intervention. Achieving
these goals is greatly influenced by the power of the neighborhood and discrepancies
between school and neighborhood goals (Lally, Mangione, Honig, & Wittmer, 1988).

Policy and cultural value conditions.   In Bronfenbrenner's terms, the **macrosystem** refers to "consistencies in the form and content of lower-order systems . . . that
exist, or could exist, at the level of the subculture or the culture as a whole, along
with any belief systems or ideology underlying such consistencies" (p. 26). When
national and state policymakers do not work to minimize conditions that predict
environmental risks for infants, they are reflecting acceptance of these conditions.
The view that each family is totally responsible for its children—and that the federal
government has no responsibility for quality childrearing—is still held by many

groups in American society. In discussing the possibilities for passage of a federal comprehensive family policy bill that would provide child care and other family services, Reder (1989) stated, "The gulf between conservatives and liberals on family policy is so wide that consensus appears almost impossible. Central to the debate are fundamental issues such as the role women should play in our society" (p. 11). These policy issues must be resolved because the power of environmental factors in shaping lives cannot be overstated. Increasing societal efforts to remove environmental risk factors, such as poverty and poor education, may help reduce such high-risk births. Demographic factors continue to influence the likelihood of risk. Demographic factors have been reported to influence cognitive diagnostic consistency more than neurologic or motor functioning (Escalona, 1982).

The federal mandate to the states to provide early intervention for at-risk infants and families is evidence that views about society's responsibility for children's development is changing to some extent. Now that P.L. 99–457 has clearly required identification of conditions causing risk to infants in the micro-, meso-, and exosystems, policymakers must examine these issues, at least for at-risk children. The breadth of each state's definition of at risk will influence its perceived responsibility for ameliorating environmental risk conditions.

IDENTIFICATION AND ASSESSMENT OF AT-RISK INFANTS AND TODDLERS

Despite what is known about the advantages of early identification of handicaps, there is no agreed-upon system in place for screening all infants. Most newborns only receive an Apgar rating and a screening for certain metabolic disorders. In general, the major methods of identifying at-risk infants include

- □ medical diagnoses
- □ developmental screening instruments
- □ family needs assessments
- □ ecological assessments

Usually assessment plans include more than one of these methods, involve personnel from a number of disciplines, and require coordination between a number of agencies such as hospitals, mental health clinics, social services, schools and child care centers, and sometimes universities.

Medical Diagnoses

Identification of biologically at-risk infants is primarily handled by medical personnel who observe, monitor, and treat prenatal, perinatal, and neonatal problems. Infants who begin their lives in neonatal nurseries are considered to be at biological risk because of prematurity, low birthweight, or various biological insults. Even though many may have essentially normal development after the intensive neonatal treatment phase is completed, their development after discharge is usually closely monitored, especially if environmental risk factors are also present. Infants with medically diagnosed established risk or biological risk conditions are referred to early intervention specialists. Infants at risk due only to environmental factors are usually not identified by medical personnel.

Because the probability of developmental delay is high for many infants who are at biological risk, transdisciplinary team interventions to prevent or treat risk conditions may be initiated early. Infants whose birthweight is less than 1,500 g, who are premature, and/or who have teenage low-income parents are often identified by many early intervention programs as appropriate for services (Badger, Burns, & DeBoer, 1982; Seigel et al., 1982).

Other infants may not be referred to an early intervention program immediately but may be referred to a monitoring agency to keep track of how well their development proceeds (National Center for Clinical Infant Programs, 1985). Some infants in this group will be subsequently identified by medical personnel when failure to thrive, specific developmental delay, or child abuse or neglect is suspected (Wolfe, Edwards, Manion, & Koverola, 1988). In a study designed to see to what extent prematurity was predictive of developmental delay, Seigel and colleagues (1982) report that when biological risk only was used as the predictor, comparisons of premature and fullterm infant development at age 2 (with the premature scores age-corrected for prematurity) showed only the motor scores as lower for the premature group. When a combination of biological and environmental predictor variables was used, however, those infants likely to have delays in cognitive, motor, and language development could be predicted accurately.

Developmental Screening Instruments

Screening instruments are typically administered by medical personnel, early interventionists, social workers, or educators. They offer a general picture of the child's delays, and require further in-depth assessment by specialists to determine precise deficits. Table 8–1 presents a sample of developmental screening instruments and their validity and reliability data. Caution should be exercised when using screening instruments because less than 10% have documented reliability and validity (Sheehan & Sites, 1989). Additional screening instruments are presented in Chapter 13.

Examples of screening instruments include the Denver Developmental Screening Test (Frankenburg & Dodds, 1968; 1981), the Minnesota Child Development Inventory (Ireton & Thwing, 1968; 1974), and the Developmental Profile II (Alpern, Boll, & Shearer, 1972; 1980). The Denver measures gross motor, fine motor-adaptive, language, and personal-social development for children between 2 weeks and 6 years, using a combined testing/observation and parent report format. The designers of this instrument initially prepared it for use by pediatricians. Validity and reliability data on the Denver are well documented.

The Minnesota Child Development Inventory (MCDI) (Ireton & Thwing, 1974) is appropriate for ages 1 to 6 years and is designed to supplement a parent interview. The MCDI requires parents to answer yes/no questions on seven developmental scales: gross motor, fine motor, expressive language, comprehension-conceptual, situation comprehension, self-help, and personal-social. Similarly, the Developmental Profile II (Alpern et al., 1980) is a maternal report instrument for children from birth

It is not uncommon for infants and their families to fall into more than one at-risk category.

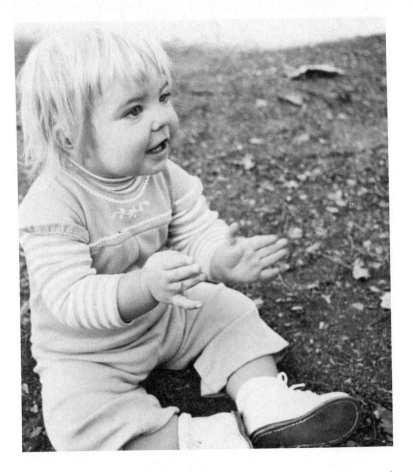

to 9 years, and provides ratings in five areas: physical, self-help, social, academic, and communication.

As indicated in Table 8–1, there is great variation in the validity and reliability of screening instruments. Although these instruments do not require a licensed psychometrician to administer them, they should only be used by people who have had training in their administration. Screening instruments are useful in providing a first indication of potential problems; however, they should never be used as the only data source for assigning infants to early intervention programs.

Family Needs Assessments

Because much of the identification of risk is based on conditions in the family system, family needs assessments are conducted when necessary. Sameroff (1983), in discussing how successful parenting can be encouraged and predicted, states that it is necessary to know parents' views because their views will "have an important impact on the way they will behave toward their children and ultimately on the developmental outcomes for those children" (p. 23).

TABLE 8–1

Sample developmental screening instruments with validity/reliability data.

Instrument Name	Age Range	Area(s) Screened	Validity/ Reliability Data
Communicative Evaluation Chart	Birth–5 yrs	Language	None available
Denver Developmental Screening Test (DDST)	2–6 wks	All	Well documented
Denver Prescreening Developmental Questionnaire	Birth–6 yrs	All	Well documented
Developmental Activities Screening Inventory Revised (DASI–R)	6–60 mos	Cognitive Fine motor	Limited evidence
Developmental Indicators for the Assessment of Learning (DIAL–R)	2–6 yrs	All	Limited evidence
Developmental Profile II	6 mos–9 yrs	All	Well documented (on I version)
Minnesota Child Development Instrument (MCDI)	1–6 yrs	All	Limited evidence
Preschool Inventory	2–6.5 yrs	Cognitive	None available

For a family needs assessment, the transdisciplinary team gathers information on a variety of environmental factors in the family system, explores the beliefs and values of the family, and develops a profile of the family's needs that might be addressed by early intervention. In addition to medical diagnosis and developmental screening information, interviews with family members, collection of data through home environmental scanning, and observations of the family's interaction patterns are often used to determine the level of risk and the most appropriate intervention strategies. Because there may be more legal disputes about judgments of environmental appropriateness, assessments must be done with reliable and valid measures that give proper documentation (Sheehan & Sites, 1989).

Instruments that assist in this type of assessment are further discussed in Chapter 12. Commonly used instruments are the Home Observation for Measurement of the Environment (HOME) (Caldwell & Bradley, 1978; 1979), the Parent Behavior Progression (PBP) (Bromwich et al., 1981), and the Parent/Family Involvement Index (Cone, DeLawyer, & Wolfe, 1985). Table 8–2 shows a sample of parent-infant interaction instruments and lists their validity and reliability data.

TABLE 8–2

Sample parent-infant interaction instruments with validity/reliability data.

Instrument	Data Collection Method	Validity/ Reliability Data
Home Observation for Measurement of the Environment (HOME)	Staff observation of parent interactions and parent self-report	Well documented
Parent Behavior Progression (PBP)	Staff checklist	None available
Parent/Family Involvement Index (P/FII)	Staff rating scale	None available

The HOME measure, Level 1 (Caldwell & Bradley, 1979) is designed for the birth to 3-year age range and requires the observer to be in the home environment. Five subscales focus on parent responsivity, acceptance, organization, involvement, and provision of play materials in the home. About one-third of the data come from parent self-report while the rest is drawn from observation.

The Parent Behavior Progression (Bromwich et al., 1981) is used with parents of infants from birth to 36 months developmental age. It measures parent responsiveness, enjoyment of the infant, play and activity provision, and sensitivity to infant cues. The information is collected after rapport has been established with the parent. Evidence can come from parental conversation or direct observation. The assessment form is not completed in the parent's presence.

The Parent/Family Involvement Index (Cone et al., 1985) is intended to be an easily administered and scored assessment of parent involvement, a potential variable of risk. Professionals who work with the family complete statements indicating contact with the teacher, participation in school and home activities, and volunteer efforts in fund raising and advocacy. Although the instrument may be useful for identifying parent needs and interests, there are numerous technical flaws in the method and, thus, it must be used with caution until reliability and validity data are added.

Whatever instrument may be used, information about a family should be collected with their cooperation, and goals of intervention should be jointly planned (Bailey, 1987; Bailey & Simeonsson, 1988). Family needs assessments are often helpful in ecological assessments as well.

Ecological Assessments

Attention to the ecology of the family system is necessary for planning and managing complex intervention strategies. Ricciuti (1983) addresses ecological issues in his multiple-risk-factor model. In this model, the parent-child interaction system is the core but it is surrounded by factors within the child (e.g., temperament, type of risk), parent factors (e.g., age, health, parenting skills), and family factors (e.g., housing conditions, level of conflict). These factors, in turn, are surrounded by the molar environment (e.g., job prospects, health care services). In an ecological assessment, all these factors must be considered.

However, to conduct sound ecological assessments interventionists must possess the ability to monitor their own value sets while trying to understand the values of high-risk families and their communities (Weinstein, 1981). To achieve this, interventionists must use the following strategies to increase the appropriateness of their efforts with culturally diverse families (Anderson & Fenichel, 1989):

1. Recognize and understand the family's cultural paradigm, attempting not to force the family into any preconceived cultural model so stereotyping may be avoided.
2. Consider all culturally defined family members as full partners in the intervention process when primary caregivers so desire.
3. Recognize the family as a unique source of insight regarding its children and culture.
4. Demonstrate a clear willingness to learn from the family and the family's community as well as offer professional expertise.

Generally, cultural errors are less alienating if families know that professionals are committed to providing services in a culturally acceptable manner.

Agency collaboration is essential in ecological assessments because information collected by each agency, using its own assessment methods, is then shared with other agency team members. The case manager is then able to draw upon all these resources in developing and implementing the most appropriate referral and/or family service plan (IFSP). Figure 8–1 presents principal factors that must be considered

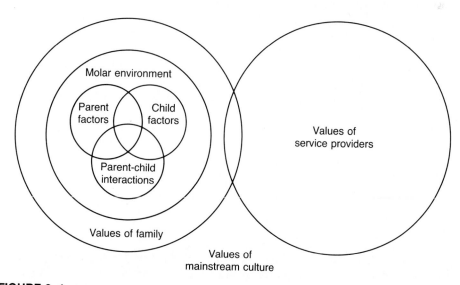

FIGURE 8–1

Ecological factors to be considered in assessment and intervention with at-risk young children and high-risk/multi-risk families. Areas that do not overlap can be a source of misunderstanding and/or conflict.

when conducting ecological assessments and planning interventions for at-risk infants and high-risk/multi-risk families.

Since 1977, Massachusetts has operated a model statewide community assessment model for providing early intervention services for children and their families from birth to 3 years of age. Under the direction of the Department of Mental Health and Public Health, identification of children who are at established, biological, and/or environmental risks is determined by regional communities' transdisciplinary teams. This community-based assessment system allows teams to be more sensitive to local norms (Smith, 1988). Information from medical diagnoses, developmental screening instruments, family assessments, and ecological assessments are all used to determine eligibility for local services.

PREVENTION OF AT-RISK CONDITIONS

Early intervention has always had a prevention orientation, and most recently programs have addressed infants who have multiple risk conditions such as biological and environmental risks (Guralnick & Bennett, 1987). Prevention is considered to be **primary prevention** if it can prevent the condition of risk from occurring at all. For example, good health practices before and during pregnancy, such as immunizations, genetic counseling, and avoidance of drugs, and health or social/economic practices after birth such as neonatal intensive care, accident prevention, and reducing dysfunctional parenting are primary prevention strategies. Attention to mesosystem factors such as health, parent employment, and increasing educational opportunities can eliminate many at-risk conditions for children.

Secondary prevention is that which improves the prognosis for infants who have been identified through prenatal, perinatal, neonatal, or early infant screening as having a high risk of disability. With early assessment and treatment, approximately 20 to 30% of the causes of developmental disability can be prevented (Guralnick & Bennett, 1987). However, even if preventive measures are implemented, programs for at-risk infants will still be needed because the causes of cognitive impairment in at least 40% of children are unknown (Guralnick & Bennett, 1987). Further, many other disabling conditions are not well understood, predictable, or completely preventable.

Odom, Yoder, and Hill (1988) suggest prevention efforts focus on potential parents, on neonatal units, and on early programs for infants. They identify three groups of high-risk mothers:

- those with medical or biological risks
- those from low socioeconomic groups
- those who are adolescents

They suggest counseling, educational, medical, and nutritional interventions in clinic and community-based settings to prevent risk conditions for infants and toddlers.

Prevention at the secondary level also includes home-based and center-based programs for infants. Because interventions that affect parental interaction styles and relationships can prevent developmental delay, most intervention programs focus on parents and other family members, as well as the child (Cappleman et al., 1982).

Parent information must be tailored to the age level of the parent (e.g., younger teens may need more concrete caregiving skills). In the case of adolescent parents, peer support tends to be a critical factor for successful programs (Helm, 1988). Any parent education/information should include efforts to

- □ change knowledge and attitudes (e.g., increase self-respect, parenting skills)
- □ impart information
- □ increase communication and support
- □ increase life options (e.g., facilitate education, vocational guidance, job training) (Nickel & Delaney, 1985)

Generally, research suggests that low socioeconomic levels, maternal smoking, later birth order, previous reproductive failure, and apnea are signals of potential risk for developmental problems (Seigel et al., 1982). Although the results of prevention efforts with at-risk conditions are still unclear, limited evidence supports the effectiveness of multi-faceted programs (Odom, Yoder, & Hill, 1988). State tracking systems will undoubtedly be valuable in monitoring both short- and long-term effects of early intervention efforts directed toward primary and secondary prevention.

LEAST-RESTRICTIVE APPROACHES TO EARLY INTERVENTION

Children with different handicapping conditions and families with various resources and needs require services that are individually tailored in nature and intensity. Federal law mandates that children with special needs be educated in least-restrictive environments. Educational and care settings for at-risk and handicapped children should be as much like the settings in which most normally developing children are educated as possible. Decisions about which models of early intervention are most appropriate for at-risk infants are often influenced by what decision makers believe is the least restrictive environment. For example, Smith (1988) argues that integrating at-risk children into generic community-based programs is the least restrictive alternative. Other early intervention planners view the home as the least restrictive environment and recommend home visiting and parent relationship-focused intervention programs as the most appropriate first intervention choice for at-risk infants (Affleck, McGrade, McQueeney, & Allen, 1982).

For many biologically and environmentally at-risk children, however, there is no clear indication of developmental delay in their first few months of life. To improve the chances that the development of these children continues to be within the normal range, tracking systems that monitor the infant's progress are necessary.

Monitoring At-risk Infants and Toddlers

Approximately 25% of the states have statewide tracking systems in place (National Center for Clinical Infant Programs, 1985). Because P.L. 99–457 requires states to locate and identify eligible children, assessment and tracking systems are now being developed throughout the nation (Hochman, 1987). State-wide tracking systems are designed to "ensure that disabled and at-risk infants and their families receive continuous and appropriate services to improve health and developmental outcome" (National Center for Clinical Infant Programs, 1985, p. 4).

The majority of states that have tracking systems have implemented procedures that include prenatal identification, focus on child and family strengths, and link to various agencies and services that can assist the family. The goals of tracking systems include

□ early identification and referral to appropriate diagnostic and treatment services
□ monitoring needs
□ providing information for planning service delivery
□ documenting outcomes of services

Each state determines the criteria for at-risk infants included in its tracking system and the appropriate time of discharge from the system. Entry is usually during the first year of life but may occur before birth. Discharge usually occurs as the child enters public school but, in some cases, may continue through adulthood.

Bricker and Squires (1989) outline four reasons for well-organized, cost-effective tracking systems. First, roughly 30 to 70% of infants classified as at risk at birth eventually develop problems that require some form of intervention. The exact percentage is influenced by the level of severity of the initial condition.

Second, most infant tests and other assessment procedures are not able to provide sufficiently valid diagnoses of early developmental problems and, consequently, many false positives and negatives occur (Bricker & Littman, 1985). It is still often impossible to detect infants who will be functioning normally by age 2 from those who will display serious developmental delays (Bricker & Squires, 1989).

Third, at-risk infants often have variable or non-normative growth rates so that testing at different age levels is required to get an accurate picture of their development (Shonkoff, 1983). For this reason, tracking programs tend to be useful in identifying failure to thrive infants since these children have severe growth failure that is not explained by organic problems or lack of food (Ricciuti, 1983).

The fourth reason for monitoring the development of at-risk infants is to increase the chances of early referral to services and thereby increase chances for optimal development.

For some children who start life identified as having treatable biological or minimal environmental risk, monitoring of developmental progress through a tracking system is probably a sufficient method of assuring that developmental delay does not occur. These children and their families may need few, if any, referrals to resources because the children's development will proceed within the normal range.

Most children who are at risk, especially those with multiple risk conditions, will need more intensive direct intervention. Children with multiple risk conditions tend to receive intervention before their birth or shortly after birth because they have a greater likelihood of developmental delay. A tracking/monitoring approach for this population of children usually is not sufficient to prevent or lessen developmental delay. Least restrictive options for these children may include early intervention through home- and/or center-based programs. It is essential that tracking systems include parents in information collecting and management roles, as well as involve parents in all decision-making processes.

Oregon has a model cost-effective tracking system that relies on periodic parental self-reports based on their infant's development (Bricker & Squires, 1989). This model, which uses the Infant Monitoring Questionnaire (IMQ), permits referral to services at the first sign of a problem. The authors of the IMQ report a high level of agreement between assessments using the IMQ and those using the Gesell Developmental and Neurologic Examination (Knobloch, Stevens, & Malone, 1980).

Service Delivery

At whatever point the infant, parent, and/or family are identified as needing direct intervention, the options for services are affected by the availability of services and recommendations of the assessment team. Generally, service delivery options include center/group programs and home/parent interventions.

Center/group programs. McLean and Odom (1988) list least restrictive options as

- ☐ mainstreamed educational programs (i.e., those that have education as the major purpose)
- ☐ mainstreamed noneducational programs (i.e., those that have child care as the major purpose)
- ☐ integrated special education or reverse mainstreamed programs (i.e., those that are set up for special needs children but that purposely include nonhandicapped children)
- ☐ nonintegrated special education programs

Because of the assistance offered by early intervention programs, more community programs for nonhandicapped children are including at-risk infants and toddlers. Most often children who are environmentally at risk, and/or children with established risks but who are developing close to normal levels, are considered for such arrangements. In these cases, the primary service provider and/or case manager monitor the at-risk child's progress, provide assistance to program staff as necessary, and serve as a resource for accessing other services needed by the child and family.

Despite the desire for mainstreamed placements, most at-risk children participate in nonintegrated special education programs. Examples of programs of this type that have demonstrated effectiveness include the Carolina Abecedarian Project (Ramey & Campbell, 1984) and the Family Development Research Program (Lally et al., 1988). Center/group approaches often include some type of parent education or counseling components, as well as a range of interdisciplinary family and child services. Table 8–3 lists the basic characteristics of some projects designed for environmentally at-risk infants and their families.

Home/parent interventions. Many intervention programs for at-risk families and infants do not stress out-of-home programming for infants. Rather, they focus on enhancement of the home situation and on parent education and therapy. Often the families for these programs are identified before the child's birth based on young maternal age or other significant environmental risk conditions. It is generally accepted that it is not a single risk factor that creates problems for children, but the

TABLE 8–3

Characeristics of projects designed for environmentally at-risk infants and multi-risk families (pp. 218–222).

Name of Study	Intervention Site	Primary Target(s)	Duration	Intensity	Activities
Infancy programs 1. Center-based, child- and parent-focused					
Milwaukee Project	Home and Center	Child and mother	Home = 4 months Center = 6 years for child; 2 years for mother	Many hours of HVs[a] in 1st 4 months, then full-day daycare year-round	Children in educational program having a cognitive-language orientation in a structured environment using prescriptive teaching techniques. Vocational and social education program for mothers including job training and remedial education.
Project CARE	Center and Home	Child and mother in Center/HV group; mother in home group	5 years; project continues to age 8	Full-day daycare, year-round plus weekly HVs to Center/HV group; weekly HVs to home group	Children in educational daycare program with focus on language and cognitive development and adaptive social behavior. All medical care provided. HVs to both E groups with focus on responsive parenting, learning activities, behavior management, and problem solving.
Carolina Abecedarian Project	Center	Child	8 years	Full-day daycare, year-round	Children in educational daycare program with focus on language and cognitive development and adaptive social behavior. All medical care provided.

Field's Center—Home Visit Comparison	Center or home	Mother and child for Center group; mother for home group	12 months	Center = 20 hours/week: home = $\frac{1}{2}$ hour HV biweekly	Curriculum items modeled by HV; activities designed from the Denver and Bayley test items. Parent training in child development and in job skills via CETA employment.
2. Center-based parent-focused					
Birmingham PCDC	Center	Mother and child	31–33 months	To 11 months = 12 hours/week; 12–17 months = 20 hours/week; 18–36 months = 40 hours/week	To 11 months = Training in parenting and child development; mothers cared for own child with assistance from center staff. 12–17 months = 4 half-days as understudies to teaching mothers; 1 half-day training in child development and family topics. 18–30 months = 4 mornings as teaching mothers, remaining time in training, taking care of own child, class preparation, and social groups.

TABLE 8–3
(continued)

Name of Study	Intervention Site	Primary Target(s)	Duration	Intensity	Activities
2. Center-based parent-focused Houston PCDC	Year 1, home; year 2, center	Mother, child, and family	24 months	Year 1 = $1\frac{1}{2}$ hour HVs for 30 weeks plus 4 family workshops; Year 2 = 3-hour sessions for 4 days/week for 8 months plus nightly meetings	Year 1 = HV topics in child development, parenting, home as learning environment, parent-child activities. Family workshops for problem solving and communication skills. Year 2 = Training in home management, child development, and parenting; videotape and discussions of parent-child interactions. English classes offered weekly.
New Orleans PCDC	Center	Mother and child	34 months	3 hours, 2 times/ week	One weekly session to counsel on child development with 1-hour discussion group and 2-hour parent-child laboratory experience. One weekly session focused on adult and family life.

3. Home visit, parent-focused

Program	Setting	Participants	Duration	Schedule	Description
Mobile Unit for Child Health	Home and mobile health unit	Mother and child	3 years	At least 20 health-related and 24 infant education 1-hour HVs over 3 years	Prenatal counseling; well-baby care; infant stimulation activities with emphasis on language; educational toy given to family often. 1st cohort received training on child development and family problems.
Florida Parent Education Project	Home	Mother for 1st 2 years, mother and child in last year	3 years for 1 group, 2 years for 3 groups, and 1 year for 3 groups	Weekly 1-hour HVs for 3 years plus playgroup for 2 hours twice a week in 3rd year	HVs used infant stimulation activities with child and mother to help mother become more effective teacher of her child. Home Learning Center in 3rd year, supervised by experienced parents, was a backyard playgroup for socialization skills.
Ypsilanti—Carnegie Infant Education Project	Home	Mother and child	16 months	Weekly 60–90 minute HVs	Focus on mothers as teachers of their children. Piagetian-based formal set of infant activities to support objectives for mothers; emphasis on fine and gross motor skills.

TABLE 8–3
(continued)

Name of Study	Intervention Site	Primary Target(s)	Duration	Intensity	Activities
3. Home visit, parent-focused					
Family-Oriented Home Visiting Program	Home	Mother	9 months	30 weekly 60–90 minute HVs	Activities were based on DARCEE principles and materials for mothers of toddlers. Intervention tailored to each family, but emphasized teaching style, competence, language, and behavior management. Used inexpensive homemade materials.
Field's Home Visit Study	Home	Mother	12 months	Biweekly $\frac{1}{2}$-hour HVs	Curriculum items modeled by HV; activities designed from the Denver and Bayley test items. Goals to educate mothers on developmental milestones and to facilitate mother-child interaction.

[a]HV = Home Visit

Source: "An Analysis of the Effectiveness of Early Intervention Programs for Environmentally At-risk Children," by D. M. Bryant & C. T. Ramey, 1987. In M. J. Guralnick & F. C. Bennett (Eds.), *The Effectiveness of Early Intervention for At-risk and Handicapped Children* (pp. 50–54). Orlando, FL: Academic Press. Copyright © 1987, Academic Press. Reprinted by permission of the publisher and the authors.

balance between prenatal and perinatal risk factors and stressful life events that heighten children's vulnerability (Werner, 1988). For example, offering assistance in securing transportation and child care for low-SES parents may increase participation in services (Lally et al., 1988). When stressful life events outweigh the protective factors in life, even the most resilient child may develop problems.

Interventions must, therefore, be conceived as attempts to shift the balance from vulnerability to resilience, either by decreasing exposure to risk factors or stressful life events, or by increasing the number of available protective factors (e.g., parenting competencies, sources of support) in the lives of vulnerable children (Werner, 1988). The goal of most programs is to assist parents in becoming more effective at providing nurturing and interactive communication for their infant, and in developing coping skills that will ameliorate some of the environmental risk factors present in the family.

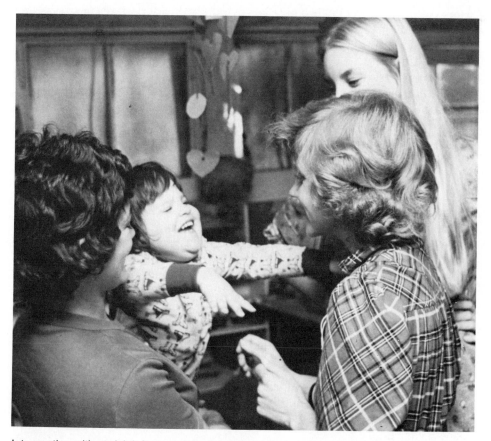

Intervention with at-risk infants and their families strives to assist parents in becoming more effective at providing nurturing and interactive communication with their child, and to develop coping skills that may ameliorate some environmental risks in the family.

Intervention may emphasize the infant, the parent(s), or both infant and parent(s). Working with families at risk and infants at environmental risk requires interventionists to acquire special skills and sensitivities. Some parents may be unwilling to attend parenting skills or counseling groups because most of their energy is focused on their own multiple problems such as substance abuse, poor mental health, or dysfunctional personal skills. Unfortunately, it is exactly these problems that contribute to their infants' risk conditions. Interventionists function as counselors, resources, consultants, enablers, mediators, and teachers to meet the needs of multi-risk and at-risk families.

MODEL PROGRAMS

Many of the model programs developed over the past 20 years for at-risk infants and their families have collected long-term evaluation data showing a range of effects that positively change the lives of the children and families who participated. Bryant and Ramey (1987), Bennett (1987), and Dickin et al. (1983) have reviewed and compared a number of these programs. Although targeted populations and results vary, it seems clear that multiple pathways for encouraging optimal development in children at risk are needed.

The emphasis on working within the ecological parameters of the culture with at-risk infants has grown out of the experiences of early intervention professionals who have come to realize that the context of family and culture influences the effectiveness of every strategy. The need to offer a variety of approaches, flexibility in meeting family needs, comprehensive services, and enhancement of family empowerment are exemplified by the following four programs.

Infant Stimulation/Mother Training Project (Badger et al., 1982). Beginning at birth, and for the first 12 months of life, low birthweight infants and their primarily low-income minority parents received a range of coordinated services, including initial in-hospital intervention. In the first year of the child's life, weekly home visits or weekly mother-infant group meetings were provided. The type of participation was based on parent-identified need, and involved other services such as transportation and assistance in gaining access to community resources. Results indicated that developmental delay was prevented during the first year of life, apparently due to a combination of the model's components. In this program, young mothers group meetings, rather than home visits, seemed to be more likely to increase infants' cognitive abilities.

Although intervention stopped at the end of the infants' first year, assessment of results continued. By 18 months, some of the at-risk infants had begun to show language delay. This type of delay, manifesting itself in the beginning of the second year of life, is reported in a number of other studies. Because modern medicine is assisting tiny infants to survive, equal emphasis needs to be placed on assuring these infants a certain quality of life.

Infant Care Center (Phillips, 1982). This community-based program was designed to "correct developmental deviation and prevent physical and emotional impairment"

(p. 586) among children from birth to 3 and their families. It included three approaches: a therapeutic child-care center, with intensive counseling services for families; long-term therapy programs for families of children younger than 3, without child-care services; and mother-child interaction groups for non child-care children. The model included a network of social, health, and educational services. Crisis intervention and long-term intensive therapy options, using the resources of the community, were offered.

A major challenge faced by the transdisciplinary team of this project was learning to work effectively with the Black and Hispanic community that the program served. The program began after assessing the needs of the community and "it has been able to continue only with the sanction of the community" with "continual and mutual sharing of customs, values, and approaches to childrearing" (Phillips, 1982, p. 591).

Clinical Infant Development Program (Weider, Poisson, Lourie, & Greenspan, 1988). This model program focused on providing comprehensive, long-term services to multi-risk families, including teen and older mothers. The families were selected on the basis of having an older sibling who was developmentally delayed. The infants served had no identified biological risk at birth. Multidimensional services included home visits, an infant center, individual and group therapy, and social/educational parent activities. Responsive parenting skills and concern for individual infant needs were stressed. Transitional services, such as referrals to preschool programs, were also provided.

The staff attempted to develop a "sustained therapeutic relationship with parents" (Weider et al., 1988, p. 6). Because many of the parents mistrusted mental health and educational systems and had a history of failure in coping with problems, they presented many challenges to staff commitment and persistence during the 6 years of the program.

Five year follow-up results indicated that the program was successful in lessening environmental risk conditions for both children and parents. Only 17% of the children in the sample had been referred to special education services (in contrast to 49% of the parents who had had impaired school functioning), and for the majority of children behavioral and emotional adjustment were within the normal range. There was a low subsequent birth rate among program participants and many obtained education and/or employment.

Family Development Research Program (Lally et al., 1988). This program provided a comprehensive approach that included education, nutrition, health, safety, and human development components from the prenatal to elementary age period. The population served was primarily Black, low-income women with less than a high school education. From birth to age 5, the children attended a full-year group program that incorporated Piagetian views on the importance of play and active child experiences. Other curriculum components included an Eriksonian emphasis on promoting emotional stages (e.g., developing trust, autonomy, and initiative), an emphasis on choice, creativity, and providing a responsive language environment stressed by linguistic theorists.

As discussed, there are many variables that may place children at risk for developmental problems. The following case study is an example of a multi-risk family whose circumstances place the children at environmental and biological risk.

ANGELA AND CARLY

Angela, age 25, was brought to the attention of the agency when her two children Nicky, age 9, and David, age 7, were removed from the home and placed in foster care after neglect was determined. The man living with Angela (not the children's father) had been charged with drug abuse and Angela was suspected of using drugs as well. Also living in the home was Danny, age 4, who was kept with his mother because of his age. Danny was already showing signs of developmental delay. Angela appeared to have a low-normal intellectual level, and expressed difficulty in knowing how to manage her life.

When the agency began working with Angela she was 7 months pregnant with a fourth child and had received no prenatal care. Angela and the agency jointly decided these intervention goals for the family

- □ to attempt to prevent developmental delay in the fourth unborn child by providing prenatal care and developmental intervention during the first years of life
- □ to assist the mother in learning appropriate nutrition and childrearing skills
- □ to assist the mother in developing job skills

Angela entered the prenatal medical and nutritional care program willingly. When her child, Carly, was born she appeared to be within the normal range developmentally, although she was slightly below average in birthweight. During the first year of Carly's life, mother and daughter attended a once-a-week program at the agency (which was the site of the family's case manager) in which Carly participated in a play group and her mother observed the children and received information on child nutrition and home care skills. Additionally, Angela attended a parent educational/support group offered by another community agency which had been arranged by her case man-

ager. Danny participated in a preschool program during this time. Carly's progress was monitored by a transdisciplinary team through regular observations and frequent developmental assessments. Carly did not evidence developmental delay during her first year of life.

About 6 months after the intervention began, Angela had progressed so well in mastering home and parenting skills that the two older children were returned to the home. Angela exhibited pride in this accomplishment and expressed enjoyment in Carly's development. She indicated that she had not experienced this enjoyment with her other three children when they were younger. She began to take note of Carly's achievements and to more effectively support Danny and Carly.

Carly's development continued to be within the normal range during her second year. Participation in the two programs continued through Carly's second year, although the agency play group was reduced to only monthly contacts. Angela was then encouraged to make contact with other appropriate community support services. She was referred to job counseling/training and was assisted in becoming a better planner of her financial resources.

At the age of 3, Carly was placed in a preschool program that continued until she was 5 years old. At about this time, Angela began working part-time. Because she wished to keep all her children in the home, Angela made use of some of the community activities and resources that could help her with her older boys.

Carly is now in kindergarten. She is functioning at age level; however, the transition to the public schools has not been an easy one for her. Angela continues to communicate with the initial agency so her family may be monitored in how they cope with new experiences. Angela has not had any more children.

The case management for this family involved six agencies and schools over the 5 years of Carly's prenatal to preschool development. Further, numerous other community resources became short-term supports for the family. The initial agency handled the family's case management throughout the 5 years of services. Case management involved direct services for Carly and her family in the first 2 years, while the last 3 years primarily involved monitoring the family on a prearranged schedule.

Ten year follow-up results indicated that children in the program had a lower incidence of delinquency, more positive self-concepts, and higher expectations about completing their education. Parents who had participated in the program were more likely to have higher goals for their children and to feel proud of their children's attitudes and behaviors. Although school achievement was higher for girls who had been program participants, this finding did not apply to boys. The researchers recommended careful planning of transitions, use of community resources, and program flexibility in meeting family needs.

These programs have certain features that seem to be important in efforts to prevent developmental delay in young children who present biological, environmental, and/or other multi-risk factors. First, one-stop educational, health, employment, and counseling services tend to be most useful with multi-risk children and their families. Second, flexible and culturally sensitive service options are productive in assisting parents' understanding of the needs of their children and in developing responsive interactions. Third, parent education information should be tailored to the needs of the family and encourage parents' feelings of self-control and competence. And fourth, any intervention with families must acknowledge the family's values and customs. These features are illustrated in the case study.

SUMMARY OF PROCEDURES

The prevention of at-risk conditions for infants discussed in this chapter focused on three types of intervention: preventing high-risk births; preventing high-risk conditions during the prenatal, perinatal, and neonatal period; and preventing developmental delay for those infants who are at biological, environmental, or multi-risk after birth. Some of the principal strategies discussed in this chapter follow.

1. To prevent high-risk births, interventionists may:
   □ Increase efforts to reduce teenage pregnancy through in-school and/or out-of-school clinics that provide birth control, health information, and intensive follow-up services.
   □ Increase societal efforts to remove environmental risk factors (e.g., poverty, drug abuse, poor education) that contribute to high-risk births for parents of all ages.
   □ Encourage pre-pregnancy genetic counseling to increase awareness of biological risk factors.
2. To prevent high-risk conditions during the prenatal, perinatal, and neonatal periods, interventionists may:
   □ Access good prenatal care for all pregnant women to reduce infant illness, death, and prematurity.
   □ Offer parent support groups during hospitalizations and transitions between services.
   □ Offer assistance in securing transportation and child care for low-SES parents to increase participation.
   □ Enable families to feel in control of their lives during crisis periods as well as during periods of stability.

3. To prevent developmental delay in infants who are at biological, environmental, and/or multi-risk, interventionists may:

   □ Arrange one-stop educational, health, employment, and counseling services for teenage and low-SES parents of at-risk children at least until their children are 3 years of age.

   □ Permit flexibility, choice, and culturally sensitive options in parent intervention services for at-risk infants and their families (e.g., tracking/monitoring only, support groups, counseling, group programs for children, home visits).

   □ Offer caregiving, nutritional, educational, and other community support services to parents of at-risk infants (e.g., child care for other children, sources for infant food and clothing, job training).

   □ Assist parents in understanding the needs of their at-risk infants and in developing responsive interactions through modeling of appropriate behaviors and offering support for any parental demonstration of positive change in behavior.

   □ Tailor parent education information to the age level of the parent and include efforts to change knowledge and attitudes, share information, increase communication and support, and increase life options.

   □ Systematically monitor variables that can negatively affect the child and family's well-being (e.g., nutrition, transportation, health care), and revise program components in response to the expressed needs of families, allowing special consideration of families' values and customs.

   □ Access long-term services at the first sign of developmental delay.

SUMMARY

In order to develop programs to serve the needs of at-risk infants, each state must define characteristics of risk and initiate a tracking or monitoring system to identify eligible infants and their families. This chapter described three categories of risk: established, biological, and environmental. Established risks are physical and/or mental abnormalities that predict developmental problems. Biological risks include infants who have suffered a biological trauma or insult before, during, or after birth that puts normal development at risk. Environmental risks are conditions in the ecological setting that are likely to compromise the infant's development and life chances. Risk conditions often overlap and interact. The variability among premature infants, for instance, illustrates the interaction of biological and environmental factors in determining the course of development.

Assessment of at-risk infants involves a comprehensive evaluation using medical diagnoses, developmental screening instruments, family needs assessments, and culturally responsive ecological assessments. Prevention of at-risk conditions that might lead to developmental delay include primary methods that focus on keeping the risk conditions from occurring, and secondary methods that improve the prognosis for infants who have been identified as being at risk.

Intervention approaches for at-risk infants and their families focus on using the least restrictive environment, which may include tracking or monitoring only, home-based intervention only, group placement in community settings with nonhandicapped children, or group placement with other children with special needs. Intervention with high risk and multi-risk families tends to focus on parent support, education, and therapy. Although the approaches for serving these families are diverse, the goal is to improve the life chances of at-risk infants and their families.

DISCUSSION QUESTIONS

1. Why should multiple methods of assessment be used to identify biologically and environmentally at-risk infants?
2. In what ways could value/cultural conflicts complicate intervention efforts with multi-risk children and their families?
3. What components should be included in a program to prevent risk during the prenatal period? Why has prevention of risk before birth been less likely to receive funding support than neonatal intervention?

APPLIED ACTIVITIES/PROJECTS

1. Interview the parents of two children who were diagnosed as being at biological risk (e.g., premature, low birthweight, respiratory distress) when they were born. Ask them to discuss their experiences with the neonatal unit, transitions from hospital to home, referral and support services they received, extent of their use of parental support groups and/or other services, and their involvement with advocacy.
2. Imagine you are assigned to be the case manager of a transdisciplinary team that works with infants from multi-risk families. Design a plan of action that answers the following questions: What organizational and communication plan would you propose for the team? What type of training should the team have? What composition of disciplines would you wish the team members to represent? How would you facilitate team operations? What type of training would you provide the team and how would you evaluate their work?
3. Plan a comprehensive program that includes both home and group care components for environmentally at-risk infants of teenage mothers. Describe the curriculum for infants and the parent involvement activities. Tell what community resources you would bring into the comprehensive plan and how you would gain access to those resources. Identify problems you might expect to encounter and how your program would try to solve those problems.

SUGGESTED READINGS

Anderson, P. P., & Fenichel, E. S. (1989). *Serving culturally diverse families of infants and toddlers with disabilities*. Washington, DC: National Center for Clinical Infant Programs.

Feldman, R., Stiffman, A., & Jung, K. (1987). *Children at risk: In the web of parental mental illness*. New Brunswick, NJ: Rutgers University Press.

Frohock, F. M. (1986). *Special care: Medical decisions at the beginning of life*. Chicago: University of Chicago Press.

Garber, H. L. (1988). *The Milwaukee Project: Preventing mental retardation in children at risk.* Washington, DC: American Association on Mental Retardation.

Guralnick, M. J., & Bennett, F. C. (Eds.). (1987). *The effectiveness of early intervention for at-risk and handicapped children.* Orlando, FL: Academic Press.

Harrison, I., & Harrison, D. (1971). The Black family experience and health behavior. In C. Crawford (Ed.), *Health and the family: A medical-sociological analysis* (pp. 175–198). New York: Macmillan.

Johnson & Johnson. *Minimizing high-risk parenting: A review of what is known and consideration of appropriate preventive intervention.* Skillman, NJ: Author.

Raising Kids. A monthly newsletter that focuses on the many aspects of normal development in young children, and often includes articles on disabilities and health problems (Available: P. O. Box 273, Braintree, MA 02184).

Sasserath, V. J. (1983). *Focus on the first 60 months: A handbook of promising prevention programs for children 0 to 5 years of age.* (Publication from the National Governors' Association Committee of Human Resources and Center for Policy Research. Available: NGA, Hall of the States, 444 North Capital Street, Washington, DC 20001–1572.)

Simon-Ailes, S. (1983). *The growing path: Traditional infant activities for Indian children.* Bernalillo, NM: The Pueblo Infant Education Project, Southwest Communication Resources, Inc.

REFERENCES

Affleck, G., McGrade, B. J., McQueeney, M., & Allen, D. (1982). Promise of relationship-focused early intervention in developmental disabilities. *Journal of Special Education, 16*(4), 413–430.

Alpern, G. D., Boll, T. J., & Shearer, M. S. (1972, 1980). *Developmental Profile II.* Indianapolis, IN: Psychological Developmental Publications.

Anderson, P. P., & Fenichel, E. S. (1989). *Serving culturally diverse families of infants and toddlers with disabilities.* Washington, DC: National Center for Clinical Infant Programs.

Badger, E., Burns, D., & DeBoer, M. (1982). An early demonstration of educational intervention beginning at birth. *Journal of the Division of Early Childhood, 5,* 19–30.

Bailey, D. B. (1987). Collaborative goal-setting with families: Resolving differences in values and priorities for service. *Topics in Early Childhood Special Education, 7*(2), 59–71.

Bailey, D. B., & Simeonsson, R. J. (1988). *Family assessment in early intervention.* Columbus, OH: Merrill.

Bailey, L., & Slee, P. T. (1984). A comparison of play interactions between non-disabled and disabled children and their mothers: A question of style. *Australia and New Zealand Journal of Developmental Disabilities, 10*(1), 5–10.

Barnard, C. P., & Corrales, R. G. (1979). *The theory and techniques of family therapy.* Springfield, IL: Charles C. Thomas.

Beckwith, L. (1984). Parent interactions with their preterm infants and later mental development. *Early Child Development and Care, 16,* 27–40.

Beckwith, L. (1985). Parent-child interaction and social-emotional development. In C. C. Brown & A. W. Gottfried (Eds.), *Play interactions: The role of toys and parental involvement in children's development* (pp. 152–159). Skillman, NJ: Johnson & Johnson.

Bennett, F. C. (1987). The effectiveness of early intervention for infants at increased biological risk. In M. J. Guralnick & F. C. Bennett (Eds.), *The effectiveness of early intervention for at-risk and handicapped children* (pp. 79–112). Orlando, FL: Academic Press.

Blackman, J. (1986). *Basic criteria for tracking at-risk infants and toddlers*. Washington, DC: National Center for Clinical Infant Programs.

Bricker, D., & Littman, D. (1985). Parental monitoring of infant development. In R. McMahon & R. Peters (Eds.), *Childhood disorders: Behavioral-developmental approaches* (pp. 90–115). New York: Brunner/Mazel.

Bricker, D., & Squires, J. (1989). Low-cost system using parents to monitor the development of at-risk infants. *Journal of Early Intervention, 13,*(1), 50–60.

Bromwich, R. M., Khokha, E., Fust, L. S., Baxter, E., Burge, D., & Koss, E. W. (1981). Parent behavior progression. In R. M. Bromwich, *Working with parents and infants: An interactional approach* (pp. 341–359). Baltimore: University Park Press.

Bronfenbrenner, U. (1979). *The ecology of human development: Experiments by nature and design*. Cambridge: Harvard University Press.

Bruner, J. S., & Sherwood, V. (1976). Peek-a-Boo and the learning of rule structures. In J. S. Bruner, A. Jolly, & K. Sylva (Eds.), *Play: Its role in development and evolution* (pp. 277–285). New York: Basic Books.

Bryant, D. M., & Ramey, C. T. (1987). An analysis of the effectiveness of early intervention programs for environmentally at-risk children. In M. J. Guralnick & F. C. Bennett (Eds.), *The effectiveness of early intervention for at-risk and handicapped children* (pp. 33–78). Orlando, FL: Academic Press.

Caldwell, B., & Bradley, R. (1978; 1979). *Home Observation for Measurement of the Environment* (HOME). Little Rock: University of Arkansas at Little Rock.

Cappleman, M. W., Thompson, R. J., DeRemer-Sullivan, P. A., King, A. A., & Sturm, J. M. (1982). Effectiveness of a home-based early intervention program with infants of adolescent mothers. *Child Psychiatry and Human Development, 13,* 55–65.

Cone, J. D., DeLawyer, D. D., & Wolfe, V. V. (1985). Assessing parent participation: The parent/family involvement index. *Exceptional Children, 51,* 416–424.

Crnic, K. A., Greenberg, M. T., Robinson, N. M., & Ragozin, A. S. (1984). Maternal stress and social support: Effects on the mother-infant relationship from birth to 18 months. *American Journal of Orthopsychiatry, 54,* 1199–1210.

Dickin, K. L., McKim, M. K., & Kirkland, J. (1983). Designing intervention programs for infants at risk: Considerations, implementation, and evaluation. *Early Child Development and Care, 11*(2), 145–163.

Escalona, S. (1982). Babies at double hazard: Early development of infants at biologic and social risk. *Pediatrics, 70,* 670–676.

Field, T. M. (1979). Games parents play with normal and high-risk infants. *Child Psychiatry and Human Development, 10,* 41–48.

Frankenburg, W., & Dodds, J. (1968; 1981). *Denver Developmental Screening Test*. Denver: University of Colorado Medical Center.

Frodi, A., & Lamb, M. (1980). Child abuser's responses to infant smiles and cries. *Child Development, 51,* 238–241.

Frohock, F. M. (1986). *Special care: Medical decisions at the beginning of life*. Chicago: University of Chicago Press.

Garber, H. L. (1988). *The Milwaukee Project: Preventing mental retardation in children at risk*. Washington, DC: American Association on Mental Retardation.

Graham, M. A., & Scott, K. G. (1988). The impact of definitions of high risk on services to infants and toddlers. *Topics in Early Childhood Special Education, 8*(3), 23–38.

Guralnick, M. J., & Bennett, F. C. (Eds.). (1987). *The effectiveness of early intervention for at-risk and handicapped children*. Orlando, FL: Academic Press.

Haynes-Seman, C., & Hart, J. S. (1987). Doll play of failure to thrive toddlers: Clues to infant experience. *Zero to Three, 7*(4), 10–13.

Helm, J. M. (1988). Adolescent mothers of handicapped children: A challenge for interventionists. *Journal of the Division of Early Childhood, 12*(4), 311–319.

Hochman, J. (1987). *Planning programs for infants*. State Series Paper for Technical Assistance Development System (TADS). Chapel Hill: University of North Carolina.

Hutinger, P. (1988). Stress: Is it an inevitable condition for families of children at risk? *Teaching Exceptional Children, 20,* 36–39.

Ireton, H. R., & Thwing, E. J. (1968, 1974). *Minnesota Child Development Inventory*. Minneapolis: Behavior Science Systems.

Kagan, J., & Segal, J. (1988). *Psychology: An introduction* (6th ed.). New York: Harcourt Brace Jovanovich.

Kirshbaum, M. (1988). Parents with physical disabilities and their babies. *Zero to Three, 8*(5), 8–15.

Klein, M. D., & Briggs, M. H. (1987). Facilitating mother-infant communicative interaction in mothers of high-risk infants. *Journal of Childhood Communication Disorders, 10,* 95–106.

Knobloch, H., Stevens, F., & Malone, A. (1980). *Manual of developmental diagnosis: The administration and interpretation of the revised Gesell and Armatruda developmental and neurological examination*. Hagerstown, MD: Harper & Row.

Lally, J. R., Mangione, P. L., Honig, A. S., & Wittmer, D. S. (1988). More pride, less delinquency: Findings from the 10-year follow-up study of the Syracuse University Family Development Research Program. *Zero to Three, 8*(4), 13–18.

Landerholm, E. (1982). High-risk infants of teenage mothers: Later candidates for special education placements? *Journal of the Division for Early Childhood, 6,* 19–30.

McLean, M., & Odom, S. (1988). *Least restrictive environment and social integration*. White Paper, Division of Early Childhood. Reston, VA: The Council for Exceptional Children.

Murphy, L. B., Heider, G. M., & Small, C. T. (1986). Individual differences in infants. *Zero to Three, 7*(2), 1–8.

National Center for Clinical Infant Programs. (1985). *Keeping track: Tracking systems for high-risk infants and young children*. Washington, DC: Division of Maternal and Child Health.

Nickel, D., & Delaney, H. (1985). *Working with teen parents: A survey of promising approaches*. Chicago: Family Focus and the Family Resource Coalition.

Odom, S. L., Yoder, P., & Hill, G. (1988). Developmental intervention for infants with handicaps: Purposes and programs. *Journal of Special Education, 22*(1), 11–24.

Ortiz, J. M. (1981). *Cultural pluralism in the delivery of services to high-risk minority children*. Papers from The Experiences of the Infant-Parent Project, Phoenix, AZ. (ERIC Document Reproduction Service No. ED 224 862, pp. 17–22)

Phillips, N. K. (1982). Intervention with high-risk infants and toddlers. *Social Casework: The Journal of Contemporary Social Work, 63*(10), 586–592.

Ramey, C. T., & Campbell, F. C. (1984). Preventive education for high-risk children: Cognitive consequences of the Carolina Abecedarian Project. *American Journal of Mental Deficiency, 88*(5), 515–523.

Reder, N. D. (1989). Single parents/dual responsibilities. *National Voter, 39*(1), 9–11.

Ricciuti, H. N. (1983). Interaction of multiple factors contributing to high-risk parenting. In V. J. Sasseratte (Ed.), *Minimizing high-risk parenting* (pp. 75–79). Skillman, NJ: Johnson & Johnson.

Rogers, S. J., & Puchalski, C. B. (1984). Social characteristics of visually impaired infants' play. *Topics in Early Childhood Special Education, 3*(4), 52–56.

Sameroff, A. J. (1983). Factors in predicting successful parenting. In V. J. Sasseratte (Ed.), *Minimizing high-risk parenting* (pp. 16–23). Skillman, NJ: Johnson & Johnson.

Seigel, L., Saigal, S., Rosenbaum, P., Morton, R., Young, A., Berenbaum, S., & Stoskopf, B. (1982). Predictors of development in preterm and fullterm infants: A model for detecting the at-risk child. *Journal of Pediatric Psychology, 7*(2), 135–148.

Shapiro, V. (1983). Growing hand in hand: Infants and parents at risk. In V. J. Sasseratte (Ed.), *Minimizing high-risk parenting* (pp. 44–50). Skillman, NJ: Johnson & Johnson.

Sheehan, R., & Sites, J. (1989). Implications of P.L. 99–457 for assessment. *Topics in Early Childhood Special Education, 8*(4), 103–115.

Shonkoff, J. (1983). The limitations of normative assessments of high-risk infants. *Topics in Early Childhood Special Education, 3*(1), 29–43.

Silber, S. (1989). Family influences on early development. *Topics in Early Childhood Special Education, 8,* 1–23.

Smith, B. (Ed.). (1988). *Mapping the future for children with special needs: P.L. 99–457.* Iowa City: University of Iowa.

Stern, D. N. (1977). *The first relationship.* Cambridge, MA: Harvard University Press.

Tjossem, T. (Ed.). (1976). *Intervention strategies for high risk infants and young children.* Baltimore: University Park Press.

Weider, S., Poisson, S., Lourie, R., & Greenspan, S. (1988). Enduring gains: A 5-year follow-up report on the Clinical Infant Development Program. *Zero to Three, 8*(4), 6–12.

Weinstein, V. (1981). *An ecological model for intervention with inner-city poor and/or minority handicapped infants and their families.* Papers from The Experiences of the Infant-Parent Project, Phoenix, AZ. (ERIC Document Reproduction Service No. ED 224 862, pp. 27–29)

Werner, E. E. (1988). Individual differences, universal needs: A 30-year study of resilient high-risk infants. *Zero to Three, 8*(4) 1–5.

White, B. (1975). *The first three years of life.* Englewood Cliffs, NJ: Prentice-Hall.

Wolfe, D. A., Edwards, B., Manion, I., & Koverola, C. (1988). Early intervention for parents at risk of child abuse and neglect: A preliminary investigation. *Journal of Consulting and Clinical Psychology, 56,* 40–47.

9

Techniques for Infants and Toddlers with Multiple or Severe Disabilities

Mary E. McLean, Mary Beth Bruder, Samera Baird, and Carl J. Dunst

OVERVIEW

This chapter describes assessment and intervention strategies to promote the development of infants and toddlers with multiple or severe handicaps, including:

- □ the importance of family-focused intervention for the provision of support, information, and involvement for family members
- □ formal and informal procedures for assessment
- □ responsive interaction procedures that capitalize on infant-initiated learning in natural environments
- □ factors that influence environmental responsiveness

Infants and toddlers with multiple or severe disabilities are most easily identified as needing early intervention services at an early age. Many begin to manifest developmental delays of sufficient magnitude during the first year of life to qualify them for services according to their state's definition of developmental delay. State's definitions commonly include designations such as a 25% delay in development or 1.5 standard deviations below the mean on a standardized assessment instrument (Ziegler, 1989). Other infants, with certain physiological or medical conditions (e.g., Down Syndrome) have a high probability that severe and multiple delays will develop.

Infants and toddlers with significant special needs have three essential characteristics: they have a severe handicap, they need an educational program requiring greater resources than traditionally provided, and they need programming that focuses on independent functioning (Dollar & Brooks, 1980). These children require intervention efforts that focus on the family as well as the child.

FAMILY INVOLVEMENT

Parents of infants and toddlers with multiple or severe disabilities rarely assume their parenting roles with any preparation for the special challenges they will face. Rather, the early days, weeks, and months of parental responsibility may be spent repeatedly visiting the hospital, the physician's office, or a special clinic, with little or no opportunity to adapt to the significant change that has taken place in their lives. Most parents report an increase in stress as a result of the birth of a child. The parents of an infant with multiple or severe disabilities must deal with unanticipated demands and responsibilities that can make their parenting role appear to be an overwhelming endeavor.

Higher levels of parental stress are generally associated with the presence of increased caregiving demands, slower rates of child progress, difficult child temperament, stereotypic child behavior patterns, and less social responsiveness from the child (Beckman-Bell, 1981). Increased financial responsibilities and the perception of stigma attached to the disability may also be sources of increased stress for the parents of a child with a severe disability (Barber, Turnbull, Behr, & Kerns, 1988; Fewell, 1986). Professionals providing services to families with a child with multiple handicapping conditions must be very careful to ensure that their actions work to reduce parental stress, rather than add to it.

As stated earlier, family-centered interventions must be individualized to the personal needs of parents and their children. Just as children with severe disabilities are not a homogeneous group, neither are their families. The early intervention professional working with young children with severe disabilities will no doubt encounter a diversity of families who vary in their cultural and economic conditions as well as their family structure (Vincent & Salisbury, 1988; Vincent, Salisbury, Strain, McCormick, & Tessier, 1989). Each family brings different resources to the task of parenting their child with special needs. Current thinking in the field emphasizes the importance of developing interventions that are based on parent identified needs and parent developed goals, instead of goals imposed upon families by professionals (Dunst, Trivette & Deal, 1988). This is perhaps particularly important for families with infants with multiple or severe disabilities because these families often are the recipients of a number of services. Services for these families should support families in "both *being* and *feeling* competent in their roles as parents and advocates" (Johnson-Martin, Davis, Goldman, & Gowen, 1989, p. 316).

Early intervention programs have several avenues for implementing family-focused intervention with their infants and toddlers with severe disabilities. Among these are case management, providing information, and providing instrumental and emotional support.

Case Management

For infants and toddlers with severe disabilities, case management can, and should, require considerable time and effort. Dunst and Trivette (1989) warn that the manner in which case management is approached can have major implications for the success of intervention. They propose an "enablement and empowerment" perspective of case management that puts the professional in a role of facilitating the family's ability to identify and access resources for their child. Families tend to be strengthened by this approach to case management because it does not usurp parent decision making, but rather supports active parent input and involvement.

Information Sharing

Families of children with severe disabilities frequently have a strong, and often urgent, need for information about the nature of their child's disabilities, specific caregiving or teaching strategies for their child, and predictions about what they might expect for their child in the future (Featherstone, 1979; Turnbull & Turnbull, 1990). Such information may be provided to families in a variety of ways.

For example, it is valuable for interventionists to ask families about their preferred manner of receiving information. The *Family Information Preference Inventory* (Turnbull & Turnbull, 1990) is one means of doing this. Possibilities for sharing information include written materials, consultation with a variety of professionals, group parent meetings, and discussion with other parents who have experienced similar situations. Remember, the desire for further information should originate with the parent. Professionals can be a helpful ally in securing the information parents desire, at the time parents desire it.

Instrumental and Emotional Support

A major aspect of family-focused intervention is facilitating positive family coping strategies through the provision of support (Dunst, 1985; Turnbull & Turnbull, 1990). There is evidence that social support reduces stress and feelings of inadequacy commonly reported in studies of parents of children with special needs (Vadasy, Fewell, Meyer, Schell, & Greenberg, 1984). For the families of infants with significant involvement, social support may be especially important and may take many forms. Participation in parent support groups and making provision for **respite care** can be very helpful. Parent to Parent is another type of support group which has been widely implemented in early intervention programs as a means of providing emotional and information support (Reynolds & Shanahan, 1981). This program trains parents of children with handicaps to serve as mentors for parents who have recently discovered their child has a disability. Many early intervention programs have witnessed the positive influence this form of support can have on both the parents receiving the support and those providing it.

For many families of children with significant disabilities, a major need is finding the time to do everything that must be done for their child and still have time to spend with other family members. Instrumental support such as providing regular respite care can make a tremendous impact on family well being. If formal respite care facilities are not available, early intervention programs may be able to organize volunteers for regular respite services and to provide the training volunteers might need to take care of infants with significant needs. Other options include helping parents organize child care exchanges, or supporting or helping parents use members of their extended family or friends to help with occasional child care. Other instrumental support may involve providing transportation, making appointments, arranging interagency conferences, and assisting with issues related to siblings in the home.

Parents can also help each other through membership in advocacy services or organizations. In some states, Parent Coalitions are now mounting advocacy activities. The activities of these groups range from assisting in the organization of state early intervention conferences to the development of state legislation.

These and other strategies are ways to offer informational, instrumental, and emotional support to families. However, perhaps the most necessary ingredient in supporting families is the development of a trusting, compassionate relationship between the professional and the family—a relationship that is designed to serve the best interests of the infant *and* the family, whatever they may be.

ASSESSMENT

Assessment is defined as the process of gathering information for decision-making purposes (Bailey & Wolery, 1989). Assessment of infants and toddlers with multiple or severe disabilities is done to make decisions about eligibility (**diagnostic assessment**), program planning, and program monitoring. As discussed in Chapter 2, assessment is more likely to be effective if it involves the collaborative efforts of a transdisciplinary team and involves the infant's family in meaningful ways.

Diagnostic Assessment

Diagnostic assessment includes information gathering and assessment activities undertaken by all members of the transdisciplinary team from the time of the child's initial referral. The importance of team assessment for the infant with multiple or severe disabilities cannot be overstated. Professionals, working closely from a variety of disciplines during this phase of assessment, examine the child's strengths and weaknesses to obtain information on the child's sensory functioning, motor condition, communication skills, and cognitive level. Clinical advancements in assessment of sensory functioning such as the Auditory Brainstem Response procedure (electrodes are used to record the brainstem response to auditory stimuli) and Visually Evoked Potential procedure (electrodes are used to determine brain activity in response to the reception of visual information) (Kinney, Ouellette, & Wolery, 1989) make it now possible to obtain sensory functioning information on many children previously thought to be untestable. Recent advances in pediatric assessment in the areas of physical and occupational therapy and communication disorders will, in the future, become part of the repertoire of many professionals in the early intervention field. All these types of team information are especially critical for the initial diagnostic assessment of infants with significant impairments.

Diagnostic assessment tends to use norm-referenced testing instruments (e.g., Bayley Scales of Infant Development [1969] and Griffiths Scales of Mental Development [1976]) that rely heavily on items requiring sensory and motor responses. Many infants with multiple or severe disabilities are unable to respond to such test items. Resulting scores on these assessments are likely to be quite low and, most frequently, do not accurately reflect the abilities of the infant (Simeonsson, Huntington, & Parse, 1980).

Program Planning and Monitoring

There is a growing dissatisfaction with the use of norm-referenced and criterion-referenced developmental assessment instruments for designing and evaluating educational programs for infants with significant disabilities. Gradel (1988) describes the problem this way:

> Assessment activities rarely correspond closely to interventions conducted in infant programs (Sheehan & Gallagher, 1984). Both norm-referenced instruments and criterion-referenced tools often meet neither the basic needs of the interventionist nor the demands presented by the heterogeneous skills and deficits of the baby with mild, moderate, or severe disabilities.... Examples abound in practice in which standard administrations of a developmental scale such as the Bayley Scales and the subsequent use of a skill profile generated from the test result in a list of intervention objectives consisting primarily of failed items. This is a highly restrictive pool of items on which to base an intervention. (p. 374)

Dissatisfaction with assessment instruments is perhaps strongest when such instruments are applied to the task of program planning and monitoring for infants with significant disabilities. Because these instruments rely on sensory and motor behavior, their use with the child with significant impairments in these areas may be useless. With some infants it is not uncommon to find that even the first items on a test cannot be passed, and yet apparent abilities go unexplored.

Process assessment methods.   The **process assessment approach** or the **child-referenced approach** to assessment, an alternative to traditional assessment, has as its goal an evaluation of strengths and deficits in order to provide a basis for intervention (Robinson & Fieber, 1988). Rather than documentation of level of development as the goal of assessment, the process assessment approach yields information on the learning processes used by the child and the child's ability to perform tasks in different settings and with different people (DuBose, Langley, & Stagg, 1977; Robinson & Fieber, 1988; Simeonsson, Huntington, & Parse, 1980; Stagg, 1988). The *Adaptive Performance Instrument (API)* (Gentry et al., in press) is an example of a process assessment that provides a good link between assessment and intervention. Items are task analyzed; adaptations can be made for different handicapping conditions and situations. Robinson and Fieber (1988) compare the process assessment approach to hypothesis testing:

> One tries a strategy and notes performance, tries another strategy and notes performance, and this cycle continues until the examiner is satisfied that the best possible performance has been obtained. (p. 136)

Robinson (1987) offers strategies for the assessment of cognitive development in motorically impaired children that employ a process assessment approach. Robinson's strategies include making adaptations in how a task is presented and in how a child responds when administering the Uzgiris-Hunt Scales of Infant Psychological Development (Uzgiris & Hunt, 1975). For example, some adapted task presentations include positioning the child to facilitate responses, positioning materials for easy accessibility, and modifying materials such as adding a bead to the end of a string to facilitate grasping. Some adapted response forms include accepting movement approximations, allowing adult-assisted movement, and observation of affective responses as an indication of cognitive stage. Robinson and Fieber (1988) remind professionals that performance on the specific items of the Uzgiris-Hunt Scales is not the most useful outcome from this assessment. Instead, the value lies within establishing the "overall stage organization as a framework for interpreting child behavior" (p. 135).

Similarly, Dunst and McWilliam (1988) propose an alternative to traditional assessment with infants with significant disabilities that is based on a developmental model of interactive competencies. The model, called the OBSERVE, is designed to measure a child's ability to learn new behavior by closely matching learning conditions to the response capabilities of the child. This is in contrast to traditional assessment procedures that require children to match their behavior to the response demands of a specific test item. By observing the child in response to environmental demands across contexts, this system identifies the type of developmental interactions the child has with the social and non-social environment. The OBSERVE is divided into five levels, following Piaget's sequence of cognitive development. The child is evaluated on responses to each level as the child moves through daily routines. An example of the use of this assessment system for an infant with severe disabilities is presented in Table 9–1. This assessment process permits the delineation of functional behaviors that are relevant and appropriate for difficult-to-test infants.

The gathering of information for making decisions about the appropriate targets and contexts of intervention is perhaps one of the most important functions of assessment practices. A number of characteristics and considerations for translating assessment information into intervention practices are described in the following section.

INTERVENTION

The strategies viewed as best practice in intervention with infants with significant disabilities has been evolving for a period of years. The emerging philosophy has come from theories of normal child development and research with both typical and atypical infants and their families. It is possible to summarize current thinking and research around four major tenets of intervention:

1. Intervention should incorporate strategies that encourage social reciprocity.
2. The infant should be actively involved in learning to control the environment.
3. Intervention should focus on the infant's functional use of behavior in typical social settings.
4. Intervention should use a combination of structured and responsive intervention strategies which depend on the characteristics of the infant, the intervention target, and the learning environment.

In general, intervention efforts that incorporate these principles work toward making infants *active* learners as opposed to passive recipients of environmental stimuli. To successfully promote development in young children with multiple impairments, interventionists must understand how to structure these principles into the infant's regular environment.

Enhancing Social Reciprocity

Interventions that promote social reciprocity are especially important for children with severe disabilities and their families (Rose, Calhoun & Ladage, 1989). Infants with multiple or severe disabilities often display behavior patterns that are atypical to such an extent that the development of normal infant-caregiver interactions may be difficult. The presence of increased irritability or nonresponsiveness, atypical motor responses, and the need for special procedures such as suctioning and tube feeding, all work against the development of typical parent-child interactions. Assessment and intervention strategies have been developed which allow the interventionist to facilitate more normalized, and rewarding, social interactions between parents and their infant with severe disabilities.

Als (1986) has developed a model of neonatal behavior, the Synactive Model of Neonatal Behavioral Organization, that holds promise for helping parents of premature or neurologically impaired babies read their infant's behavior and respond appropriately. Additionally, interventionists frequently use videotaped segments of

The young child with multiple and/or severe disabilities must be actively involved in learning to control the environment.

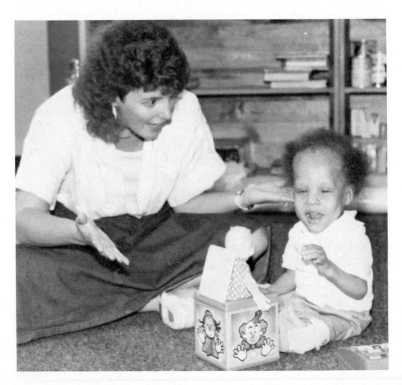

TABLE 9–1

Selected findings from using the OBSERVE to map a child's topography of behavior (pp. 241–243).*

CONTEXT OF ASSESSMENT

Levels of Development	Circle Time	Free Play	Group Time	Meals	Outside Play	Bathroom
Attentional interactions: The capacity to attend to and discriminate between stimuli	1. Looks at caregiver when she's talking or singing. 2. Orients toward different caregivers and children when they talk.	1. Attends to caregiver's actions. 2. Laughs at funny events. 3. Tracks objects moving in and out of visual field.	1. Smiles when talked to. 2. Attends to other children. 3. Looks with interest at toys placed on his travel chair tray.	1. Watches other children at the table. 2. Searches for sources of sounds.	1. Orients toward voice when his name is called. 2. Pays attention to sights and sounds on the playground.	1. Tracks children and caregivers as they come and go.
Contingency interactions: The use of simple, undifferentiated forms of behavior to initiate and sustain control over reinforcing consequences	1. Reaches for child to initiate interaction. 2. Vocalizes to get adult's attention.	1. Makes kite (suspended from ceiling) move using a string attached to his arm. 2. Swipes at wind chimes to make them move. 3. Rolls over to reinitiate social interaction.	1. Smiles or laughs to get adult to continue activity. 2. Picks up toys and "examines" them.	1. Finger-feeds self with some difficulty.	1. Vocalizes to have an adult continue activity (e.g., swinging).	

241

TABLE 9–1
(continued)

CONTEXT OF ASSESSMENT

Levels of Development	Circle Time	Free Play	Group Time	Meals	Outside Play	Bathroom
Differentiated interactions: The coordination and regulation of behavior that reflects elaboration and progress toward conventionalization	1. Responds to "What do you want to sing now?" using arm movements to indicate which song he wants to hear (nonconventional gestures). 2. Imitates actions of other children and caregivers. 3. Engages in reciprocal turn-taking during interactive episodes.	1. Moves toward play activity in walker. 2. Points to items on shelf. 3. Uses objects and toys to initiate play with caregiver. 4. Demonstrates complex motor action with objects (rolls car). 5. "Talks" and holds pretend phone conversations.	1. Chooses "favorite" activity among several options. 2. Points to items he wants if out of reach. 3. Associates sound with action (attempts car sounds). 4. Hands toys and objects to adults to have them activated. 5. Shows ability to feed doll using spoon and bottle.	1. Uses head shake or facial expression to indicate yes or no. 2. Reaches for or grasps spoon to help with feeding. 3. Uses spoon to eat with (although with considerable difficulty).	1. Moves toward children (in walker) to engage in play episodes. 2. Will imitate motor actions made by other children. 3. Plays cooperatively with other children (takes turns trying to throw ball).	1. Indicates yes or no when asked if he has to go to the bathroom.

Encoded interactions: The use of conventionalized forms of behavior that are context bound and that depend on referents as a basis for evoking the behaviors	1. Engages in pretend play (makes hotdogs, puts them in the oven to cook). 2. Pretends to "drive" car, vocalizations in attempt to make a motor sound. 3. Uses communication board to indicate desired activity. 4. Engages in pretend eating and drinking in doll corner.	1. Displays problem-solving abilities in getting objects and activities he wants. 2. Puts dolls in appropriate situations when playing house (e.g., baby in bed in bedroom, car in garage, stove in kitchen).	1. Uses symbol board to select food item he wants.	1. Chooses from approximately 10 outside activities on communication board. 2. Follows series of two related commands.
Symbolic interactions: The use of conventionalized forms of behavior to communicate a message in the absence of reference giving cues			1. Uses symbol board to signal desire to go to kitchen and eat.	

*Many of the behaviors displayed were approximations of those described because of the child's physical impairments.

Source: From *Assessment of Young Developmentally Disabled Children* (pp. 230–231) by T. Wach & R. Sheehan, 1988, New York: Plenum. Copyright © 1988, Plenum Publishers. Reprinted by permission.

243

parent-child interaction to help parents identify their child's meaningful behavior and to identify the effect parents' interaction style has on their child (Baird & Hass, 1989; McCollum & Stayton, 1985). For instance, using information gathered from an assessment of parent-child interaction in which the parent and child were observed in an unstructured play situation, an intervention goal may be to help the parent/caregiver wait until the infant makes eye contact before talking to the child. A program developed by Calhoun and Rose (1988) specifically targets crying and smiling, behaviors which dramatically influence parent-child relationships, to increase positive caregiver-child interactions. Clearly, any intervention which promotes positive social interactions between the infant with severe disabilities and the parents can profoundly improve the quality of life for both the infant and family.

Factors influencing social responsivity.   Infants with severe and multiple handicaps frequently manifest impaired motor and sensory abilities which interfere with their capacity to act upon and interact with their social and physical environment. In addition, their disabilities may interfere with or undermine a perception of competence that may further characterize interactions infants have with their environment.

Discrepancies between parental expectations and child performance theoretically lead to increases in parental direction (Hanzlik & Stevenson, 1986). Parents who are frustrated with their child's level of performance or who want to assist their infant to "catch up" have been found to adopt a directive teaching style as an attempt to encourage their infant to achieve higher level skills (Mahoney & Robenalt, 1986; Hanzlik & Stevenson, 1986). This adult-directed interaction style, in which parents "run the show," has been correlated with less developmental progress in nonhandicapped infants than an interaction style that is responsive to the child's interests (Mahoney, 1985). In general, families with severely handicapped young children often need to be trained to recognize infant-initiated behaviors and to encourage as well as reward these actions.

Infant-initiated learning.   A growing body of theoretical and empirical evidence suggests that responsive teaching styles are related to optimal development for normally developing, preterm, high-risk, and handicapped infants and children (Dunst, 1983; Goldberg, 1977; Linn & Horowitz, 1983; Mahoney, 1985). Specifically, parental responsivity has been found to be related to security of attachment (Smith & Pederson, 1988); compliance (Roberts & Strayer, 1987); and measures of mental development (Mahoney, 1985). Watson's (1976) seminal research on infant awareness of **contingency experiences** suggests that parents come to be endeared by infants because parents provide infants with contingent experiences which consequently promote infant feelings of efficacy and competence.

Contingency experiences, experiences that occur because of the infant's actions or behavior, enable infants to learn that they can effectively exert an influence or control various aspects of their social and physical world (Lewis, 1978). Conversely, exposure to repeated noncontingent experiences are thought to have a negative effect on infant learning, readiness to initiate and respond, motivation, and affective behavior. Although there is some controversy regarding whether infants display true signs of learned helplessness, the negative impact of repeated exposure to noncontingent experiences has been documented by negative facial expression and decreased response rate (Trad, 1986; Fincham & Cain, 1986).

Contingency experiences can be either social or nonsocial in nature. The most important social contingency experiences for infants occur in the context of infant-parent/caregiver interaction. Linn and Horowitz (1983) define **responsivity** in parental behavior as a tendency for a parent to quickly follow infant signaling behaviors with a behavior by the parent. **Contingent responsivity** in infant-parent interaction has been defined as parental behavior that is temporally and functionally related to the infant's signals. The degree to which parents observe their infant's behavior, notice cues or signaling behavior, interpret those behaviors, and respond according to their interpretations, is an indication of parental contingent responsivity to infants' behavior (Nover, Shore, Timberlake, & Greenspan, 1984). Through these experiences, infants encounter their world and create mental representations of themselves and their environment.

Nonsocial contingency experiences are also important for infant learning. These experiences provide infants with opportunities to learn the extent to which they can effectively exert an influence over, or control, aspects of their physical environment. Nonsocial contingency experiences occur when an infant obtains feedback about the effectiveness of an action upon the environment. For example, helium balloons tied to an infant's wrist, mobiles that are voice activated, and mirrors that provide visual images provide nonsocial contingency experiences which afford infants opportunities to learn the relationship between their behavior and its consequences on their environment.

Learning that outcomes are uncontrollable, which is often associated with repeated exposure to noncontingent experiences, leads to decreased awareness of an ability to exert an influence on the environment, decreased motivation to act, and depressed affect (Abramson, Seligman, Martin, & Teasdale, 1978).

Learning to Influence the Environment

Research in early infant development reminds us that nonhandicapped infants learn at a very early age that they can control various aspects of their environments (Watson, 1971; Brinker & Lewis, 1982). Only recently, however, have we begun to view intervention efforts from this perspective.

Dunst and Lesko (1988) advocate an approach to intervention they call providing *active learning episodes*. They state:

> Ironically, the inability of children with handicaps to learn to control their environments may have less to do with the lack of any inherent capabilities of the children and more to do with the types of interventions and experiences they are often afforded. It is not uncommon to find interventionists working with young handicapped children attempting to *elicit* behaviors like looking, listening and vocalizing by *stimulating* the children. Eliciting behaviors like visually tracking an object by moving it back-and-forth across the child's midline or shaking a rattle to the side of the child's head to elicit sound localization are examples of these types of experiences. This type of

TABLE 9–2
Active learning episodes for facilitating the acquisition of response-contingent behavior.

Behavior Target	Active Learning Episodes
Head rotation/visual fixation	1. Rotating the head from the side to midline (while supine) in order to activate lights using a head switch. 2. Rotating the head from the side to midline while being held in a nursing position in order to be talked to.
Head movements	1. Lifting the head off the floor while prone in order to view a visual display. 2. "Peeking" around a barrier in order to have a person say "peek-a-boo".
Sucking	1. Sucking on a nipple in order to produce a nutritive substance. 2. Sucking from a straw in order to produce a nutritive substance.
Arm movements	1. Swiping at a mobile or roly-poly in order to produce a reinforcing consequence. 2. Shaking the arm in an up-and-down movement in order to move a helium-filled balloon attached to a child's wrist. 3. Splashing in tub of water in order to produce an interesting spectacle.
Generalized excitement	1. Getting excited and bright-eyed in order to initiate and sustain social interactions. 2. Vigorous shaking of the body, arms, and legs in order to move a cradle to make a mobile attached to the cradle move.

Source: From "Promoting the Active Learning Capabilities of Young Children with Handicaps" by C. Dunst & J. Lesko, 1988, *Early Childhood Intervention Monograph*, No. 1. Morganton, NC: Family, Infant and Preschool Program, Western Carolina Center. Copyright © 1988, Family, Infant and Preschool Program, Western Carolina Center. Reprinted by permission.

stimulation is called *noncontingent* because the stimulation is presented independent of the child's own behavior. . . . Ironically, LARGE DOSES OF NONCONTINGENT STIMULATION OVER EXTENDED PERIODS OF TIME PROBABLY MAKE HANDICAPPED CHILDREN MORE PASSIVE AND MORE DIFFICULT TO TEACH TO BECOME ACTIVE LEARNERS. (p. 1)

These authors propose using **response-contingent learning episodes,** experiences that offer interesting consequences as a result of the child's actions on the environment. Response-contingent activities enable children to learn that their behavior has an impact on the environment. This understanding, which occurs rather easily for the nonhandicapped infant, may not occur or may occur in very limited form for the infant with significant motor, sensory, or cognitive delays.

Dunst and Lesko (1988) designed a program for children with handicaps who are functioning developmentally between birth and 6 to 8 months. This program is built around responses and contingencies that naturally occur in the child's environ-

TABLE 9–2
(continued)

Behavior Target	Active Learning Episodes
Grasping movements	1. Squeezing soft, pliable toys in order to produce auditory feedback. 2. Grasping and holding onto an adult's finger in order to play "pull-to-sit."
Directed gaze/visual	1. Looking toward a person in order to be talked to and played with. 2. Orienting toward a sight or sound in order to be able to see an interesting spectacle.
Smiling/laughter	1. Socially instigating and maintaining adult attention in order to have the adult continue playing lap games like "I'm gonna get you."
Cooing/babbling	1. Vocalizing in order to elicit and sustain an adult's attention. 2. Activating a visual display (e.g., slide projector) using a voice-activated microphone/switching device in order to view interesting pictures.
Foot/leg kicking	1. Kicking the legs in order to make a mobile move by a ribbon attached to the child's ankle and mobile. 2. Pushing against a hard surface or an adult's hand in order to move forward while supine or prone on the floor.

ment. The program begins with observation of the child to determine which behaviors in the child's repertoire should be selected for response-contingent learning. Potential behaviors include sucking, head rotations, directed gaze and visual fixations, smiling and laughter, cooing and babbling, gross body movements, arm movements and arm flexion/extension, grasping movements, and foot and leg kicking. After selecting reinforcers for the child, which are used as contingencies, active learning episodes are developed and used to promote the child's active learning capabilities. Table 9–2 presents examples of active learning episodes that may be used to develop response-contingent behaviors. As can be seen, unlike traditional intervention strategies, the infant must first perform some behavior (such as lifting the head) before some consequence (such as observing a desired toy) is consistently offered.

Functional Behavior in Typical Environments

Educators of students with severe handicaps have long advocated instruction that targets the development of functional skills in natural environments such as the home or center. This principle, which is used to select teaching goals for older students, also has utility for the selection of goals for severely handicapped infants. **Functional skills** are abilities that will be immediately useful to the infant and that will have relatively frequent opportunities for use in the infant's typical environment. Given the severity of learning deficits of most children with multiple or severe disabilities, it is difficult to justify the selection of any goal which will not be almost immediately useful for the infant in home, school, and community environments.

Choosing behavior targets that occur rather frequently during typical routines allows the provision of intervention that is **dispersed** or **distributed**, rather than **massed**. This means that teaching takes place in several different situations during the day, rather than in one situation with a specified number of trials. Dispersed intervention results in better generalization of learning to new situations and people (Holvoet, Guess, Mulligan, & Brown, 1980). For example, the child can be encouraged to manipulate and visually explore objects during dressing (e.g., exploring shoes), during feeding (e.g., examining the bottle or fabric of the mother's dress), and during bathing (e.g., placing floating balls in bath water).

However, interventionists must be careful to select goals which do not place excessive demands on the child's parent/caregiver. It is important that objectives are tasks that family members are able to implement without feeling overworked. The selection of excessive, complicated, or demanding procedures reduces the likelihood that the procedures will be implemented. Selecting goals that can be implemented easily during routine activities at home and in other settings facilitates their implementation. Table 9–3 provides a sample **intervention matrix** presented by Dunst and Lesko (1988) as an example of a strategy for combining intervention targets with daily routines so intervention will occur naturally throughout the day. Desired behaviors such as increasing social bids (e.g., social initiations) and intentional motor activity are elicited and regularly rewarded. Thinking of intervention in this way allows caregivers and interventionists to move away from the teaching-time model of intervention for severely disabled young children.

Responsive Intervention Techniques

Intervention strategies for teaching children with severe disabilities have traditionally encompassed highly structured, adult-directed techniques that emphasized bringing the child under stimulus control so desired behavior might be elicited in the presence of particular stimuli prompts and/or correction procedures. However, the generalization of skills taught in this manner has long been of concern (Guess, Keogh, & Sailor, 1978; Stokes & Baer, 1977). There is now considerable evidence to indicate that intervention that is responsive to child interests and is child-initiated will be more effective (Dunst & Lesko, 1988; Mahoney, Powell, Finnegan, Fors, & Wood, 1986). As a result, many early interventionists are advocating the use of incidental teaching (Hart & Risley, 1975), milieu teaching (Halle, 1987) and active learning episodes (Dunst & Lesko, 1988) for early intervention practices. As discussed in Chapter 4, the commonality among these approaches is the implementation of intervention strategies in a child-initiated context that occurs naturally during a relatively unstructured time. In using these approaches, interventionists must be keen observers

TABLE 9-3

Example of an intervention matrix for promoting the active learning capabilities of an infant with handicaps at home.

CHILD'S NAME _____ SETTING _____ PROGRAM PLAN _____ to _____

OBJECTIVES	ROUTINES					
	Wake-up	Dressing	Feeding	Playtime	Riding in the Car	Bathtime
Lifts head when prone to view visual displays and/or be responded to socially						
Uses social bids (e.g., smiling & vocalizations) to initiate adult-child interactions						
Uses kicking movements to produce movement of a mobile						
Lifts head up to midline position while in travel chair to observe goings-on						
Uses cooing sounds to evoke adult responsiveness						
Shakes arm up and down to produce movement of bells attached to child's wrist						
Activates a music box using a voice-activated microphone						

Source: From "Promoting the Active Learning Capabilities of Young Children with Handicaps" by C. Dunst & J. Lesko, 1988, *Early Childhood Intervention Monograph*, No. 1. Morganton, NC: Family, Infant and Preschool Program, Western Carolina Center. Copyright © 1988, Family, Infant and Preschool Program, Western Carolina Center. Reprinted by permission.

of child behavior, be aware of ways to arrange the environment to facilitate child initiations, and maximize adult responsiveness to child-initiated interactions with the social and nonsocial environment.

Interventionists do not have to forfeit all claim to structure in order to provide a responsive learning environment. It is possible, and often advisable, to implement procedures such as prompting and time-delay within a responsive learning environment. The key to utilizing these procedures in naturalistic teaching situations lies in tailoring intervention to the needs of each child while being careful to use the least intrusive teaching strategies needed to promote the learning of skills.

Prompts.   Instructional procedures for children with significant disabilities commonly include systematically applied **antecedent prompts** (cues, signals, or other assistance to get the child's attention) or **correction procedures** (demonstrating, cueing, or moving child through a task) in an effort to elicit desired behavior (Ault, Wolery, Doyle, & Gast, 1989). It is highly likely that there will be situations when using responsive teaching procedures that prompts are necessary. Dunst, Cushing, and Vance (1985), for example, investigated the response-contingent learning capabilities of six profoundly retarded, multihandicapped children. They used a visual display that illuminated contingent upon head turns made by the children. With these

Interventionists can be helpful to families in identifying ways to arrange the environment that facilitate child-initiated actions.

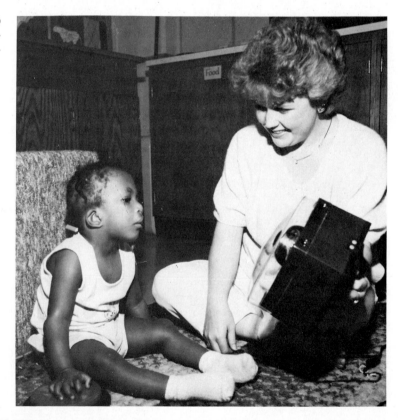

subjects, **conditioning latencies** occurred. That is, learning did not occur for several trials. When physical prompts were provided for head turns (the children's heads were physically moved to activate the display), the conditioning latency time was greatly reduced. Environmental arrangements for teaching severely handicapped infants, then, may necessitate some antecedent prompts or correction procedures. These may include an auditory stimulus, a physical prompt, or a visual stimulus to focus the child's attention.

Time delay.   Time-delay procedures can be used in naturalistic teaching to encourage infants to respond to physical or sensory cues without adult verbalization or direction (Halle, Marshall, & Spradlin, 1979). At the point in an interaction where the infant is to emit a particular behavior, the interventionist delays the prompt, waiting expectantly for the infant. If the infant performs the behavior before the end of the designated time delay period (usually a matter of seconds), the infant is rewarded and the activity continues. If not, the infant is prompted to perform the desired behavior. Time delay techniques promote independent actions in children.

The approaches to assessment and intervention described view developing children as embedded within their families. The nature of child-parent/caregiver interactions are an important context for infants to learn about their own capabilities as well as the behavior of others. The extent to which this "family system as context of infant learning" perspective can become a reality depends upon the program models used to guide assessment and intervention practices.

PROGRAM MODELS

Generally, programs for infants with severe disabilities consist of those services that are already available. Many families will require services delivered by different agencies, such as therapy or medical services, some of which may be difficult to obtain (Shelton, Jeppson, & Johnson, 1987). For example, an infant may be required to participate in a hospital follow-up clinic, hospital or home-based therapy services, home health services (including equipment maintenance services), and intervention program services. To make it more complicated, these agencies may have differing goals, orientations, funding sources, services, and eligibility requirements that further limit their availability. Although it is clear that few agencies have the resources to provide a total continuum of services to deal with all the needs that infants with severe disabilities and their families may have, services should be organized to maximize coordination among services, and reduce family stress.

The Niños Especiales Program (N.E.P.), for example, is an early intervention project funded by the Handicapped Children's Early Education Program to develop a culturally sensitive model of early intervention for infants with severe disabilities (Bruder, Anderson, Sheetz, & Caldera, in press). The Niños program serves the Puerto Rican community in Hartford, Connecticut. Staff are bilingual and familiar with the cultural heritage of the Puerto Rican population. As suggested in Chapter 8, such cultural sensitivity may enhance the results of intervention efforts. Services to children and families are provided by an early interventionist who makes weekly home visits.

TRANSDISCIPLINARY CASE

THE CASAS FAMILY

Rosa Casas is of Puerto Rican heritage. She is 23 years old, single, and has completed the 10th grade. English is her preferred language. She has lived all her life in the United States and has spent the last 12 years in Connecticut. Her socioeconomic situation is one of extreme poverty. She shares a one-bedroom apartment in a housing project with her two sisters and their three young children. Rosa is not employed and receives all financial assistance from the Department of Income Maintenance.

Juanita is Rosa's only child. Rosa enjoys children and has expressed disappointment about two previous miscarriages. Juanita was born to Rosa at 26 weeks gestation, weighing 1 pound 12 ounces. After birth, the child was hospitalized for 3 months due to complications that included severe respiratory distress, bronchial pulmonary dysplasia, retinopathy grade 1, apnea, anemia, jaundice, and reflux.

Juanita was referred to the Niños Especiales Program (N.E.P.) when she was 6 months old (3 months corrected age) by a project that offers follow-up to NICU infants. The N.E.P. is an early intervention project funded by the Handicapped Children's Early Education Program to develop a culturally sensitive model of early intervention. At the time of referral, Juanita's motor tone was spastic, visual tracking was inconsistent, and she was not smiling spontaneously. Juanita was followed medically by a pediatric clinic, a neonatal follow-up clinic, and by an ophthalmologist.

During the initial needs assessment, Rosa expressed a strong desire to have her own two-bedroom apartment that would enable her to remain close to her sisters (a needed source of support for her) and medical care providers. She had no transportation and needed access to the emergency room due to Juanita's frequent respiratory illnesses. Rosa also requested assistance during Juanita's frequent medical visits because she was feeling overwhelmed dealing with so many professionals. She requested ongoing information and clarification regarding Juanita's test results (medical and educational) as well as information on feeding and nutrition. Juanita's test results from the transdisciplinary team showed significant developmental delays, with delays in the motor domain being most significant.

The interventionists from N.E.P. addressed needs related to family support, parent information, and early intervention. The Individualized Family Service Plan (IFSP) for Juanita and Rosa had the following goals:

1. Rosa will attend medical visits for Juanita with the interventionist's assistance.
2. Rosa will obtain a housing certificate with the interventionist's assistance.
3. Rosa will read and utilize information on feeding and nutrition provided by the interventionist.
4. Rosa will be able to explain Juanita's test results to the interventionist.
5. Rosa will demonstrate these motor activities with Juanita—facilitation of independent sit-

The interventionist works with the family to help them identify and acquire the resources and information needed to manage the medical and educational needs of their child. An example of services provided by the N.E.P. is provided in the case study.

PROGRAM EVALUATION

The efficacy of evaluating programs for severely and multiply handicapped infants has received much attention (Bricker, Bailey, & Bruder, 1984; Dunst, 1986; Guralnick, 1988; Hanson, 1984). The result of this scrutiny has been an increased awareness of the importance of viewing evaluation as a means of improving early intervention service systems.

ting, rolling, rocking on hands and knees, and reaching for objects in front of her—with assistance from the physical therapist.

Ninety-minute home visits by the early interventionist in Rosa's home occurred weekly. A typical home visit began by addressing the support and information goals in the IFSP. For example, the interventionist followed up on the housing issue by finding out how many apartments Rosa had visited. Next, the interventionist observed Rosa feeding Juanita to check her understanding of the nutritional information previously received. Each session typically ended with both Rosa and the interventionist playing with Juanita to increase Rosa's enjoyment of her child and to model naturalistic teaching tactics. During these play times, social interaction and communication activities were also emphasized. The play interactions were responsive, reciprocal, and mutually pleasurable. Juanita laughed frequently.

A physical therapist from the Visiting Nurse Association also made home visits twice a week, and the interventionist and physical therapist made joint visits at least once a month. (Because so many professionals were involved, careful coordination of services and training on cultural issues and preferences were systematically arranged.) Therapy sessions included neurodevelopmental treatment techniques, facilitation of dynamic movement patterns within a developmental sequence, facilitation of weight bearing with mobility, providing sensorimotor and vestibular input, and helping Rosa in home intervention. During home visits, Rosa was assisted in carrying out these activities within her daily routine.

One year after referral to N.E.P., Rosa is living in her own apartment in a safer neighborhood, within walking distance of her sisters and medical care providers. This was the most difficult goal to achieve, due to a severe housing shortage. She successfully applied for public housing with support and transportation provided by N.E.P. As head of the household, Rosa now qualifies for her own Food Stamps and other forms of financial assistance (before this, her older sister listed her as a dependent for those services). Prior to the move she enrolled in Job Connection and is receiving secretarial training on a half-time basis. Rosa's cousin, who lives nearby, was willing to care for Juanita. Rosa is now comfortable taking Juanita to her various medical appointments, so assistance in this area was reduced.

Juanita is now 17 months old (14 months corrected age). She has a visual defect in her left eye and continued hypertonicity. Juanita is eating table foods with no further reflux, and beginning to verbally communicate her needs.

Success at meeting the child's needs were, in part, dependent upon responsiveness to the concerns and needs of the mother. It is often difficult to separate the needs of the family from those of the child. A broad-based social context of early intervention practices is often necessary and may produce the most lasting positive outcomes for the child.

Program evaluation is an objective, systematic process for gathering information about a program or set of activities that can be used to ascertain the program's ability to achieve stated goals; suggest modifications that might lead to improvement in quality and effectiveness; and lead to well-informed decisions about the worth, merit, and level of support a program warrants (Bickman & Weatherford, 1988). For program evaluation to be effective, it must be designed with specific purposes in mind. Few early intervention programs have well-developed purposes and evaluation plans prior to the beginning of service, and therefore, compromise their program's ability to document outcomes (Sheehan & Gallagher, 1983).

Early intervention programs that serve severely disabled infants and families must consider a number of issues when designing evaluation plans. The first is the heterogeneity of this population. This factor may limit the types and scope of variables that can be measured across the group of program participants. The second factor relates to the first, in that few standardized tools are available that either meet the diverse developmental needs of the population, or measure small rates of growth over time. A third factor relates to the inherent methodological limitations that may compromise evaluation efforts with the severely disabled or any other children.

In order to remedy these problems, it has been suggested that evaluation for early intervention programs be multidimensional (Sheehan & Gallagher, 1983). For the most severely disabled infants, the measurement of program effectiveness should match the specific goals of each child's interventions. This means that information that reflects the infant's attainment of goals (such as increases in interactional competence, contingency awareness, and engagement with the environment) are used to evaluate the effectiveness of intervention.

In addition, programs should measure the outcomes of various family variables such as independent resource management or mobilization of support networks. Finally, program evaluation should be conducted using both **formative** (during program operation) and **summative** (at the completion of services) schedules. Proper attention to these considerations will increase the likelihood that program activities will achieve intended goals.

The preceding case study illustrates how a broad-based and culturally sensitive service delivery system influences the outcomes of meeting both child and family needs.

SUMMARY OF PROCEDURES

Because of the wide range of functioning levels in infants and toddlers designated as having severe and multiple disabilities and the equally diverse needs of their families, it is difficult to discuss intervention techniques for this population as a group. However, some of the key procedures that have been discussed in this chapter follow:

1. Use special sensitivity when providing parents of children with severe disabilities information and support because these parents tend to experience extreme stress levels, often prompted by their child's caregiving responsibilities.
2. Provide families with options about the way in which they would like information to be shared with them.
3. Use process assessment methods and instruments, such as the OBSERVE, to better plan and monitor intervention programs for infants and toddlers with multiple handicaps. Use adapted task presentations and adapted child responses for better evaluation of child competence and learning.
4. Use social contingency experiences (e.g., tickling each time a child vocalizes or touching the child after a look) and nonsocial contingency experiences (e.g., helium balloon tied to the child's wrist or a mirror in the crib) to encourage social responsivity.

5. Use waiting for the child's response, turn-taking, and arrangement of active learning episodes to encourage infant-initiated, response-contingent learning.
6. Use responsive intervention strategies, such as naturalistic teaching techniques, to advance the child's development in typical structured and unstructured daily routines.
7. Use functionality as a guide in the selection of teaching goals for children and their families.
8. Emphasize interagency communication in case management to increase uneventful coordination of services. Families with severely handicapped infants, requiring services from a number of disciplines, are especially at risk to become overwhelmed by the flow of professionals in their lives.

SUMMARY

Intervention programs serving infants with multiple or severe disabilities begin by focusing on family needs as well as the needs of the child. Higher levels of parental/family stress have been found to be associated with characteristics typical of severely handicapped infants such as increased caregiving demands, slower rates of child progress, and reduced social responsiveness. Providing information and instrumental and emotional support can promote positive coping strategies in families. Any service provided to families should be undertaken with the intention of strengthening families' active involvement and decision making with regard to their child's educational program.

Theoretical and empirical evidence support intervention strategies that focus on the child's social and nonsocial interactions with the environment. Responsive teaching styles, which allow for infant-initiated rather than adult-directed interactions, are important for the learning of severely handicapped young children. Interventionists working with these infants and toddlers are challenged to identify situations, throughout the children's daily routine, that facilitate the development of appropriate interactions with both people and objects in their environment.

DISCUSSION QUESTIONS

1. How does an enablement and empowerment approach to case management differ from case management that is primarily concerned with the delivery of intervention services? How might you evaluate the success of the former approach?
2. What are the potential benefits of process assessment methods for designing intervention programs for infants with multiple or severe disabilities?
3. What is the philosophical rationale for intervention strategies that emphasize infant-initiated learning versus teacher-directed learning?

APPLIED ACTIVITIES/PROJECTS

1. Observe an infant with multiple or severe disabilities during three daily routines (home- or center-based program) and record examples of each of the five types of interactions used in the OBSERVE.
2. Observe an infant who is functioning at younger than 8 months of age and design a strategy for using contingency interactions to promote infant learning.
3. Interview a family with a severely handicapped toddler. Ask a family member to describe: the advantages and disadvantages of the family's circumstances, the most useful coping mechanism the family employs, and the way the family's social context has responded to their situation. Explain what this family's experiences mean to an interventionist who provides both professional and emotional support.

SUGGESTED READINGS

Cross, T., Bazron, B., Dennis, K., & Isaacs, M. (1989). *Towards a culturally competent system of care: A monograph on effective services for minority children who are severely emotionally disturbed*. Washington, DC: CASSP Technical Assistance Center, Georgetown University Child Development Center.

Dunst, C. J., & Lesko, J. (1988). Promoting the active learning capabilities of young children with handicaps. *Early Childhood Intervention Monograph, 1,*(1). Morganton, NC: Family, Infant and Preschool Program, Western Carolina Center.

Wachs, T., & Sheehan, R. (1988). *Assessment of young developmentally disabled children*. New York: Plenum.

REFERENCES

Abramson, L. Y., Seligman, M., Martin, E. P., & Teasdale, J. D. (1978). Learned helplessness in humans: Critique and reformulation. *Journal of Abnormal Psychology, 87,* 49–74.

Als, H. (1986). A synactive model of neonatal behavioral organization: Framework for the assessment and support of neurobehavioral development of premature infants and their parents in the environment of the NICU. In J. K. Sweeney (Ed.), *Physical and occupational therapy in pediatrics* (Vols. 3 & 4) (pp. 3–55). New York: Haworth.

Ault, M., Wolery, M., Doyle, P., & Gast, D. (1989). Review of comparative studies in the instruction of students with moderate and severe handicaps. *Exceptional Children, 55,* 346–356.

Bailey, D., & Wolery, M. (1989). *Assessing infants and preschoolers with handicaps*. Columbus, OH: Merrill.

Baird, S., & Haas, L. (1989). *Maternal interpretation of prelinguistic infant behavior*. Unpublished manuscript: Auburn University.

Barber, P., Turnbull, A., Behr, S., & Kerns, G. (1988). A family systems perspective on early childhood special education. In S. Odom & M. Karnes (Eds.), *Early intervention for infants and children with handicaps: An empirical base* (pp. 179–198). Baltimore: Paul H. Brookes.

Bayley, N. (1969). *Bayley Scales of Infant Development*. New York: Psychological Corporation.

Beckman-Bell, P. (1981). Child-related stress in families of handicapped children. *Topics in Early Childhood Special Education, 1,* 45–53.

Bickman, L., & Weatherford, D. (1988). *Evaluating early intervention programs for severely handicapped children and their families*. Austin, TX: PRO-ED.

Bricker, D., Bailey, E., & Bruder, M. B. (1984). The efficacy of early intervention and the handicapped infant. In M. Wolraich & D. Routh (Eds.), *Advances in developmental and behavioral pediatrics* (Vol. 5) (pp. 373–423). Greenwich, CT: JAI Press.

Brinker, R., & Lewis, M. (1982). Discovering the competent handicapped infant: A process approach to assessment and intervention. *Topics in Early Childhood Special Education, 2,* 1–16.

Bruder, M. B., Anderson, R., Sheetz, G., & Caldera, M. (In press). Niños Especiales Program: A culturally sensitive model of early intervention. *Journal of Early Intervention.*

Calhoun, M. L., & Rose, T. L. (1988). Promoting positive parent-child interactions. *TEACHING Exceptional Children, 21*(4), 44–45.

Dollar, S., & Brooks, C. (1980). Assessment of severely and profoundly handicapped. *Exceptional Educational Quarterly, 1,* 87–101.

DuBose, R., Langley, B., & Stagg, V. (1977). Assessing severely handicapped children. *Focus on Exceptional Children, 9,* 1–13.

Dunst, C. J. (1983). Communicative competence and deficits: Effects on early social interactions. In E. McDonald & D. Gallagher (Eds.), *Facilitating social-emotional development in young multiply handicapped children* (pp. 93–140). Philadelphia: HLM Press.

Dunst, C. J. (1985). Rethinking early intervention. *Analysis and Intervention in Developmental Disabilities, 5,* 165–201.

Dunst, C. J. (1986). Overview of efficacy of early intervention programs. In L. Brickman & D. Weatherford (Eds.), *Evaluating early intervention programs for severely handicapped children and their families* (pp. 79–148). Austin, TX: PRO–ED.

Dunst, C. J., Cushing, P. J., & Vance, S. (1985). Response-contingent learning in profoundly handicapped infants: A social systems perspective. *Analysis and Intervention in Developmental Disabilities, 5,* 33–47.

Dunst, C. J., & Lesko, J. (1988). Promoting the active learning capabilities of young children with handicaps. *Early Childhood Intervention Monograph,* 1. Morganton, NC: Family, Infant and Preschool Program, Western Carolina Center.

Dunst, C. J., & McWilliam, R. A. (1988). Cognitive assessment of multiply handicapped young children. In T. Wachs & R. Sheehan (Eds.), *Assessment of young developmentally disabled children* (pp. 213–238). New York: Plenum.

Dunst, C., & Trivette, C. (1989). An enablement and empowerment perspective of case management. *Topics in Early Childhood Special Education, 8,* 87–102.

Dunst, C. J., Trivette, C. M., & Deal, A. G. (1988). *Enabling and empowering families: Principles and guidelines for practice.* Cambridge, MA: Brookline Books.

Featherstone, H. (1979). *A difference in the family.* New York: Penguin.

Fewell, R. (1986). A handicapped child in the family. In R. Fewell & P. Vadasy (Eds.), *Families of handicapped children: Needs and supports across the life span* (pp. 3–34). Austin, TX: PRO-ED.

Fincham, F. D., & Cain, K. M. (1986). Learned helplessness in humans: A developmental analysis. *Developmental Review, 6,* 301–333.

Gentry, D., Bricker, D., Brown, E., Hart, V., McCartan, K., Vincent, E., & White, O. (in press). *Adaptive Performance Instrument.* Moscow: University of Idaho Press.

Goldberg, S. (1977). Social competence in infancy: A model of parent-infant interaction. *Merrill-Palmer Quarterly, 23,* 163–177.

Gradel, K. (1988). Interface between assessment and intervention for infants and preschoolers with disabilities. In T. Wachs & R. Sheehan (Eds.), *Assessment of young developmentally disabled children* (pp. 373–396). New York: Plenum.

Griffiths, R. (1976). *The abilities of babies.* High Wycombe, England: The Test Agency Ltd.

Guess, D., Keogh, W., & Sailor, W. (1978). Generalization of speech and language behavior: Measurement and training tactics. In R. L. Schiefelbusch (Ed.), *Bases of language intervention,* (Vol. 2) (pp. 373–396). Baltimore: University Park Press.

Guralnick, M. (1988). Efficacy research in early childhood intervention programs. In S. Odom & M. Karnes (Eds.), *Early intervention for infants and children with handicaps: An empirical base* (pp. 75–88). Baltimore: Paul H. Brookes.

Halle, J. W. (1987). Teaching language in the natural environment: An analysis of spontaneity. *Journal of the Association for Persons with Severe Handicaps, 12,* 28–37.

Halle, J. W., Marshall, A. M., & Spradlin, J. E. (1979). Time delay: A technique to increase language use and facilitate generalization in retarded children. *Journal of Applied Behavior Analysis, 12,* 431–439.

Hanson, M. (1984). The effects of early intervention. In M. Hanson (Ed.), *Atypical infant development* (pp. 385–406). Baltimore: University Park Press.

Hanzlik, J. R., & Stevenson, M. B. (1986). Interaction of mothers with infants who are mentally retarded, retarded with cerebral palsy, or nonretarded. *American Journal of Mental Deficiency, 90,* 513–520.

Hart, B., & Risley, T. (1975). Incidental teaching of language in the preschool. *Journal of Applied Behavior Analysis, 8,* 411–420.

Holvoet, J., Guess, D., Mulligan, M., & Brown, F. (1980). The individual curriculum sequencing model (II): A teaching strategy for severely handicapped students. *Journal of the Association for Persons with Severe Handicaps, 5,* 337–351.

Johnson-Martin, N., Davis, B., Goldman, B., & Gowen, J. (1989). Working with families in early intervention. In C. Tingey, *Implementing early intervention* (pp. 303–318). Baltimore: Paul H. Brookes.

Kinney, P., Ouellette, T., & Wolery, M. (1989). Screening and assessing sensory functioning. In D. Bailey & M. Wolery (Eds.), *Assessing infants and preschoolers with handicaps* (pp. 144–165). Columbus, OH: Merrill.

Lewis, M. (1978). The infant and its caregiver: The role of contingency. *Allied Health and Behavioral Sciences, 1,* 469–492.

Linn, L., & Horowitz, F. (1983). The relationship between infant individual differences and mother-infant interaction during the neonatal period. *Infant Behavior and Development, 6,* 415–427.

Mahoney, G. (1985, April). *Mother-child interaction: Research and intervention with young handicapped children.* A presentation at The Council for Exceptional Children 63rd Annual Convention, Anaheim, CA.

Mahoney, G., Powell, A., Finnegan, C., Fors, S., & Wood, S. (1986). *The transactional intervention program: Theory, procedures and evaluation.* Unpublished paper, Department of Special Education, School of Education, University of Michigan.

Mahoney, G., & Robenalt, K. (1986). A comparison of conversational patterns between mothers and their Down Syndrome and normal infants. *Journal of the Division for Early Childhood, 10,* 172–180.

McCollum, J., & Stayton, V. (1985). Infant/parent interaction: Studies and intervention guidelines based on the SIAI model. *Journal of the Division for Early Childhood, 9,* 125–135.

Nover, A., Shore, M., Timberlake, E., & Greenspan, S. I. (1984). The relationship of maternal perception and maternal behavior: A study of normal mothers and their infants, *Journal of the American Orthopsychiatric Association, 54,* 210–223.

Reynolds, K., & Shanahan, V. (1981). *The Parent to Parent Program: Organizational handbook.* Athens: University Affiliated Facility, University of Georgia.

Roberts, W., & Strayer, J. (1987). Parents' responses to the emotional distress of their children: Relations with children's competence. *Developmental Psychology, 23,* 415–422.

Robinson, C. (1987). A strategy for assessing motorically impaired infants. In I. Uzgiris & J. Hunt (Eds.), *Infant performance and experience: New findings with the ordinal scales* (pp. 311–339). Urbana: University of Illinois Press.

Robinson, C., & Fieber, N. (1988). Cognitive assessment of motorically impaired infants and preschoolers. In T. Wachs & R. Sheehan (Eds.), *Assessment of young developmentally disabled children* (pp. 127–162). New York: Plenum.

Rose, T., Calhoun, M. L., & Ladage, L. (1989). Helping young children respond to caregivers. *Teaching Exceptional Children 21,* 48–51.

Sheehan, R., & Gallagher, R. (1983). Conducting evaluations of infant intervention programs. In S. G. Garwood & R. Fewell (Eds.), *Educating handicapped infants: Issues in development and intervention* (pp. 352–424). Rockville, MD: Aspen.

Sheehan, R., & Gallagher, R. J. (1984). Assessment of infants. In P. Mittanson (Ed.), *Atypical infant development* (pp. 495–524). Austin, TX: PRO-ED.

Shelton, T. L., Jeppson, E. S., & Johnson, B. H. (1987). *Family-centered care for children with special health care needs* (2nd ed.). Washington, DC: The Association for the Care of Children's Health.

Simeonsson, R., Huntington, G., & Parse, S. (1980). Assessment of children with severe handicaps: Multiple problems—multivariate goals. *Journal of the Association for the Severely Handicapped, 5,* 55–72.

Smith, P. B., & Pederson, D. R. (1988). Maternal sensitivity and patterns of infant-mother attachment. *Child Development, 59,* 1097–1101.

Stagg, V. (1988). Clinical considerations in the assessment of young handicapped children. In T. Wachs & R. Sheehan (Eds.), *Assessment of young developmentally disabled children* (pp. 61–74). New York: Plenum.

Stokes, T. F., & Baer, D. M. (1977). An implicit technology of generalization. *Journal of Applied Behavior Analysis, 10,* 349–367.

Trad, P. V. (1986). *Infant depression: Paradigms and paradoxes.* New York: Springer–Verlag.

Turnbull, A. P., & Turnbull, H. R. (1990). *Families, professionals, and exceptionality: A special partnership* (2nd ed.). Columbus, OH: Merrill.

Uzgiris, I., & Hunt, J. (1975). *Assessment in infancy: Ordinal Scales of Psychological Development.* Urbana: University of Illinois Press.

Vadasy, P. F., Fewell, R. R., Meyer, D. J., Schell, G., & Greenberg, D. (1984). Siblings of handicapped children: A developmental perspective on family interactions. *Family Relations, 33,* 155–167.

Vincent, L. J., & Salisbury, C. L. (1988). Changing economic and social influences on family involvement. *Topics in Early Childhood Special Education, 8,* 48–59.

Vincent, L. J., Salisbury, C. L., Strain, P. S., McCormick, K. C., & Tessier, A. (1989). A behavioral-ecological approach to early intervention: Focus on cultural diversity. In S. Meisels & J. Shonkoff (Eds.), *Handbook of early intervention* (pp. 173–195) London: Cambridge University Press.

Wach, T., & Sheehan, R. (1988). *Assessment of young developmentally disabled children.* New York: Plenum.

Watson, J. S. (1971). Cognitive-perceptual development in infancy: Setting for the seventies. *Merrill-Palmer Quarterly of Behavior and Development, 17,* 139–152.

Watson, J. S. (1976). Smiling, cooing, and "the game." In J. S. Bruner, A. Jolley, & K. Sylva (Eds.), *Play—Its role in development and evolution* (pp. 268–276). New York: Basic Books.

Ziegler, D. (1989). *Definitions and eligibility criteria.* Division for Early Childhood White Paper. Reston, VA: The Council for Exceptional Children.

10

Techniques for Infants and Toddlers with Hearing Impairments

Marilyn Sass-Lehrer

OVERVIEW

This chapter discusses issues relating to providing services to hearing-impaired infants and toddlers and their families, including:

- ☐ effects of hearing loss on perceptual, social-emotional, cognitive, and communication and language development
- ☐ communication methodologies for hearing-impaired infants and toddlers
- ☐ family involvement and education
- ☐ assessment and intervention strategies for transdisciplinary teaming with hearing-impaired young children

THE EFFECTS OF HEARING LOSS

Although hearing loss does not cause any delays in cognitive, social-emotional, or motor development (Furth, 1966; Rosenstein, 1961; Vernon, 1967), the inability to hear has a profound impact on the acquisition of communication skills. Delays or barriers to communication may, in turn, inhibit the development of some cognitive abilities, and may have a negative impact on self-concept and social interactions (Allen, 1986). Effective early interventionists working with families and other specialists can help minimize or prevent the occurrence of delays or disabilities which may result from the inability to hear and communicate.

Many factors influence the effects of hearing loss. For some children a hearing loss has minimal consequences for overall development, communication, educational achievement, or social interactions. For others, the impact is devastating. To understand why hearing loss affects different children in different ways, it is important to consider the factors related to hearing loss, the characteristics of each child, and the uniqueness of each family.

Causes of Hearing Loss

The cause, type, and degree of severity of a hearing loss have significant repercussions on development. Hearing loss may occur at any time in life. A **congenital hearing loss,** one which is present at birth, is potentially more devastating to communication and spoken language acquisition than a loss which occurs **postlingually,** after one has developed communication skills.

Since 1980 the major causes of deafness identified in young children are heredity, **cytomegalovirus** (CMV), **meningitis,** and complications of prematurity (Moores, 1987). Genetic factors or heredity are the known causes of approximately 50% of all cases of hearing loss. Parents and professionals may be unaware of a genetic cause of a hearing loss because family members may be carriers of deafness genes and yet have normal hearing. Approximately one-third of all cases of genetic hearing loss are related to syndromes such as Waardenburg's Syndrome and Usher's Syndrome (Vernon, 1982). Refer to Batshaw and Perret (1981) for information about these syndromes.

Complications during pregnancy or at birth that may result in a hearing loss include maternal rubella, a major cause of deafness in the mid 1960's; mother-child blood incompatibility such as Rh-factor complications; **hyperbilirubinemia;** cytomegalovirus, a herpes virus; infections; prematurity; or birth complications which result in anoxia or injuries incurred during the birth process. Postnatal causes of hearing loss include **otitis media;** meningitis, the most common postnatal cause of hearing loss in school-age children; and accidents resulting in head trauma.

Genetic counseling is recommended for families with a hearing-impaired child. Parents are often concerned about the chance of another child in the family having a hearing impairment, but the knowledge of the cause of deafness may also provide parents and professionals with critical information about the medical and educational implications of hearing loss for their child. Vernon (1982) describes additional handicapping conditions associated with the major origins of deafness. Parents and infant interventionists need to be aware of conditions related to certain causes, and which etiologies require specialized intervention strategies.

Types of Hearing Loss

Hearing loss may be described as either sensorineural, conductive, or mixed. A **sensorineural hearing loss** is caused by damage to the inner ear. Damage to the cochlea or the auditory nerve generally cannot be corrected medically or surgically and often results in a significant loss of hearing. A sensorineural hearing loss is characterized by a decreased sensitivity to sound and impaired word recognition abilities. Hearing aids and intensive instruction on the development of listening skills is often required.

A **conductive hearing loss** is characterized by a decreased sensitivity to sound but does not generally affect word recognition abilities. Conductive hearing loss results from problems in the middle or outer ear such as otitis media or middle ear fluid. Conditions associated with a conductive hearing loss may be corrected medically or surgically. However, if correction is not possible or must be delayed, consistent and appropriate amplification and development of listening skills may be needed.

Mixed hearing losses have both a sensorineural and conductive component. An individual with a mixed loss may experience difficulties with both loudness and distortion.

Another way to describe hearing loss is by the severity of the loss, or how loud a sound must be at different pitches before an individual can hear it. To determine this, an audiologist assesses responses to different sounds and plots the results on an audiogram. Figure 10–1 shows an audiogram with the relative loudness and pitch of common environmental and speech sounds. Loudness, or intensity of sound, is measured in decibel (dB) units. These are shown on the horizontal lines of the audiogram. The average decibel level at which people with normal hearing are first able to detect sounds is 0 dB Hearing Level (HL).

FIGURE 10–1

Audiogram with relative loudness and pitch of common environmental sounds. (Source: From *Picture Audiogram* by M. A. Kinsella-Meier & F. C. Vold, 1989, University Park, MD: Audiology Communication Counseling. Copyright © 1989 by M. A. Kinsella-Meier and F. C. Vold. Adapted by permission. Reproductions of this color 18″ × 24″ poster can be obtained by writing to 6822 Pineway, University Park, MD 20782.)

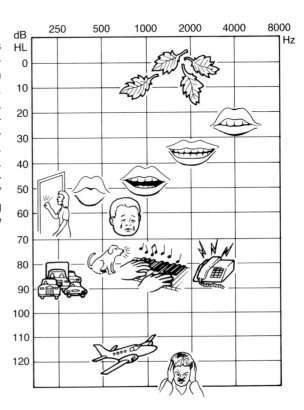

Pitch or frequency of sound is measured in **Hertz (Hz)**. The range of response to pitch measured on an audiogram is between 250 and 8000 Hz. An audiogram measures responses to pure tones that are single-frequency sounds. Most sounds in everyday life, however, are multi-frequency, with both low- and high-frequency components. The rumbling of thunder and the beat of a drum are examples of sounds that have strong low-frequency components. The chirping of birds and the sound of a spoon tapping a glass are sounds with strong high-frequency components. The frequencies most important for speech recognition are between 500 and 4000 Hz. Responses to pitch are shown on the vertical lines of the audiogram in Figure 10–1.

Degrees of severity of hearing loss are categorized as normal hearing, mild, moderate, severe, and profound hearing loss. Table 10–1 describes these categories and the difficulties that may be experienced with a particular severity of hearing loss.

It is important for infant interventionists to be able to understand the basic information provided in an audiogram in order to develop appropriate intervention plans. Deaf education specialists and audiologists should work with all team members, including families, to explain the nature and severity of the hearing loss and to discuss the implications for each child's development. Hearing impaired specialists and audiologists should closely monitor the child's auditory behaviors and develop auditory intervention strategies appropriate for the child's hearing abilities. Families, hearing specialists, and other team members need to understand the implications of the child's impairment to insure provision of appropriate services including an effective plan for **auditory habilitation**.

Perceptual Development

Hearing-impaired children experience the same rate and sequence of development in motor areas as normally hearing children. In the absence of additional disabilities all sensory avenues, with the exception of hearing, are unaffected. Often infants with hearing impairments appear to be very alert, active, and curious because they depend upon vision and physical interaction with the environment to learn about their surroundings.

A severe or profound loss of hearing, however, results in a lost opportunity to use hearing to acquire information about the environment and the people in it. Studies of both animals and humans suggest that early auditory deprivation may result in prolonged decreased sensitivity or responsiveness to sound (Northern & Downs, 1984). Although there is controversy concerning the impact and alterability of early auditory deprivation, researchers and practitioners agree that auditory stimulation during the first year of life is critical.

Without hearing, the infant is unable to acquire spoken language through normal interactions with parents and significant others. The abilities to process spoken language, interpret the emotional messages conveyed through tone of voice, and make sense of many events in the environment are affected by a loss of hearing. Early auditory deprivation may prevent the infant from perceiving the world as secure, predictable, and responsive in the same way that a normally hearing infant does.

TABLE 10–1
Classification and characteristics of hearing loss.

Group	Threshold Range[1]	Description of Hearing Loss	WITHOUT AMPLIFICATION			WITH AMPLIFICATION		
			Audibility of Conversational Speech	Discrimination Capacity for Speech	Learning Modality	Audibility of Conversational Speech	Discrimination Capacity	Learning Modality
I	15–30 dB	Mild	Normal	Normal	Auditory	Normal	Normal	Auditory
II	31–60 dB	Moderate	Partial	Almost normal	Auditory w. support from vision	Normal	Almost normal	Auditory
III	61–90 dB	Severe	None	Irrelevant	Visual	Normal	Good[2]	Auditory w. support from vision
IV	91–120 dB	Profound	None	Irrelevant	Visual	Partial	Poor[3]	Visual w. support from audition
V	121 dB or more	Total	None	Irrelevant	Visual	None	Irrelevant	Visual

[1]Average of pure tone thresholds at 500, 1000 and 2000 Hz in dBHL using the standard for normal threshold set by the American National Standards Institute (ANSI) in 1969.
[2]Main problems are with discrimination of voice quality differences and place of articulation of consonants.
[3]Main benefits of hearing are in recognition and control of rhythm and intonation and discrimination of certain vowel differences.

Source: From *Hearing Impairments in Young Children* (p. 54) by A. Boothroyd, 1982, Washington, DC: Alexander Graham Bell Association, Inc. Copyright © 1982, Alexander Graham Bell Association, Inc. Reprinted by permission.

Social-emotional Development

Infants need a trusting and responsive environment to develop healthy self-concepts and relationships with others. Hearing provides infants with cues to help them organize and classify their environment. Voices and sounds can be classified into the familiar and the unfamiliar as well as the friendly or unfriendly. Infants recognize sounds that signal danger and those that are calming, allowing them to feel safe and secure.

A hearing-impaired infant experiences events that appear to occur without warning or explanation. Sounds alert normally hearing individuals to the approach of others so that their appearance is neither startling nor unpredictable. Sounds signal people to respond in predictable ways, such as answering the telephone, going to the door when someone knocks, or turning to look at the person who is talking. Lack of predictability or explanation of events may cause an infant to feel insecure or powerless.

Infants' perceptions of self-worth and security also depend upon the quality and consistency of interactions with their family and others in their environment. In turn, parents are dependent upon the responsiveness of their babies to fuel and maintain a mutually rewarding and reinforcing relationship. Before diagnosis, parents of infants with impaired hearing are often confused by their infant's inconsistent or apparently unresponsive behaviors. Parents' attempts to interact with the baby (sing to calm the baby, coo, or play other vocal games) typically do not bring the expected responses. Infants with hearing losses may be perceived as unresponsive, resistant, or defiant. Parents may interpret these responses as rejection and begin to feel less competent as parents.

After parents suspect that something is amiss with their infant's development, they may respond by withdrawing or avoiding contact with their child. Parents may consciously or unconsciously diminish the quantity of their interactions with their babies by playing, holding, and talking to them less, which may affect the children's social-emotional development.

The diagnosis of hearing loss may come as a relief to some parents who feared additional handicapping conditions, but to most parents, the diagnosis is devastating. Many parents experience extreme sadness, anxiety, stress, guilt, anger, or fear. Although a period of mourning may be essential to adapt to the reality of a hearing loss (Luterman, 1979), grieving may have a negative impact on parents' sensitivity and responsiveness to the needs of their infants. Prolonged grieving may threaten the development of a secure parent-child bond and may negatively affect the parents' responses to their child for years (Meadow, 1980).

Cognitive Development

Infants learn about their environment through sensorimotor exploration and their relationships with significant others. Early experiences and stimulation form the framework for the development of early cognitive processes, which in turn affect the quality of higher-level cognitive and communicative abilities. The interrelationship between cognition and language suggests that the development of each accelerates and supports the development of the other. Concepts provide children with a structure for organizing their experiences and provide the basis for understanding and expressing early language, so a lag in language acquisition may delay the formation of some concepts.

The child with limited hearing develops a view of the world in which sound has no meaning; sight, movement, touch, and smell are the avenues through which experiences are gained. Although the absence of hearing does not impede sensorimotor development (Best & Roberts, 1976), the early interventionist needs to be aware of the impact of hearing loss and needs to provide guidance to families to assist children in acquiring important cognitive skills through sensory modalities salient to the child. For example, the development of object permanence, the recognition that objects or people continue to exist when they are no longer within view, is facilitated by the ability to hear. The sounds of voices, airplanes, birds, and trains signal the existence of people or objects even when they are not visually present. In the mind of a hearing-impaired child, however, an object or person that is not in view may not exist. Alerting hearing-impaired children to the presence of sounds when the source of the sound is no longer visible may facilitate the acquisition of this concept.

Goal-directed behavior aids infants in understanding that something can be obtained as a result of their actions. Early vocal communicative behaviors assist in the development of goal-directed behaviors. The infants' cries are a powerful tool for learning that vocalizations can bring mom or dad to their side, satiate hunger, or bring comfort. Children with a severe or profound hearing loss may not be aware of the powerful link between their vocalizations and the subsequent response of an adult. Adults who respond consistently to the infant's vocalizations and indicate that they heard them (by pointing to their own ears) will enable infants to grasp the consequences of their vocal behaviors.

Similarly, the development of cause and effect relations requires that infants understand not only the consequences of their own actions, but also the impact of others' actions, and the relationship among a series of events. Many cause and effect relationships can be observed through vision; others rely on hearing. For example, the telephone rings; dad answers it and talks; dad calls to mom and she appears; she talks briefly; mom disappears and returns with her coat. The source of many events and the consequent actions or responses may be confusing to the child who is unable to hear and may require special intervention.

Positive parent-child interactions such as warmth and affection, contingent responsiveness, sensitivity, and stimulation have been linked to early cognitive competence in nonhandicapped infants (Clarke-Stewart, 1973; Yarrow, Rubenstein, Pedersen, & Jankowski, 1972). As a result of parents' feelings about their infants and the hearing loss, as well as the frustrations that may result from their inability to affect their infant's behavior in anticipated ways, parents may have difficulty establishing positive nurturing relationships with their children. A lack of understanding of the effects of hearing loss on communication and other areas of development may prevent parents from establishing realistic goals, or result in overprotective or oversolicitous behaviors toward their children (Quigley & Kretschmer, 1982). Parents who are overprotective may discourage exploration of the environment and inhibit their child's natural curiosity, which are fundamental to the acquisition of early cognitive development.

Although the infant with severe or profound hearing loss is likely to have early experiences that differ from those of normally hearing infants, the infant interventionist can work with families to support positive and nurturing interactions and atmospheres which stimulate the cognitive growth of their children. By providing stimulating environments that encourage infants to explore, and that heighten infants' curiosity for learning, families can facilitate the development of concepts fundamental to language acquisition and more complex cognitive development.

Communication and Language

The development of spoken (oral) language depends not only on the ability to hear but also on the development of social-emotional and cognitive skills and early communicative behaviors. Communication acquisition is built on a foundation of sensorimotor experiences that provide opportunities for learning and skills for interacting successfully with the environment and the people in it. Like the development of early cognitive schema, preverbal communication is stimulated by a secure and trusting environment that builds the infant's self-esteem. Mutually responsive parent-child relationships establish a facilitative framework for optimal development of social-emotional, cognitive, and communicative competence.

The auditorily stimulating and responsive environment essential to the natural acquisition of spoken language may not be accessible to the infant with a severe to profound hearing loss. If, in addition to a loss of hearing, there is a disruption in the parent-child bond, the development of a positive self-concept and enriching early cognitive experiences may be negatively affected. This, in turn, may further delay the growth of communication skills. Trusting and mutually satisfying parent-child relationships and stimulating environments provide a framework for children with impaired hearing to develop early communicative behaviors.

The early interventionist must understand the relationship between communication, language, and speech (spoken language). Although communication involves nonverbal as well as verbal means of sharing information, language requires the ability to use a recognized symbol system to communicate thoughts and ideas. Language may be expressed through speech, signs, or written symbols, and is built upon a strong foundation of preverbal and presymbolic communication. The infant cry, initially involuntary, is the earliest oral communicative behavior. Other early communications include facial expressions, body movements, eye gazes, smiles, touches, points, gestures, and extensive vocalizations. Infants whose early communications are reinforced tend to be more motivated to expand and use additional communication strategies. A rich and varied presymbolic communication system is necessary for the development of symbolic language.

For one group of hearing-impaired children, the acquisition of sign language is as natural as the acquisition of spoken language for their normally hearing peers. Deaf children with deaf parents who sign with them from birth obtain sign language skills at a rate comparable to that of normally hearing children's acquisition of oral language (Newport & Meier, 1985). For most of these families there is minimal disruption in the parent-child relationship and communication occurs from birth without interruption. Hearing-impaired children who have parents who are fluent signers develop sign language skills naturally and spontaneously through parent-child interactions.

Speech is one way in which language is expressed and thus it is dependent on the ability to use symbolic communication. The acquisition of speech, spoken language, is difficult for most severely and profoundly hearing-impaired children because vision offers limited access to the sounds and prosody of language. Speech production involves the ability to produce and combine sounds to form words that are understood by others.

A severe to profound hearing loss occurring in infancy will have a significant impact on the development of speech. Although the early vocalizations of many infants with impaired hearing appear to be very much like those of their normally hearing peers, by 6 to 8 months of age differences in the amount and type of vocalizations begin to be noticeable. Without an effective auditory feedback system, hearing-impaired children do not develop internal auditory reinforcement for their vocalizations. Hearing-impaired infants may either decrease the quantity of their vocalizations (Stark, 1983) or modify their vocalizations to create tactile or kinesthetic feedback (Oller, Eilers, Bull, & Carney, 1985; Stoel-Gammon & Otomo, 1986). Normally hearing infants begin babbling between 7 and 10 months of age; infants with severe hearing loss may not babble until well into their second year of life (Oller, 1978).

The ability to use speech as a means to communicate depends on many factors. Given a reasonably intact cognitive and perceptual structure and a reasonably supportive environment, the amount and quality of an individual's hearing strongly influences the quality of an individual's speech (Ling, 1976b). In addition, the age of onset of the hearing loss, the ability of the child to use residual hearing and visual cues to understand and produce spoken language, the extent to which speech is used as a means of communication in the child's environment, and the consistency and quality of responsiveness to the child's vocalizations and speech attempts influence the acquisition of speech. There is little evidence to suggest that the use of signs impedes the development of speech. In fact, several studies suggest that children in programs using oral-plus-visual communication have equivalent spoken language skills and enhanced achievement when compared with children using oral-only communication (Meadow-Orlans, 1987).

More than 90% of infants with impaired hearing have normally hearing parents who do not have the communication skills to enable their children to acquire communicative competence naturally and spontaneously in the home. The acquisition of language (signed or spoken) for all hearing-impaired children depends on the degree to which family members are responsive to their children's communication needs and to the extent that children are able to process language visually or auditorily.

Hearing-impaired children of both deaf and hearing parents need extensive exposure to language and the opportunity to use it in meaningful ways. Interaction with parents and caregivers using communicative behaviors and language structures appropriate to the developmental level and interests of the child is fundamental to the development of a symbolic communication system, signed or spoken. Early interventionists need to work closely with specialists trained and experienced in working with hearing-impaired infants and their families to facilitate the development of communication and spoken language skills.

Additional Disabilities

Other disabilities affect approximately 20% of hearing-impaired children under age 6 (Schildroth, 1986). These children may experience motor disabilities, developmental delays, neurological, emotional, or other disorders. Although medical advances may eventually reduce the prevalence of nongenetic causes of deafness, such as rubella and meningitis, medically fragile and premature infants who survive are increasing the number of hearing-impaired children with additional handicaps (Moores, 1987). The early interventionist needs to be alert to behaviors that may indicate the presence of an additional disability.

The child who is considered multihandicapped with a hearing loss is a child who has physical, mental, emotional, or behavioral disorders that significantly add to the complexity of educating the child (Gentile & McCarthy, 1973). The effect of an additional disability on the child with a hearing loss is often more than simply additive. For example, developing functional communication and social relationships become significantly more difficult for a child with a visual impairment in addition to a hearing loss. A deaf-blind child may only be aware of events and communication that can be directly experienced through touch, movement, or smell. Vision, the major channel for developing communication for a hearing-impaired child, is impaired. The early interventionist needs to explore alternative modalities as well as residual visual and auditory abilities to help the deaf-blind child acquire communication and learn about the environment, self, and others.

The identification and development of appropriate intervention strategies for a child with additional handicaps and the family often involves the expertise of other professionals. The early interventionist may need to identify appropriate resources and coordinate an array of services to meet the needs of the multihandicapped hearing-impaired child and the child's family. It is imperative that professionals involved in the diagnostic process understand the implications of impaired hearing to insure selection and administration of appropriate assessment tools, interpretation of results, and identification of effective goals and strategies for intervention. Schuyler and Rushmer (1987) list several tools and techniques that are helpful in assessing and planning interventions for the child with additional disabilities.

Three potential effects of disabilities in addition to a hearing loss are multisensory deprivation (such as reduction in the ability to acquire experiences through channels other than hearing), learned helplessness, and insufficient parent-child attachment (Schuyler & Rushmer, 1987). **Learned helplessness** refers to the belief that the individual lacks control of life and life's events (Seligman, 1975). This condition can result when others focus on the inabilities, rather than the abilities, of the multihandicapped child. If family members or others treat the child with pity or communicate a sense of powerlessness, the child may respond with apathy, depression, and an overall lack of motivation.

Poor attachment between infant and parents, in combination with hearing loss, may affect an infant's temperament, ability to respond to affection, communicate nonverbally, or achieve developmental milestones. Difficulties in calming or stimulating may cause parents to feel inadequate. Feelings of hopelessness, anger, fear, guilt, or powerlessness may also be expressed by parents of multihandicapped children. The early interventionist needs to be sensitive to the increased emotional burdens and demands a multihandicapped hearing-impaired child places on the family, and be prepared to work closely with families and other professionals and agencies who are able to provide appropriate services.

COMMUNICATION METHODOLOGIES

Nothing in the field of education of the deaf stirs more controversy than the discussion of which communication methodology is best for children with a hearing loss. Despite strong opinions of professionals, deaf adults, parents of hearing-impaired children, and others, no one methodology is best for everyone. Professionals working with families of children who have hearing losses must be knowledgeable about the different communication options and be able to present information to parents accurately and objectively. Families need opportunities to discuss concerns and questions openly, to meet a variety of hearing-impaired adults and school-age children, and to share their feelings with other families who have hearing-impaired children. The role of the professional is to provide information and support families in the selection of a communication mode that most appropriately meets the cognitive, linguistic, and social demands of the children and their families.

Total Communication

Total communication, a philosophy adopted by the majority of school programs for hearing-impaired children, involves listening, speaking, speechreading, signing, gestures, fingerspelling, reading, and writing (Bodner-Johnson, 1987). (**Speechreading** refers to recognizing spoken words by watching the speaker's lip and mouth movements and facial expressions. **Fingerspelling** refers to hand and finger shapes used to represent each of the 26 letters of the alphabet to form words, phrases, and sentences.) Total communication implies the choice of any one method or a combination of methods to communicate effectively in a given situation. While total communication is a philosophy of communication, **simultaneous communication** is a method of communication which refers to the simultaneous use of both speech and signs. This method includes listening, speechreading, and reading signs and fingerspelling for understanding; and speaking, signing, and fingerspelling for expression. Simultaneous communication is based on English word order using the signs of **American Sign Language** and the structure of the English language.

Signs are based on concepts, rather than English words, and therefore, there is not always a direct correlation between spoken words and signs. For example, one basic sign is used for the concept *hungry* (represented by several English words, i.e., famished, starving, ravenous). Emphasis and facial expressions are used in sign language to differentiate among these words. On the other hand, there are signs that represent American Sign Language idioms and are difficult to express through standard patterns of English. For example, the sign for *finish,* when used with the sign for *eat,* means "Have you eaten yet?" When the sign *finish* is used following the sign for *play* it means, "Stop playing around." American Sign Language, like any language, contains expressions and idioms that must be translated to make sense in English (Madsen, 1987).

Manually Coded English systems modify or create signs to provide a more complete visual representation of English using a direct correlation between English and sign. These invented sign systems use American Sign Language signs as a base and create signs to mark grammatical structures such as pronouns, verb tenses, affixes, and articles (Moores, 1987). Two of the most frequently used English sign communication systems are **Signing Exact English** (SEE II) (Gustason, Pfetzing, & Zawolkow, 1972) and **Signed English** (Bornstein & Saulnier, 1981; Bornstein, Saulnier, & Hamilton, 1980).

Families considering using signs with speech should understand that signing requires a significant amount of time and commitment. Sign classes for parents, as well as video tapes to help parents learn signs at home, are available in most communities. Families need the opportunity to practice and use signs with hearing-impaired individuals in order to develop adequate communication skills. Early interventionists may facilitate family sign communication by arranging opportunities for families to interact with adults who sign.

American Sign Language

American Sign Language, ASL or Ameslan, is a visual, gestural, and non-oral method of communication used by a majority of deaf adults and many children who have deaf parents. American Sign Language has, like all other languages, its own vocabulary, grammatical structures, and idioms (Moores, 1987). ASL is very different from English and, therefore, cannot be used simultaneously with speech.

Proponents of the use of ASL as the first language of children who are hearing impaired believe that it is a natural language for children who cannot hear. Some linguists suggest that once the child acquires ASL, the acquisition of a second language, such as English, will be easier (Johnson, Liddell, & Erting, 1989). Others have suggested that American Sign Language and English be acquired in a bilingual fashion (Quigley & Kretschmer, 1982). Learning American Sign Language, like learning any foreign language, requires intensive exposure and opportunity to communicate with individuals using ASL.

Auditory-oral Communication

Auditory-oral communication, also known as auditory/verbal or aural-oral, is a communication methodology requiring listening and speechreading to process spoken language and speech for expression. Hearing-impaired individuals who use auditory-oral communication acquire information from the environment without the use of signs or other manual communication systems. Because auditory-oral communication relies on the accessibility of spoken language, this methodology requires families and professionals to pay maximum attention to the acoustic and visual components of speech and the environment.

Appropriate and consistent amplification is essential to the ability to process auditory information for most severely and profoundly hearing-impaired children. Careful monitoring of the child's hearing aids, the acoustics of the environment, the distance between the speaker and the listener, and background noises are needed to ensure an optimal listening environment. The deaf education specialist and audiologist need to guide the family and other involved professionals in determining ways to check hearing aids and the child's responses to speech and environmental sounds daily. In addition, arranging the environment to ensure optimal visibility of the speaker's lips and facial expressions is important. Lighting, glare from windows or the sun, and distance between speaker and receiver will affect the relative ease or difficulty for receiving information. Regular consultations with the child's audiologist and the deaf education specialist are essential to assist the infant interventionist and family and help them maintain an environment conducive to auditory-oral communication.

The ability to communicate auditorily-orally is not dependent upon the degree and type of hearing loss alone, but also age of onset of deafness, age when intervention began, English language competence, quality of auditory and oral intervention, presence of additional disabilities, and family constellation. However, the more severe the impairment, the less information one is likely to obtain through the auditory channel and the more one is dependent upon manual or other visual cues for receiving and transmitting information.

Cued Speech

Cued speech is a system of hand signals used in combination with speech to make speechreading more visible. Cued speech uses eight different handshapes and four hand positions to clarify sounds that cannot be distinguished through speechreading alone (Williams-Scott, 1987). Speechreading is very difficult. Speech sounds range from being visible but ambiguous to completely invisible. More than 40% of all speech sounds look alike on the lips (Ling, 1976a). For example, the words pat, mat, and bat, although very different in meaning, look the same on the lips.

Cues are based on groups of consonant and vowel sounds and can be learned by a fluent speaker of English in a short period of time. Idiomatic expressions, puns on words, and rhymes that are not easily communicated to a child with impaired hearing may be communicated through cued speech. Because cued speech is a visual representation of the sounds of speech, it can be useful for demonstrating correct pronunciation and may be helpful when used with a phonetic approach to reading.

A disadvantage of this approach is the limited extent to which it is available as a teaching or communication tool with hearing-impaired children. Few educational programs have teachers, interpreters, and other professionals who use cued speech. Cued speech users need to rely on either auditory-oral or sign communication to communicate with the majority of hearing and hearing-impaired individuals. Families considering using cued speech must be committed and prepared to become long-term advocates for the use of this approach.

Selecting an Approach

The communication methodology most appropriate for a child depends upon a number of factors including the degree and type of hearing loss, the age of onset of the loss, the child's cognitive and social development, the rate at which the child acquires language, the child's learning environment, available educational resources, and the family's values and beliefs. Families should have the opportunity to explore all options, to discuss their feelings, and to receive professional input in their decision. By learning about the advantages and disadvantages of each option in an objective manner, families can make informed decisions based on their unique situations. Families should be aware that any decision that they make is not forever, and that as a team, the professionals and the family should continue to assess the child's rate of communication, social, and academic development to ensure that the methodology is meeting the needs of the child and family. Whether an auditory-oral communication approach or a total communication approach is selected, families must work to ensure that the child consistently has access to the clearest communication possible. Whatever communication option is selected by a family, it is imperative that interventionists without formal training in deaf education seek regular guidance and training from specialists. Only cohesive teamwork can provide the support families must have.

FAMILY INVOLVEMENT

Reactions to Hearing Loss

Parental reactions to the diagnosis of their child's hearing loss vary, and range from devastation to relief that the problem is nothing more than a hearing loss. Some families may adapt quickly, by learning about deafness, modifying their communication behaviors, and seeking professional advice and support; others may struggle for years trying to cope with the adjustments required. Reactions may depend upon the medical state of their child. For example, the family facing medical complications that threaten the life of their child may, understandably, be less concerned about the impact of a hearing loss. Families struggling to meet the basic needs of their families (health, housing, food, or clothing) may be overwhelmed by survival concerns that consume their energy and attention.

Parents who are hearing impaired typically have less difficulty than parents with normal hearing in adjusting to a hearing loss of a child (Meadow-Orlans, 1987; Quigley & Kretschmer, 1982). Normally hearing parents often report that their first encounter with deafness was when they discovered their child had a hearing loss. Consequently, the effects of a hearing loss and the interventions required are unknown to most parents. Parents who have impaired hearing are likely to be familiar with the communicative, educational, and social implications. They typically have friends who are also hearing impaired and can envision a productive future for children despite the hearing loss. Deaf parents may feel a sense of comfort when they discover their child is also deaf. For many deaf parents, communicating with their deaf children is as natural as it is for hearing parents to communicate with normally hearing children.

In addition to differences in families' reactions, the early interventionist will also note different reactions within the family. Spouses may disagree about the consequences of the hearing loss on their child's future; they may disagree about the type of intervention, the use of hearing aids, or the communication methodology. The grandparents of the child may have difficulties accepting the permanence of the condition or may disagree about the decisions that the parents of the child make. Siblings may create additional tension by responding negatively to the attention their hearing-impaired sibling receives or the changes that have occurred in the family. These conflicts increase the stress in the family and may prolong or intensify feelings of despair.

Early interventionists must be sensitive to the varying emotions families may experience from the time of discovery of the hearing loss to the realization and acceptance that the loss is permanent. For many families, the diagnosis of a hearing loss is a family crisis. When parents express feelings of shock, disbelief, or denial, the helpful professional will recognize these feelings as a natural part of a grieving process and will respond by listening and communicating acceptance of their feelings. (Chapter 12 discusses specific communication skills for helping families through stress and grief.)

The diagnosis of a hearing loss often follows many months of parents' suspicion that something is wrong (Meadow-Orlans, 1987; Schuyler & Rushmer, 1987). Despite the suspicion, many parents have difficulty believing the diagnosis, or accepting the severity or permanence of the loss. Because the consequences of a severe or profound loss are often not evident until there is an obvious delay in the development of communication, parents, as well as members of the medical community, may not recognize the existence of a hearing loss.

Parents of children who have less severe hearing losses may have a difficult time believing the diagnosis, especially if they have received conflicting reports from professionals or if their child has some residual hearing and is able to hear some spoken language and environmental sounds. Parents of children with disabilities may initially believe that the condition will improve, or that there will be a cure. Because a hearing loss is invisible, parents of children with hearing losses may be tempted to pass them as having normal hearing, and shun hearing aids, special communication methodologies, or recommendations for special educational services that are tangible signs of hearing loss.

As the habilitation process begins and professionals enter their lives, families may also sense a loss of control over the parenting of their children. Professionals, eager to provide advice for parents, may inadvertently cause parents to feel inadequate. As families recognize the irreversibility and permanence of the situation they may also begin to realize that children with hearing loss will demand significant time, energy, and financial resources for many years. Early interventionists should be in touch with each family's readiness and receptiveness to additional demands. They may need to adjust the amount and content of information presented to families who are struggling to cope with the impact of their child's hearing loss. Skilled professionals understand that frequent repetition of basic information is often necessary, because parents of newly identified children are often overwhelmed and unable to respond in constructive ways. Parents, siblings, and other family members need opportunities to explore and share their feelings in supportive environments.

Critical to a family's adaptation to a child's disability is the establishment of an effective parent-professional relationship. Listening and communicating acceptance of the parents' feelings is just the beginning. Early interventionists must also communicate respect for the beliefs and values that are an integral part of each family. Understanding the expectations and goals that the family has set for themselves and their children, and encouraging families to become true partners, are fundamental to the process of successful intervention.

Unrecognized and unresolved feelings of resentment, guilt, or sadness may interfere with a family's ability to participate fully in the intervention process. Professionals and families working together may need to identify resources to assist the families in adapting, in order to facilitate their child's development. Families who have accepted their children's hearing loss are able to focus on ways to adapt their communicative behaviors and develop realistic expectations and positive interactions that form the foundation of effective parent-child relationships.

Parent-child Communication

A major challenge of the early interventionist is to guide families in developing skills needed to communicate effectively with their children. The significance of early positive stimulation and responsiveness to communication poses a challenge to professionals to facilitate families' acceptance of the reality of the hearing loss and develop strategies for effective interaction. Through observations of parent-child interaction, professionals can assist parents in recognizing their child's stage of communication development and together identify behaviors that will promote the development of communication. Schuyler and Rushmer (1987) have compiled several strategies parents can use to foster communicative development. Skills that promote presymbolic communication interactions are listed in Table 10–2. Skills for promoting symbolic language learning are presented in Table 10–3.

Recent evidence has revealed that the application of the processes used by parents of normally hearing infants for establishing communication may not be appropriate for severely and profoundly impaired infants. Instead, these infants may learn better with an emphasis on visual and gestural input rather than on auditory and vocal input. A series of studies conducted by a team of researchers at the Center for Studies in Education and Human Development at Gallaudet University in Washington, D.C. indicate that deaf parents of deaf infants use different strategies than hearing parents of hearing children to respond to their babies, gain and maintain attention, and converse. Interest in deaf parents' communicative behaviors has in-

TABLE 10–2
Skills to promote presymbolic communication interactions.

1. Acknowledge and respond to the infant's non-verbal communication attempts.
2. Include non-verbal signals in conversations with the infant: peek-a-boo; smiles; a variety of facial expressions (eye-widening, eye-blinks, "surprised" look, "funny" mouth positions, tongue wiggling); hiding face; touching (poking, tapping, tickling, "creepy-crawling"); body movement.
3. Entice infant to look when directing conversation to him.
4. *Avoid forcing* infant's visual attention in intrusive ways.
5. Be dramatic and visually interesting in order to hold the infant's attention.
6. Take turns "conversing" with the infant; avoid interrupting his "conversation."
7. Avoid overtalking. Use pauses and give the infant time to rest and respond.
8. Imitate the infant's vocal and body movement communication.
9. Imitate the baby's rhythmic movements and vocalization and initiate rhythmic movement patterns for the baby to imitate.

Source: From *Parent-infant Habilitation: A Comprehensive Approach to Working with Hearing-impaired Infants and Toddlers and Their Families* (p. 351) by V. Schuyler and N. Rushmer, 1987, Portland, OR: Infant Hearing Resource. Copyright © 1987 by Infant Hearing Resource. Reprinted by permission.

TABLE 10–3
Skills to promote symbolic language learning.

1. Use appropriate methods of gaining the child's auditory and visual attention.
2. Use effective methods of maintaining the child's attention.
3. Make communication relevant and interesting.
4. Use voice effectively.
5. Use repetition.
6. Encourage the child to use language to express his feelings, wants, and needs.
7. Use short sentences initially.
8. Emphasize the one or two important words in the sentence.
9. Include the child in family conversation.
10. Provide correct word when the child mispronounces or misnames.
11. Expand the child's incomplete words or sentences into complete words or sentences.
12. Once a language concept has been learned, help the child broaden it and generalize it to other situations.
13. Pose questions that elicit thinking and problem-solving.
14. Use active listening techniques in communicating with the child.

Source: From *Parent-infant Habilitation: A Comprehensive Approach to Working with Hearing-impaired Infants and Toddlers and Their Families* (p. 369) by V. Schuyler and N. Rushmer, 1987, Portland, OR: Infant Hearing Resource. Copyright © 1987 by Infant Hearing Resource. Reprinted by permission.

creased as a result of mounting evidence that shows that deaf children with deaf parents acquire language at faster rates, experience higher levels of academic achievement, and are socially better adjusted than deaf children with hearing parents (Meadow, 1980; Meadow, Greenberg, Erting, & Carmichael, 1981).

Deaf parents modify their communicative behaviors to allow the infant to process a language that is visually based. Many of the behaviors differ significantly from the normally hearing model as well as the traditional techniques espoused by early intervention programs for hearing-impaired infants (John Tracy Clinic, 1983; Pollack, 1970). For example, deaf mothers tend to

- □ use touch, stroking, tickling, and moving of infant's feet and hands to get or maintain attention (Maestas y Moores, 1980; Schlesinger & Meadow, 1972)
- □ position infants so that they can see their mothers' faces and signs as well as focus on objects or people of interest (Maestas y Moores, 1980)
- □ use positive and interesting facial expressions (Erting, Prezioso, & Hynes, 1989)
- □ sign within baby's visual space, or sign directly on the baby or the object that has the baby's attention (Harris, Clibbens, Tibbitts, & Chasin, 1987)
- □ sign short and simple messages rather than complete or complex structures (Kyle & Ackerman, 1987)
- □ use frequent repetition of signs (Launer, 1982)

Deaf adults are an important resource to the early interventionist and can help professionals and families adopt strategies for developing effective communication skills. Together, families and professionals can examine their communicative behaviors and systematically identify behaviors which will enhance the quality and enjoyment of parent-child communication.

ASSESSMENT

Transdisciplinary assessment, a key component of P.L. 99–457, requires professionals to blend their expertise in different areas to describe the nature of the child's disability and to identify strengths and areas of need for the child and the child's family. The purposes of assessment of infants and preschoolers with handicaps include screening, diagnosis, placement, planning, and evaluation.

Hearing Screening

Early and accurate identification of hearing loss is critical for the ability to comprehend and use spoken language, and can produce exponential effects. Newborns can be screened for hearing loss while still in the hospital through high-risk registers, devices such as the Crib-O-Gram Neonatal Hearing Screening Audiometer (Simmons, 1977), and Auditory Brain Stem Response testing. Hearing loss in newborns and infants can also be identified by pediatricians during well-baby visits in the first year of life.

The Joint Committee on Infant Hearing (1982) developed seven risk criteria that have been used by many states to establish high-risk registers for infant screening. However, less than half of the states have operational or planned hearing screening and follow-up for high-risk infants (Mahoney & Eichwald, 1987). Despite the fact that hearing loss can be detected as early as the first day of birth, infants with hearing losses may not be identified until after their second birthdays. This situation is deplorable given present technology, high-risk screening, and follow-up procedures which are capable of detecting 50 to 75% of all newborns with severe hearing impairments (Mahoney & Eichwald, 1987).

The American Speech-Language-Hearing Association recently established guidelines for audiologic screening of newborn infants (ASLHA, 1989). The guidelines establish recommendations for audiometric evaluation, follow-up, and management of hearing-impaired infants, and recommend that all infants who evidence one or more of the seven risk criteria identified by the Joint Committee on Infant Hearing (1982) should receive audiologic screening. The seven factors include:

- a family history of childhood hearing impairment
- congenital perinatal infection (e.g. cytomegalovirus [CMV], rubella, herpes, toxoplasmosis, syphilis)
- anatomic malformation involving the head or neck (e.g., dysmorphic appearance including syndromal and nonsyndromal abnormalities, overt or submucous cleft palate, morphologic abnormalities of the pinna)
- birthweight less than 1500 g
- hyperbilirubinemia at levels exceeding indications of exchange transfusion
- bacterial meningitis, especially H. influenza
- severe asphyxia which may include infants with Apgar scores of 0 to 3 who fail to institute spontaneous respiration by 10 minutes and those with hypotonia persisting to 2 hours of age

The ASLHA guidelines recommend that infants at risk for hearing loss (7 to 12% of the newborn population, according to Mahoney & Eichwald, 1987) be screened prior to discharge from the newborn nursery. Furthermore, at-risk newborns should be screened using **Auditory Brainstem Response (ABR) testing** (Ling, 1976b). Auditory Brainstem Response testing is a screening tool also recommended for infants and older children for whom a clear picture of their voluntary behavioral response to sound is not evident. By measuring electrical change in the brain in response to sound, ABR, when administered and interpreted by experienced professionals, can provide an objective measure of auditory response. This information should be coupled with behavioral testing and observations from the child's family to formulate a complete audiologic assessment (Hasenstab & Horner, 1982; Schuyler & Rushmer, 1987).

Because one-third of all children with hearing loss are presently not detected through neonatal screening or high-risk registers (Cox, 1988), it is imperative that physicians, parents, and early childhood educators are aware of normal hearing, language, and speech milestones. Only then can they identify infants and toddlers who may have impaired hearing and refer them for audiological assessment as soon as possible. When referring a family to an audiologist, the interventionist should recommend an audiologist with extensive experience assessing infants and working with families. The skillful audiologist will be familiar with techniques for assessing infants and toddlers and will be able to communicate the results of the testing in a clear and straightforward manner. Equally important is the audiologist's ability to provide support through listening in a manner which fosters mutual respect and a parent-professional partnership.

Comprehensive Assessment

After a hearing loss has been confirmed, comprehensive assessment for program planning should focus on four major areas:

1. **Audiologic assessment** includes the ability to detect and process auditory information and the potential use of amplification and other assistive devices.
2. **Developmental assessment** includes cognitive, motor, social-emotional, and self-help development.
3. **Communication assessment** includes prelinguistic communicative behaviors, vocal, gestural, and signed communication; linguistic abilities; listening skills; and speech.
4. **Family environment assessment** includes support of family members and others, resources, information and skill needs.

The first three of these are discussed here.

Audiologic assessment. An audiologic assessment includes an assessment of the child's auditory sensitivity to sounds as well as the ability to discriminate, recognize, and process the meaning of sounds. A confirmation of hearing loss is followed by a search for the most appropriate hearing aid(s) and guidance for the family in a schedule of gradual hearing aid use leading to full-time wearing (see Downs, 1966).

Auditory sensitivity of infants and toddlers is evaluated by an audiologist with the assistance of the parents and the infant interventionist. The infant interventionist who lacks training in audiologic assessment and management should work closely with the specialist in hearing impairment as well. A team approach to testing provides the audiologist with critical information concerning the child's overall development, communication abilities, and auditory responses to environmental sounds and speech. In addition, the involvement of the early interventionist reinforces the parents' understanding of the results of the tests and the educational implications for the child and family.

Assessment of newborns involves observing the child's responses to sounds through a technique called **Behavioral Observation Audiometry (BOA)**. Sound is presented in a sound-treated booth through speakers (sound-field testing). Music, speech, and some forms of pure tones are generally used. The audiologist, parents, and early interventionist observe the child's changes in behavior for indications that a particular sound was heard. Slight movements such as eye blinks, eye widening, increased respiration, or startles, when temporally related to the presentation of the sound stimulus, may be indications that the child hears the sound.

Animated Visually Reinforced Audiometry (AVRA) is a behavioral assessment technique for more mature infants and toddlers. AVRA can be used with infants as young as 4 1/2 to 5 months of age who are conditioned to look in the direction of a sound when the sound is presented through speakers (Northern & Downs, 1984). Children are reinforced for looking in the correct direction by a lighted clown, dancing bears, or similarly attractive lighted or moving objects.

Before children are ready to simply tell the audiologist that they hear a sound, **Conditioned Play Audiometry (CPA)** is used. Conditioned Play Audiometry is used successfully with children from about 2 years of age. Children indicate that they hear a sound by performing a motor act such as placing a block in a can, fitting a puzzle piece into a puzzle, or stacking rings. Parents and early interventionists can help prepare children for these tasks by playing similar auditory games at home. See Schuyler & Rushmer (1987) for techniques for play audiometry conditioning.

Another integral part of an infant's audiologic assessment is the **immittance** (or impedance) **audiometry**. Immittance testing allows the audiologist or the physician to determine whether there are physical problems in the infant's middle ear, for example, otitis media, middle ear infections, or absence of middle ear structures due to genetic abnormalities. Immittance testing, specifically the acoustic reflex subtest, gives some indirect objective evidence concerning the degree of hearing loss present. See Bailey & Wolery (1989), Hasenstab & Horner (1982), and Northern & Downs (1984) for further descriptions of immittance audiometry.

Developmental assessment.   Professionals conducting a developmental assessment of a child with a hearing loss must give careful consideration to the following assessment principles:

Ensure the domains assessed comprehensively describe the functioning of the child. Careful review of assessment tools will enable the early interventionist to determine the validity and reliability, as well as the depth and range, of the constructs the specific domains evaluate. An assessment instrument focusing on the development of the hearing-impaired child's communication abilities, for example, must be sensitive enough to describe the multiple aspects of communication including receptive and expressive ability, both verbal and nonverbal.

Consider the impact of the hearing loss on the measurement of the domain. Many assessment instruments include items that require the ability to hear and process language. For instance, a cognitive item at the 4-month level of the *Early Learning Accomplishment Profile* (E-LAP) (Glover, Preminger, & Sanford, 1978), "Turns head to source of voice," may be failed by a child with a hearing loss. Failure of items such as this does not accurately reflect a child's true abilities in the cognitive domain.

Ensure that assessments are conducted by or with early interventionists experienced in working with hearing-impaired children. Without experience or training in hearing impairment, it may be difficult to obtain, and interpret, an accurate description of the child's true abilities. The examiner must arrange the environment in a way that provides maximum auditory and visual benefit and reduces potentially distracting stimuli. The examiner must communicate effectively with the child, using the child's preferred communication system. The child who uses gestures or signs requires an examiner who is able to use and understand signed communication. Likewise, the child whose speech is severely impaired needs the expertise of a professional who is able to interpret the child's oral communication.

Ensure that the child understands and is able to perform the tasks required by the test. Many test items require children to repeat, say, or point to the correct response in order to demonstrate a particular ability. Hearing-impaired children may require several examples of the desired response before they understand what is required. Signs, pictures, or other prompts may be needed to elicit appropriate responses. In some cases, responses signed rather than spoken by the child should be accepted. The test manual should be consulted to insure that modifications to promote effective communication with a child who is hearing impaired do not invalidate the results obtained. For a description of instruments and checklists for assessing the developmental needs of hearing-impaired infants and toddlers see Hasenstab & Horner (1982).

Communication assessment.   An indepth assessment of the communication abilities of a child with a hearing loss is fundamental to an effective intervention program. A comprehensive description of communication should include both comprehension and production of multiple aspects of communication. For the child with a hearing loss this includes an analysis of the child's abilities to comprehend language auditorily through listening, as well as visually through speechreading or sign communication. Assessment of expressive communication includes the abilities to use nonvocal, as well as vocal, forms of communication including gestures and signs, vocalizations, and spoken language.

Table 10–4 lists instruments that provide useful data for assessment, planning, and monitoring progress of hearing-impaired infants' and toddlers' communication development. For descriptions of communication assessment tools for hearing-impaired children see Thompson, Biro, Vethievelu, Pious, & Hatfield (1987).

Early interventionists without experience in deafness should work closely with the hearing-impairment specialist, and, when appropriate, the speech pathologist to assess and plan communication intervention goals for the hearing-impaired child. A battery of formal and informal assessments should be selected to best assess the child's presymbolic communication, receptive and expressive sign communication, auditory comprehension, speech, and linguistic abilities.

INTERVENTION

The wide range of abilities and characteristics of infants and toddlers with hearing loss, and their families, makes individualized programs imperative. No two children have the same developmental, social, cognitive, communicative, audiological, or linguistic needs. No two families have the same needs for information or formal and informal support. Not only are differences obvious in overall rates of development, but differences in the type, degree, and age of onset of hearing loss, and family environment preclude generalizations in programming for hearing-impaired young

TABLE 10–4

Tools to assess communication development of infants and toddlers with hearing loss.

Test	Age Range	Areas Evaluated
Sequenced Inventory of Communication Development (SICD) (Hedrick, Prather, Tobin, 1975)	4 mo–4 yrs	Receptive and expressive scales; auditory awareness, discrimination, and understanding; imitation and spontaneous speech; language sample
Bare Essentials in Assessing Really Little Kids—Concept Analysis Profile (BEAR-CAPS) (Hasenstab & Laughton, 1982)	1 yr 6 mos to 5 yrs 9 mos	Conceptual understanding of relationships including position/ location, quantity, quality, size, pronouns, and body parts
CID Scales of Early Communication Skills for Hearing-impaired Children (SECS) (Moog & Geers, 1975)	2–8 yrs	Receptive and expressive language skills (verbal and nonverbal)
Communicative Intention Inventory (CII) (Coggins & Carpenter, 1981)	8 mo–2 yrs	Gestural, vocal, and verbal behaviors; 8 categories of communicative intent
SKI*HI Language Development Scale (LDS) (Watkins, 1979)	Birth–5 yrs	Receptive and expressive communication and language skills
Teacher Assessment of Grammatical Structures (TAGS) (Moog & Kozak, 1983)	Birth–9 yrs	Receptive and expressive use of grammatical structures
Phonetic and Phonologic Level Evaluation (Ling, 1976a)	Birth to adult	Voice quality, suprasegmentals, vowels, consonants, blends

children. Good intervention involves utilizing play as the context for learning, implementing an effective program of family education and guidance, and matching the most advantageous services to the needs of each family.

Play as a Medium for Communication

Play is a process that involves all aspects of growth and development. As infants mature, their play changes from reflexive movements and vocalizations to imitative behaviors and then purposeful and imaginary interactions with objects and people in their world. Play enables children to discover and acquire knowledge of the world as well as to practice newly learned skills.

Play is critical to the development of cognition, communication, social, and motor skills. Play is the context for experimenting, practicing, and developing new linguistic structures (Vygotsky, 1967), and thus is an important medium for communication intervention.

TABLE 10–4
(continued)

Test	Age Range	Areas Evaluated
Developmental Approach to Successful Listening (Stout & Van Ert Windle, 1986)	Birth to adult	Sound awareness, phonetic listening, auditory comprehension
Schedules of Development in Audition, Speech, Language and Communication (Ling, 1977)	From birth	Hearing aid use, listening skills, speech skills, language comprehension, expression, and communication
Stages of Phonetic Development (Oller, 1978)	Birth–12 mos	Infant vocalizations and speech development
Parent-Infant Communication (Infant Hearing Resource, 1985)	Birth–3 yrs	Checklist for auditory development, presymbolic communication, vocalization, receptive and expressive language
Auditory Skills Curriculum: Preschool Supplement (Lexington School for the Deaf, 1986)	Birth–4 yrs	Auditory discrimination, auditory memory, sequencing, auditory feedback, figure-ground
I Heard That! A Developmental Sequence of Listening Activities for the Young Child (Northcott, 1983)	Birth–3 yrs	Auditory comprehension, receptive and expressive speech-language

Although impaired hearing has little effect on the development of imaginary play there is some evidence that the social play of hearing-impaired children is limited (Gregory, 1976; Singer & Lenaham, 1976). Given a stimulating and supportive environment, hearing-impaired infants, like those with normal hearing, will explore, manipulate, and use objects constructively, and play imaginatively (Gregory, 1976). Social dramatic play, however, depends on the child's ability to communicate and interact appropriately with others. The communication handicaps of hearing-impaired children may interfere with the development of both cooperative and social dramatic play (Higginbotham & Baker, 1981).

A child who is unable to communicate effectively with peers may prefer solitary play activities to play involving sharing of complex information, roles, or rules. Hearing-impaired children who lack the skills or opportunities to engage in social dramatic play miss a critical opportunity to acquire or expand new cognitive and linguistic skills. This situation may result in social isolation.

Parents and early interventionists who recognize the importance of play for hearing-impaired children will be better equipped to create home and center-based environments that foster opportunities for play. The development of play can be facilitated through the following strategies:

- □ create environments to encourage and reinforce play
- □ provide materials to stimulate interactive and imaginative play
- □ provide opportunities for young hearing-impaired children to participate in play groups or other group settings
- □ observe the child's play and then model new, more complex, or more imaginative ways to use the same toys or play
- □ model communication and social skills needed to engage in symbolic and imaginative play with other children
- □ coach children who demonstrate effective play skills to involve hearing-impaired children who lack these skills in their play routines

Using play as the medium for learning will also support the development of positive parent-child, professional-child, and parent-professional relationships by weaving the development of communication, social, and cognitive skills into naturally enjoyable and intrinsically motivating experiences.

Family Education

The unique needs of the family and the developmental needs of the child will dictate the content and delivery of the educational program and specialized services for families. Without training and experience in working with families of hearing-impaired children, early interventionists need to work closely with educators of the deaf, as well as audiologists, family counselors, and other experienced professionals to provide programming for families that meets their informational and emotional support needs.

Early interventionists need to work with specialists and deaf adults to introduce families to the world of deafness, including the wide variations of linguistic, cultural, and social preferences of individuals who have a hearing loss. Opportunities to meet and interact with adults and older children who are hearing impaired are crucial for helping families understand the implications of a loss of hearing. See Hafer and Richmond (1988) for many practical activities.

Providing social and educational programs for families in which hearing-impaired adults and adolescents participate helps parents appreciate the range of skills, abilities, and talents of hearing-impaired individuals. Discussions with hearing-impaired adults about their lives, including communication, educational, and social experiences, are extremely effective ways to help parents understand deafness.

Service Delivery Models

Early intervention programs for hearing-impaired infants are found in educational settings (special schools for hearing-impaired children as well as local public school programs that have classes or special services for children who have impaired hearing), hospitals and clinics, and local or state agencies.

Typically, home-based intervention is provided for families with young children to enable families and professionals to take advantage of the child's most familiar learning environment. Children are taught to more effectively interact in their home and parents are provided support and strategies for maximizing their child's communication and development. Regular visits to child care centers or other homes in which some young children spend a significant part of the day should be included as a regular part of the intervention program.

Center-based intervention offers families the opportunity to interact with other parents, professionals, and adults and children who are hearing impaired. Visits to the center may be invaluable for families who need support from other parents or simply an opportunity to get out. Programs should consider establishing a satellite center for families living a great distance from the early intervention center. Individual or play group sessions may be arranged for families and children; and informational, support, or social events planned for families.

Families and early interventionists need to consider distance, time, and expense for travel; work and other responsibilities; and special educational or health needs of the child to arrange a schedule for intervention sessions that best meets individual situations. Balancing families' needs and preferences with resources available will result in flexible scheduling to meet the changing needs of families and encourage maximum participation from all members of the child's family and significant others.

Hearing aids need to be checked daily to ensure proper functioning.

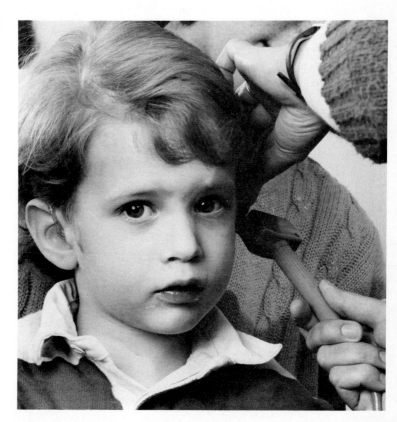

TRANSDISCIPLINARY CASE

The following case study and Individualized Family Service Plan (IFSP) are representative of the broad-based needs of hearing-impaired children and their families.

THE GREEN FAMILY

Li Green is a 14-month-old child with a bilateral sensorineural profound hearing loss. Li was born at fullterm weighing 7, 7. Ms. Green reported an uneventful pregnancy and no perinatal complications. Li is in good health, and her otologic history is unremarkable. (**Otologic history** is a medical examination by an otologist, an ear specialist, that indicates information related to ear abnormalities, middle ear infections, and other physical problems related to the ear.) Both parents have normal hearing, although Ms. Green's brother has a progressive hearing loss which began when he was a teenager.

Li is the Greens' first child. Mr. Green is an auto mechanic and Ms. Green worked for the telephone company as an operator prior to Li's birth. She now works part-time.

Audiologic Background

Ms. Green reported that she first noticed Li's lack of response to sound at 5 months of age. The family has a large dog, and Li showed no response to the dog's barking. An Auditory Brainstem Response (ABR) test conducted at 9 months of age indicated that Li had a profound bilateral sensorineural hearing loss. Further auditory behavioral observations at 10 1/2 months showed no response to broadband sounds (noisemakers, speech, and music) and frequency-specific sounds (warbled pure tones) presented through sound field at the limits of the audiometer.

Li was fitted with binaural Oticon E28P behind-the-ear hearing aids at 12 months of age. Mr. and Ms. Green report that Li adjusted to her hearing aids quickly. She wears her hearing aids during all waking hours. Presently she is using a personal **FM system** on a trial basis for structured listening activities. (An FM system is an assistive listening device that transmits the speaker's voice directly to the child's hearing aid, thereby minimizing the common problems associated with reverberation, distance, and background noise.)

Transdisciplinary Assessment

Mr. and Ms. Green were referred by the audiologist to an early intervention program serving infants and toddlers with disabilities and their families. The Greens and the program staff agreed that an accurate assessment would require the involvement of the following professional personnel: early childhood/deaf education specialist, educational audiologist, and a speech and language specialist. The program coordinator introduced the Greens to Ms. Stein, an infant interventionist on the staff with some experience working with infants and toddlers with hearing loss. Ms. Stein agreed to work with the Greens as case manager.

Results of Transdisciplinary Assessment

Cognitive Development. Based on information obtained from the Ordinal Scales of Psychological Development (Uzgiris & Hunt, 1975), Early Learning Accomplishment Profile (E-LAP) (Glover, Preminger, & Sanford, 1978), and parent observations, Li is able to perform cognitive tasks that typically develop between 12 and 15 months of age. She is able to find an object that has been hidden from her view, pull the correct one of two strings to obtain an object to which the string is attached, and imitate familiar and unfamiliar gestures and games such as Peek-A-Boo and Patty-Cake. She has begun to look at pictures in books and build a tower of 2 to 3 blocks. Tasks that require response to sounds or require spoken language, however, are not evident due to the severity of her hearing loss and the short time (2 months) that she has had her hearing aids.

Social-emotional Development. According to the E-LAP and parent observations, Li demonstrates social and emotional behaviors typical for her chronological age. She interacts with familiar adults by giving them toys or other objects. She bangs, pulls, pushes, and uses other forms to explore toys. Li has developed a strong attachment to her mother and cries when her mother leaves the room.

Motor Development and Self-help Skills. Again using the E-LAP and parent observations, Li demonstrates motor and self-help skills which are appropriate for her chronological age. Li has been walking since 11 months. She is able to stoop without falling; throw a ball; and crawl up steps using her arms and legs. She has just begun to scribble and is able to place a round block into a form board with the same shape. She has begun to use a spoon, but prefers to use her fingers. Her parents report that she is a good eater and chews most of her foods. She has begun to pull off her socks and shoes.

Communication/Language. The Communicative Intention Inventory, SKI*HI Language Development Scale, Parent-Infant Communication checklist, and parent observations indicate that receptively Li looks to her mother and father when requesting either help or information. She responds to her parents' expressions of disapproval (shaking their heads accompanied by negative facial expressions) by temporarily inhibiting her actions.

The same tools indicate that expressively Li requests help to obtain what she wants. She points, pulls, or brings her mother to the object she is requesting. Li uses a variety of facial expressions to communicate her likes, dislikes, surprise, sadness, and anger. She has begun imitating adult games and gestures such as bye-bye. She indicates no by shaking her head or kicking vigorously.

Speech/Auditory Development. Oller's stages of phonetic development (1978), the Developmental Approach to Successful Listening, and parent observations reveal that Li vocalizes frequently in both isolated play and social situations. Li will continue vocalizing when she is stimulated by an adult through imitation; however, she is not consistently aware of when she is vocalizing. Her voice quality

is normal with no noticeable strain or tension. Vocalizations are characterized by vowel-like utterances approximating the neutral and back vowels. Vocal closure of the back of the vocal tract results in some velar and epiglottal consonant-like productions. In addition, her vocalizations include low-pitch growls and high-pitch squeals, variations in loudness, and "raspberries."

Li becomes very quiet and visually searches the room when her hearing aids are first turned on, indicating that she is aware of the presence of sound. Her responses to loud environmental sounds are inconsistent, and she shows no consistent response to voice at close distances. This is true even with a personal FM system used in structured situations.

Based on the results of the assessment, the child-focused goals shown in the table on pp. 288–289 were selected by the Greens and the other members of the transdisciplinary team.

Family-focused Goals and Resources

Based on discussions with the Green family, four family strengths, needs, and interventions were identified.

1. **Family strengths**: The Greens are very knowledgeable, observant, and active participants in the assessment and development of an intervention program. **Family needs**: The Greens recognize the need for early intervention services and are anxious to initiate services. **Family intervention strategy**: Li and her mother will come to the center one day each week for a 1 1/2-hour individual session with Ms. Stein and other professionals as needed to discuss Li's progress and to develop skills to foster her development. Li's father and a deaf educator will join them on alternate weeks.

2. **Family strengths**: Li's parents have developed some excellent strategies to interact with Li nonverbally. They have a very positive parent-child relationship. **Family needs**: The Greens often feel frustrated by their

Child-focused goals and programming resources.

Goals	Resources

Cognition

Search for objects when hidden outside view	SKI*HI Curriculum Manual (Clark & Watkins, 1985)
Remove lids of containers and remove contents	Parent-Infant Communication (Infant Hearing Resource, 1985)
Activate switch toys	Ordinal Scales of Psychological Development (Uzgiris & Hunt, 1975)
Look at picture book and turn pages	Hawaii Early Learning Profile: Activity Guide (HELP) (Furuno et al., 1979)
Match identical and familiar objects	Early Learning Accomplishment Profile (E-LAP) (Glover, Preminger, & Sanford, 1978)
Build tower of 5–6 blocks	
Imitate new, unfamiliar gestures and actions	
Initiate play with toys	
Complete 3-piece form board	

Social-emotional development

Demand personal attention	Same as cognition
Demand proximity of familiar adult	
Initiate play with adults (e.g., Peek-A-Boo, Patty-Cake)	
Play near other children	
Play alone near a familiar adult for short periods of time	
Pretend to feed self, comb hair, or other familiar routine	

Motor development and self-help

Walk up steps with help	Same as cognition
Run	
Push and pull large objects	
Scribble	
Place beads, blocks, etc. in small holes	
Drink from cup with little spilling	
Use spoon with little spilling	

Language/communication

Receptive communication:	SKI*HI Language Development Scale (Watkins, 1979)
Attend when someone is communicating using words/signs	Parent-Infant Communication (Infant Hearing Resource, 1985)
Respond to name when said/signed	Presymbolic Communication, pp. 23–30.
Recognize names of family members and dog when said/signed	

Child-focused goals and programming resources (continued).

Goals	Resources

Language/communication (continued)

Goals	Resources
Recognize familiar words (e.g., bottle, doggie, more, up, stop, no, bye-bye, etc.) when said/signed	A Developmental Language Centered Curriculum for Hearing Impaired Children: Stage 0 (Texas Education Agency, 1982)
Expressive communication:	Birth to Three: A Curriculum for Parents, Parent Trainers, and Teachers of Very Young Hearing-Impaired Children (Thompson, Atcheson, & Pious, 1986).
Uses turn-taking when playing vocal/gesture communication games	
Initiates greetings by waving hi or bye-bye	
Uses pointing, gestures, and pantomime to communicate requests	
Imitates approximate signs for objects or actions	

Speech development

Goals	Resources
Accompany gestures of request for help, action, or information with vocalization	Speech and the Hearing-impaired Child, (Ling, 1976b)
Vocalize when stimulated, reinforced	Teaching Speech to Hearing-impaired Infants & Children (Stovall, 1982)
Indicate wants by differentiated vocalizations or gestures	Schedules of Development in Audition, Speech, Language and Communication (Ling, 1977)
Increase quantity of vocalizations	I Heard That! (Northcott, 1983)
Aware of own vocalizations	
Increase range of vocalizations to include variations in pitch and loudness	
Increase duration of vocalizations	
Maintain quality of vocalizations	
Imitate vocal approximations of animal, transportation, or other interesting sounds	

Auditory development

Goals	Resources
Alert to loud, low-frequency environmental sounds	Schedules of Development in Audition, Speech, Language and Communication (Ling, 1977)
Alert to name or other speech at close distance in quiet environment	Developmental Approach to Successful Listening (Stout & Van Ert Windle, 1986)
Alert to music under good listening conditions	Preschool Auditory Skills Curriculum (Lexington School for the Deaf, 1986)
Indicate when ongoing environmental sound stops	I Heard That! (Northcott, 1983)
Indicate when continuous speech syllable stops	
Aware of when hearing aid is on or off	
Put on hearing aid with help	

inability to communicate complex concepts effectively with Li. They are anxious to improve their communication skills and to investigate the use of signs to augment their communication. **Family intervention strategy**: Ms. Stein, with the assistance of the educator of the deaf, will work with the Greens to improve their communication skills and to help them respond more effectively to Li's vocalizations and gestural communication. Working closely with the deaf educator, Ms. Stein will obtain information and readings about methods of communication and arrange for the Greens to visit programs using different communication methodologies and discuss communication options with deaf adults, deaf educators, and parents of children who have hearing losses. In addition, the Greens will learn some signs to facilitate communication.

3. **Family strengths**: The home environment is supportive of Li's physical, social-emotional, and cognitive growth. The Greens have provided Li with a safe and responsive environment that encourages exploration and manipulation with developmentally appropriate toys and other household materials. The Greens check the hearing aids daily to insure proper functioning. **Family needs**: The Greens expressed a desire to meet with the audiologist and Ms. Stein to further explain what Li can hear, how the hearing aids help, and what they can do at home to help. **Family intervention strategy**: Ms. Stein will set up an appointment with the audiologist. Hearing evaluations for Li will be scheduled every 3 months. **Family needs**: The Greens recognize the need to learn about the impact of hearing loss on development, deaf culture, methods of communication, and educational programs. **Family intervention**

strategy: Ms. Stein will meet with the deaf education specialist to arrange opportunities for the Greens to meet deaf adults, attend meetings with other parents who have hearing-impaired children, and visit educational programs in special schools and regular public schools. In addition, the Greens will attend educational meetings at the center that focus on speech and language development.

4. **Family strengths**: Both of the Greens' parents and three siblings live in the area and have provided emotional support and have helped meet the time and energy demands they have faced. The childcare provider with whom Li spends several hours each week has also been very helpful to the Greens. **Family needs**: The Greens would like to involve the extended family and Li's childcare provider in the intervention program so that they can better understand the impact of hearing loss and improve their communication with Li. **Family intervention strategy**: Ms. Stein will meet with Li's childcare provider 1 hour each week in her home. Grandparents, aunts, and uncles will participate in the family information sessions and other special programs offered by the center. **Family needs**: The Greens expressed a need to discuss their fears and frustrations about Li's hearing loss. They are concerned about her ability to develop speech and language and lead a satisfying social life. They are also saddened by the prospect that her educational progress may not match that of her normally hearing peers. **Family intervention strategy**: Ms. Stein recommended that the Greens participate in a bi-weekly support group for parents at the center where they would have the opportunity to share their concerns with other parents.

SUMMARY OF PROCEDURES

A hearing loss creates special challenges for young children and their families. It often means that families have to make significant changes in their style of communication, and have to carefully consider choices in communication methodology, early intervention services, and future school placement. Children with hearing impairments and their families, like normally hearing children and families, have a wide range of abilities and needs. Nonetheless, some general techniques can be identified that appear to maximize development. Some of the key procedures from this chapter follow:

1. Help families understand the impact of their child's hearing loss on development to promote realistic expectations for their child.
2. Encourage families to understand the type, degree, and severity of their child's hearing loss and the effects of the hearing loss on how their child perceives sound. Encourage families who are unaware of the etiology of their child's hearing loss to seek genetic counseling to better understand medical and educational implications.
3. Provide opportunities for families to meet other families with hearing-impaired children to share information as well as provide support for one another.
4. Involve deaf adults in the early intervention program to provide opportunities for families to meet adults with hearing loss and to provide positive role models for children and families.
5. Assist families in understanding the importance of play as the central medium for learning and facilitating motor, social, cognitive, and communicative skills. Support families in developing positive, nurturing, and mutually enjoyable interactions with their children.
6. Help families recognize and respond to their child's communication attempts to facilitate the development of communication.
7. Meet regularly with specialists in deafness to better assist families in planning and implementing strategies for promoting communication, language, speech, and auditory development.
8. Present communication methodologies to families in an objective and non-biased manner. Support families in selecting and implementing a methodology that meets their child's and family's needs.
9. Ensure that each child with impaired hearing has a comprehensive trans-disciplinary assessment that accurately reflect the child's abilities and needs.
10. Include extended family members in the intervention process. Provide a wide range of services for families, as well as regularly assessing the family's perceptions of how the intervention process can best support their goals.

SUMMARY

The inability to hear has a profound impact on the development of communication in a world where hearing is the channel through which language is acquired. The discovery of impaired hearing often disturbs the delicate fabric that supports the complex patterns of family-child relationships. Early interventionists working with families of hearing-impaired children must examine the consequences of a child's deafness within the framework of the family as a whole. Specialists in the field of deafness and deaf adults are essential members of the transdisciplinary team working with families to promote positive perspectives and facilitative environments that enable children to grow unhampered by disabilities in communication, social interactions, or learning.

DISCUSSION QUESTIONS

1. How are infants with hearing losses similar to/different from infants with normal hearing?
2. What family and child characteristics will influence the communication methodology selected by a particular family?
3. What does comprehensive assessment for a hearing-impaired child encompass? What must the early interventionist do regarding selection, administration, and interpretation of assessments to ensure valid and useful results?

APPLIED ACTIVITIES/PROJECTS

1. Enroll in a sign language class.
2. Using an interpreter, interview a deaf adult who associates with adults who are also deaf. Ask about the individual's educational experiences, communication methodology, early life experiences, and family and social relationships.
3. Interview hearing and hearing-impaired parents of a hearing-impaired preadolescent. Ask them to share their experiences when they discovered their child's hearing loss. To what professionals did they turn? What were the professionals' responses? Who was most helpful to them during that time? Why? What advice do they have for professionals? What would they like to tell parents of newly identified hearing-impaired infants?
4. Contact an audiology clinic that assesses infant hearing. Observe the behavioral and/or electrophysiologic assessments being administered. Observe how the audiologist interacts with the family and/or other professionals. Meet with the audiologist following the session to discuss the findings and recommendations.

SUGGESTED READINGS

Chency, H., Compton, C., & Harder, K. (1988). *Developmental Language Curriculum (DLC): A comprehensive guide and recordkeeping system for hearing-impaired students, infants through 12 years.* Seattle: University of Washington Press.

Clark, T., & Watkins, S. (1985). *SKI*HI curriculum manual: Programming for hearing-impaired infants through home intervention.* North Logan, UT: Hope Inc.

Hasenstab, M., & Horner, J. (1982). *Comprehensive intervention with hearing-impaired infants and preschool children*. Rockville, MD: Aspen.

Infant Hearing Resource. (1985). *Parent-Infant Communication: A program of clinical and home training for parents and hearing-impaired infants* (3rd ed.). Portland, OR: Infant Hearing Resource.

Ling, D. (1976). Phonetic and Phonologic Level Evaluation. In D. Ling (Ed.), *Speech and the hearing impaired child* (pp. 160–169). Washington, DC: Alexander Graham Bell Association.

Northcott, W. (1983). *I Heard That! A Developmental Sequence of Listening Activities for the Young Child*. Washington, DC: Alexander Graham Bell Association.

Thompson, M., Atcheson, J., & Pious, C. (1986). *Birth to three: A curriculum for parents, parent trainers, and teachers of very young hearing-impaired children*. Seattle: University of Washington Press.

REFERENCES

Allen, T. (1986). A study of the achievement patterns of hearing-impaired students: 1974–1983. In A. Schildroth & M. Karchmer (Eds.), *Deaf Children in America* (pp. 161–206). San Diego: College Hill Press.

ASLHA. (1989). Guidelines. Audiologic screening of newborn infants who are at risk for hearing impairment. *ASLHA, 31,* 89–92.

Bailey, D., & Wolery, M. (1989). *Assessing infants and preschoolers with handicaps*. Columbus, OH: Merrill.

Batshaw, M. L., & Perret, Y. M. (1981). *Children with handicaps: A medical primer*. Baltimore: Paul H. Brookes.

Best, B., & Roberts, G. (1976). Early cognitive development in hearing-impaired children. *American Annals of the Deaf, 121,* 560–564.

Bodner-Johnson, B. (1987). Total communication: A professional point of view. In S. Schwartz (Ed.), *Choices in deafness: A parent's guide* (pp. 89–96). Kensington, MD: Woodbine House.

Boothroyd, A. (1982). *Hearing impairments in young children*. Washington, DC: Alexander Graham Bell Association.

Bornstein, H., & Saulnier, K. (1981). Signed English: A brief follow-up to the first evaluation. *American Annals of the Deaf, 126,* 69–72.

Bornstein, H., Saulnier, K., & Hamilton, L. (1980). Signed English: A first evaluation. *American Annals of the Deaf, 125,* 468–481.

Clark, T., & Watkins, S. (1985). *SKI*HI curriculum manual: Programming for hearing-impaired infants through home intervention*. North Logan, UT: Hope Inc.

Clarke-Stewart, A. (1973). Interactions between mothers and their young children: Characteristics and consequences. *Monographs of the Society for Research in Child Development, 38,* (Serial No. 153).

Coggins, T. E., & Carpenter, R. L. (1981). The Communicative Intention Inventory: A system for observing and coding children's early intentional communication. *Applied Psycholinguistics, 2,* 235–251.

Corson, H. (1967). *Comparing deaf children of oral deaf parents and deaf children using manual communication with deaf children of hearing parents on academic, social, and communicative functioning*. Unpublished doctoral dissertation, University of Cincinnati, Ohio.

Cox, L. C. (1988). Screening the high-risk newborn for hearing loss: The Crib-O-Gram v the Auditory Brainstem Response. *Infants and Young Children, 1*(1), 71–81.

Downs, M. (1966). *The establishment of hearing aid use: A program for parents* Vol. IV, Report 5. Maico Audiological Library Series.

Erting, C., Prezioso, C., & Hynes, M. (1989). The interactional context of deaf mother-infant communication. In V. Volterra & C. J. Erting (Eds.), *From gestures to language in hearing and deaf children* (pp. 97–106). New York: Springer-Verlag.

Furth, H. (1966). *Thinking without language: Psychological implications of deafness.* New York: Free Press.

Furuno, S., O'Reilly, K., Hosaka, C., Inatsuka, T., Aleman, T., & Zeisloft, B. (1979). *Hawaii Early Learning Profile (HELP).* Palo Alto, CA: VORT.

Gentile, A., & McCarthy, B. (1973). *Additional handicapping conditions among hearing-impaired students, United States: 1971–72* (Serial D, No. 14). Washington, DC: Gallaudet College Office of Demographic Studies.

Glover, M. E., Preminger, J. L., & Sanford, A. R. (1978). *Early Learning Accomplishment Profile (E-LAP).* Winston-Salem, NC: Kaplan School Supply.

Gregory, S. (1976). *The deaf child at play.* New York: Wiley.

Gustason, G., Pfetzing, D., & Zawolkow, E. (1972). *Signing Exact English.* Rossmoor, CA: Modern Signs Press.

Hafer, J., & Richmond, E. (1988). What hearing parents should learn about deaf culture. *Perspectives, 7,* 2–5.

Harris, M., Clibbens, J., Tibbitts, R., & Chasin, J. (1987, June). *Communication between deaf mothers and their deaf infants.* Paper presented at the Child Language Seminar, York, England.

Hasenstab, M., & Horner, J. (1982). *Comprehensive intervention with hearing-impaired infants and preschool children.* Rockville, MD: Aspen.

Hasenstab, M. S., & Laughton, J. (1982). Bare essentials for assessing really little kids: An approach. In M. S. Hasenstab & J. S. Horner (Eds.), *Comprehensive intervention with hearing-impaired infants and preschool children* (pp. 203–318). Rockville, MD: Aspen.

Hedrick, D., Prather, E., & Tobin, A. (1975). *Sequenced inventory of communication development (SICD)* (rev. ed.). Seattle: University of Washington Press.

Higginbotham, D. J., & Baker, B. M. (1981). Social participation and cognitive play differences in hearing-impaired and normally hearing preschoolers. *Volta Review, 83,* 135–149.

Infant Hearing Resource. (1985). *Parent-Infant Communication: A program of clinical and home training for parents and hearing-impaired infants* (3rd ed.). Portland, OR: Infant Hearing Resource.

John Tracy Clinic. (1983). *Correspondence course for parents of young deaf children.* Los Angeles: Author.

Johnson, R. E., Liddell, S. K., & Erting, C. J. (1989). *Unlocking the curriculum: Principles for achieving access in deaf education* (Gallaudet Research Institute Working Paper 89–3). Washington, DC: Gallaudet University.

Joint Committee on Infant Hearing. (1982). Position statement. *ASHA, 24,* 1017–1018.

Kinsella-Meier, M. A., & Vold, F. C. (1989). *Picture Audiogram.* University Park, MD: Audiology Communication Counseling.

Kyle, J., & Ackerman, H. (1987). *Signing for infants: Deaf mothers using BSL in the early stages of development.* Unpublished manuscript, University of Bristol, Education Research Unit, Bristol, England.

Launer, P. (1982). *A plane is not "to fly:" Acquiring the distinction between related nouns and verbs in ASL.* Unpublished doctoral dissertation, City University of New York.

Lexington School for the Deaf. (1986). *Auditory Skills Curriculum: Preschool Supplement*. North Hollywood, CA: Foreworks.

Ling, A. (1977). *Schedules of Development in Audition, Speech, Language and Communication*. Washington, DC: Alexander Graham Bell Association.

Ling, D. (1976a). Phonetic and Phonologic Level Evaluation. In D. Ling (Ed.), *Speech and the hearing-impaired child: Theory and practice* (pp. 160–169). Washington, DC: Alexander Graham Bell Association.

Ling, D. (Ed.). (1976b). *Speech and the hearing-impaired child: Theory and practice*. Washington, DC: Alexander Graham Bell Association.

Luterman, D. (1979). *Counseling parents of hearing-impaired children*. Boston: Little, Brown.

Madsen, W. (1987). *Conversational sign language II* (11th ed.). Washington, DC: Gallaudet University Press.

Maestas y Moores, J. (1980). Early linguistic environment: Interactions of deaf parents with their infants. *Sign Language Studies, 26,* 1–13.

Mahoney, T., & Eichwald, J. (1987). The ups and "downs" of high-risk screening: The Utah statewide program. In K. Gerkin & A. Amochaev (Eds.), *Seminars in Hearing, 8,* 155–163.

Meadow, K. (1980). *Deafness and child development*. Berkeley: University of California Press.

Meadow, K., Greenberg, M., Erting, C., & Carmichael, H. (1981). Interactions of deaf mothers and deaf preschool children: Comparisons with three other groups of deaf and hearing dyads. *American Annals of the Deaf, 126,* 454–468.

Meadow-Orlans, K. (1987). An analysis of the effectiveness of early intervention programs for hearing-impaired children. In M. J. Guralnick & F. C. Bennett (Eds.), *The effectiveness of early intervention for at-risk and handicapped children* (pp. 325–362). New York: Academic Press.

Moog, J., & Geers, A. (1975). *CID Scales of Early Communication Skills for Hearing-impaired Children*. St. Louis: Central Institute for the Deaf.

Moog, J. S., & Kozak, V. J. (1983). *Teacher Assessment of Grammatical Structures*. St. Louis: Central Institute for the Deaf.

Moores, D. (1987). *Educating the deaf: Psychology, principles and practices* (3rd ed.). Boston: Houghton Mifflin.

Newport, E. L., & Meier, R. P. (1985). The acquisition of American Sign Language. In D. I. Slobin (Ed.), *The crosslinguistic study of language acquisition: Vol. 1. The data* (pp. 881–938). Hillsdale, NJ: Erlbaum.

Northcott, W. (1983). *I Heard That! A Developmental Sequence of Listening Activities for the Young Child*. Washington, DC: Alexander Graham Bell Association.

Northern, J., & Downs, M. (1984). *Hearing in children* (3rd ed.). Baltimore: Williams & Wilkins.

Oller, D. K. (1978). Infant vocalization and the development of speech. *Allied Health and Behavioral Sciences, 1,* 523–549.

Oller, D. K., Eilers, R. E., Bull, D. H., & Carney, A. E. (1985). Prespeech vocalizations of a deaf infant: A comparison with normal metaphonological development. *Journal of Speech and Hearing Research, 28,* 47–63.

Pollack, D. (1970). *Educational audiology for the limited hearing infant*. Springfield, IL: Charles C. Thomas.

Quigley, S., & Kretschmer, R. (1982). *The education of deaf children: Issues, theory and practice*. Baltimore: University Park Press.

Rosenstein, J. (1961). Perception, cognition, and language in deaf children. *Exceptional Children, 27,* 276–284.

Schildroth, A. (1986). Hearing-impaired children under age 6: 1977 & 1984. *American Annals of the Deaf, 131,* 85–90.

Schlesinger, H., & Meadow, K. (1972). *Sound and sign, childhood deafness and mental health*. Berkeley: University of California Press.

Schuyler, V., & Rushmer, N. (1987). *Parent-infant habilitation: A comprehensive approach to working with hearing-impaired infants and toddlers and their families*. Portland, OR: Infant Hearing Resource.

Seligman, M. (1975). *Helplessness: On depression, development and death*. San Francisco: W. H. Freeman.

Simmons, F. B. (1977). Automated screening test for newborns: The Crib-O-Gram. In B. F. Jaffe (Ed.), *Hearing loss in children* (pp. 89–98). Baltimore: University Park Press.

Singer, D. G., & Lenaham, M. L. (1976). Imagination content in dreams of deaf children. *American Annals of the Deaf, 121,* 44–48.

Stark, R. (1983). Phonatory development in young normally hearing and hearing-impaired children. In I. Hochberg, H. Levitt, & M. J. Osberger (Eds.), *Speech of the hearing impaired: Research, training, and personnel preparation* (pp. 251–266). Baltimore: University Park Press.

Stoel-Gammon, C., & Otomo, K. (1986). Babbling development of hearing-impaired and normally hearing subjects. *Journal of Speech and Hearing Disorders, 51,* 33–41.

Stout, G., & Van Ert Windle, J. (1986). *Developmental Approach to Successful Listening*. Houston: Houston School for the Deaf.

Stovall, D. (1982). *Teaching speech to hearing-impaired infants and children*. Springfield, IL: Charles C. Thomas.

Texas Education Agency. (1982). *A Developmental Language Centered Curriculum for Hearing Impaired Children: Stage 0*. Austin: Texas Education Agency.

Thompson, M., Atcheson, J., & Pious, C. (1986). *Birth to three: A curriculum for parents, parent trainers, and teachers of very young hearing-impaired children*. Seattle: University of Washington Press.

Thompson, M., Biro, P., Vethievelu, S., Pious, C., & Hatfield, N. (1987). *Language assessment of hearing-impaired school-age children*. Seattle: University of Washington Press.

Uzgiris, E. C., & Hunt, J. M. (1975). *Ordinal Scales of Psychological Development: Assessment in Infancy*. Urbana: University of Illinois Press.

Vernon, M. (1967). Relationship of language to the thinking process. *Archives of Genetic Psychiatry, 16,* 325–333.

Vernon, M. (1982). Multi-handicapped deaf children: Types and causes. In D. Tweedie & E. Shroyer (Eds.), *The multi-handicapped hearing-impaired: Identification and instruction* (pp. 11–28). Washington, DC: Gallaudet College Press.

Vygotsky, L. S. (1967). Play and its role in the mental development of the child. *Soviet Psychology, 12,* 62–76.

Watkins, S. (1979). *SKI*HI Language Development Scale: Assessment of Language Skills for Hearing Impaired Children from Infancy to Five Years of Age*. Logan: Utah State University.

Williams-Scott, B. (1987). Cued speech: A professional point of view. In S. Schwartz (Ed.), *Choices in deafness: A parent's guide* (pp. 23–31). Kensington, MD: Woodbine House.

Yarrow, L., Rubenstein, J., Pedersen, F., & Jankowski, J. (1972). Dimensions of early stimulation and their differential effects in infant development. *Merrill-Palmer Quarterly, 18,* 205–218.

11

Techniques for Infants and Toddlers with Visual Impairments

Kay Alicyn Ferrell and Sharon A. Raver

OVERVIEW

This chapter discusses the development and assessment of children with visual impairments and blindness, including:

□ causes of visual impairments and blindness
□ effects of visual loss on development
□ assessment of visually impaired infants and toddlers
□ specialized intervention and adaptations for visually impaired infants and toddlers

The role of vision in infancy is to motivate, guide, and verify the child's interaction with the environment. The loss or limitation of vision can have a profound effect on a child's development. Children with visual impairments or blindness are at risk for significant delays in cognitive functions, exploratory behavior, and emotional development unless early intervention is provided (Warren, 1989).

TERMINOLOGY

Before examining the major issues involved in visual impairment in infancy, it is necessary to define terms used to describe aspects of this disability. For example, **visual impairment** is generally used to refer to an array of eye conditions that result in visual abilities that are less than normal. P.L. 94–142, The Education of the Handicapped Act, uses **visually handicapped** to refer to children who have "a visual impairment which, even with correction, adversely affects a child's educational performance" (20 U.S.C. 1401(b)(1)). Both of these terms are broad and cover a range of visual functioning from total blindness to minor refraction problems. When these terms are applied to infants, they become even more nebulous, particularly since methods for identification of visual impairments in young children have not been perfected.

To further complicate the situation, there are other terms currently used by the legal and educational communities. **Legal blindness,** for example, is used by federal and state governments for certain entitlement programs. It is based on specific clinical measurements of distance vision and requires that an individual have central visual acuity of 20/200 or less in the better eye with corrective lenses, or a visual field defect of 20 degrees or less in the better eye (Koestler, 1976). **Central visual acuity** of 20/200 means that the individual can see at 20 feet only as well as the individual with normal vision sees at 200 feet. Obviously, these measurements have little applicability to infants who are unable to read a Snellen chart.

Also, these terms provide little information about visual functioning. **Visual functioning** is frequently used to refer to a continuum of visual ability that ranges from normal or near-normal vision to total blindness (Barraga, 1977). Visual functioning (also described as functional vision) is how individuals use the vision they possess. That is, many individuals who are legally blind for distance are able to read regular size print at near point. Regardless of measured visual acuity, visual functioning may vary depending on the environmental conditions and the tasks required. In regular daytime room lighting, for example, an infant with a visual impairment may use vision to guide play with stacking and nesting toys. On a bright sunny day at the beach, however, the same infant may have to rely on touch to play with the same toys, or may, more likely, refuse to play at all. The tasks have not changed, but the environment makes the child **functionally blind** due to the bright sunlight and the glare from the sand.

Children with visual impairments are further described in terms of the primary learning modality by which they learn. The **blind infant** learns primarily through sensory modalities other than vision (usually, but not exclusively, touch and hearing). (The **congenitally blind** infant is a child who is blind from birth). The **low vision infant** is severely limited visually, but will be able to use vision to some extent in conjunction with other senses. The **visually limited infant** is a child who is primarily a visual learner but who is limited visually under specific everyday conditions such as bright sunlight (Barraga, 1983).

There are not only many degrees of visual impairment, but an extremely broad range of visual functioning as well. For intervention purposes, it is best to assume that any visual impairment, regardless of degree, has the potential to affect the child's ability to obtain information about the environment and the people in it.

CAUSES OF VISUAL IMPAIRMENTS

It is difficult to delineate accurately the causes of visual impairment in infancy. There are no national registers of individuals with visual impairments, and in states where mandatory reporting laws are in effect, the states often have little enforcement. Consequently, etiology estimates are based either on small samples from a limited geographic area or on national counts with recognized unreliable methods of data collection.

Nonetheless, some generalizations can be made. In general, visual impairment in infancy has three causes: inheritance, prenatal infection or injury, and peri- or postnatal insult. Ferrell (1987) reported preliminary data on a national survey of categorical programs serving 1,671 children with visual impairment younger than age 5. The leading causes of visual impairment in this sample were cortical blindness (21%); retinopathy of prematurity (20%); optic nerve hypoplasia (7%); congenital cataracts (6%); and Leber's amaurosis, albinism, and optic atrophy (5% each). A study conducted in the New York City metropolitan area by the Visually Impaired Infants Research Consortium (VIIRC) (Ferrell et al., in press) found a similar pattern. This study reports that of the 82 children currently being served, the leading causes of visual impairment are retinopathy of prematurity (23.2%), cortical blindness (13.4%), and Leber's amaurosis (12.2%).

Although figures may vary between regions and states, these two studies, regardless of their limitations, permit inferences about the current population of visually impaired infants.

Retinopathy of prematurity.   A large proportion of infants are visually impaired as a result of **retinopathy of prematurity**, a pathology that 15 years ago was predicted to disappear (Hatfield, 1975). Instead, the incidence of this disease has risen sharply with the increased survival rate of extremely low birthweight infants (Phelps, 1981; Silverman, 1982). As discussed in Chapter 6, retinopathy of prematurity (ROP) is an eye condition associated with prematurity which can lead to detachment of the retina and visual impairment or blindness. Once known as retrolental fibroplasia and thought to be caused by excessive oxygen administration after birth, medical scientists have yet to determine ROP's exact cause. At present, it appears to be associated more with low birthweight than any other factor (Flynn, 1987). However, there is also limited evidence that ROP may be influenced by: intensity of light exposure in neo-natal hospital units (Glass et al., 1985), the number of hours the infant requires ventilator assistance (Hammer et al., 1986), multiple spells of apnea and/or brady-cardia (Flynn, 1987), and the need for blood transfusions (Hammer et al., 1986). This condition creates a very difficult dilemma for medical professionals because, at present, ROP seems to be an inevitable condition of prematurity for some infants.

Cortical blindness.   The large proportion of children with cortical blindness may reflect the difficulty in diagnosing visual abilities in infants, or more likely reflects a catch-all term applied to infants with severe brain insult. **Cortical blindness** is defined as a disturbance of the visual cortex in the absence of any other known pathology. Seventy-eight percent of children described as having cortical blindness in Ferrell's (1987) study were also reported to have one or more additional handicapping con-ditions; all of the children with cortical blindness in the VIIRC study (Ferrell et al., in press) are also multiply handicapped. This appears to support the possibility that cortical blindness is being used to describe any severe brain insult that results in blindness.

Other causes.   The remaining causes of visual impairment suggest either hereditary factors such as albinism, or a disturbance in the development of the eye in utero affecting either the lens (e.g., cataracts) or the retina and associated structures (e.g., optic nerve hypoplasia, Leber's amaurosis). As Hatfield (1975) predicted, infection is no longer a major cause of eye pathology in infants in the United States.

None of the leading causes of visual impairment appear to produce a predictable developmental pattern in infants. Retinopathy of prematurity (ROP) may affect only a small portion of the retina, or it may lead to retinal detachment and total blindness. Other retinal disorders differ according to where the lesions occur. Infants with the same visual diagnosis, born on the same day, and in the same hospital will, more likely than not, have completely different patterns of visual functioning and overall development.

The variability in the etiology of visual impairments, the vicissitudes of different environments, and the difficulty of identifying and referring infants for early intervention services all work together to make it difficult to predict the developmental outcome of any young child.

Prevalence of Visual Impairment

Precise figures on the prevalence and incidence of visual impairment in infancy are also difficult to obtain. While P.L. 94–142 requires annual reports from states on the number of children being served, the count of visually handicapped children is generally thought to be inaccurate and to grossly undercount the number of children between the ages of birth and 21 years who are visually impaired (Huebner & Ferrell, 1986; Kirchner, 1989; Packer & Kirchner, 1985). The situation is further confused by the addition, in the late 1970s, of deaf-blind and multiply handicapped categories in the schools' annual count (Vaughn & Scholl, 1980). Many visually handicapped children may, in fact, be counted in these new categories.

Kirchner (1989) thoroughly discusses the various data sources and their weaknesses, including the variability of definitions, methodologies, and age ranges used. She shows that the databases that include children younger than 5 years indicate a prevalence of visual impairment of 0.42 to 0.86 per 1,000 population. (Interestingly, the highest rate is reported by the American Printing House for the Blind, which uses the more restrictive definition of legal blindness). Whatever database is used, the population of infants with visual impairment who receive early intervention services is small.

EFFECTS OF VISUAL LOSS

The low prevalence and wide functional and developmental heterogeneity of infants with visual impairment make it virtually impossible to state, with any certainty, the exact effect visual impairment has on infant and toddler development. Several studies have made generalizations about the entire population of visually impaired young children, but caution must be used when accepting conclusions drawn either from case studies or studies with larger samples that possess serious methodological weaknesses in their designs.

Developmental Research

Four major research efforts provide interventionists with general guidelines to the more significant developmental hurdles infants with visual impairment are likely to face. For example, Norris, Spaulding, and Brodie (1957) attempted to establish developmental norms for visually impaired children by administering the Cattell Infant Intelligence Scale (Cattell, 1940) to 66 children born between 1945 and 1952. Eighty-five percent of the sample experienced a preterm birth and subsequently developed retrolental fibroplasia (RLF, now known as ROP, retinopathy of prematurity). None of the subjects was identified as multihandicapped. The degree of visual functioning was not reported. These researchers concluded that the delays in developmental milestones noted in their blind sample were due primarily to the lack of experience, rather than to the visual impairment. Further, they stated that developmental delay increased geometrically with age, pointing out that the more time that passed between when the child was ready to learn and when the opportunity to learn was actually provided, the greater the time delay before the child actually acquired the skill.

The same year Maxfield and Buchholz (1957) attempted to adapt the Vineland Social Maturity Scale (Doll, 1953) by norming the test on a group of 308 visually impaired children ranging in age from 5 months to 5 years, 11 months. This work resulted in the publication of the *Social Maturity Scale for Blind Preschool Children*. Again, the majority of this sample was premature with subsequent ROP, and neither the degree of visual functioning nor the presence of additional handicapping conditions were reported.

Perhaps the best known of the developmental studies, Fraiberg's work (1977) with her colleagues at the University of Michigan is widely cited as evidence of the significant delays caused by visual impairment. Only 10 children were studied intensively, none of whom were reported to be multihandicapped, and only 3 of whom had ROP. All were involved in what Fraiberg called a home-based education and guidance program, until the age of 2 1/2 years. Fraiberg concluded:

> Blindness as an impediment to adaptation was clearly discerned in each of the areas of development in this study, even when we employed our knowledge to facilitate development and helped the child and his parents find adaptive solutions. (1977, p. 272)

Finally, Reynell (1983) studied visually handicapped children to develop the mental development portion of the *Reynell Zinkin Scales*. Reynell studied 109 partially seeing and blind children, about one-fourth of whom had additional handicapping conditions. Like the other major studies, Reynell found delays in mental development, with blind children experiencing greater delays than the partially seeing children.

Developmental Research in Progress

The Visually Impaired Infants Research Consortium (VIIRC) has developed a database for tracking the development of infants with visual impairment and is gathering information on demographic and birth information, as well as the age of acquisition of 21 milestones selected by VIIRC as indices of developmental progress (Ferrell et

TABLE 11–1

Acquisition of selected developmental milestones by young children with visual impairments (median age, in months).

Milestone	Infants without Disabilities	Infants with VI[1] (n = 39)	Infants with VI/MH[2] (n = 43)
Gross Motor			
Rolls over intentionally from stomach to back	4.0[3]	6.0	7.0
Rolls over intentionally from back to stomach	6.4[4]	5.0	9.0
Range:[3]	4–10 mos		
Sits alone without support	6.6[4]	7.0	14.0
Range:	5–9 mos		
Crawls forward on hands and knees 3 or more feet	9.0[3]	10.0	13.0[6]
Walks alone without support (10 feet)	13.0[7]	15.0	20.0
Walks up and down stairs alternating feet	30.0+[4]	24.0[6]	30.0[8]
Fine motor			
Reaches for and grasps toy	5.4[4]	6.5	9.0
Range:	4–10 mos		
Transfers object from hand to hand	5.5[4]	7.0	8.0
Range:	4–8 mos		
Searches for a dropped toy	6.0[4]	12.0	12.0[6]
Range:	5–10 mos		
Picks up and eats small foods	7.4[4]	11.0	15.0
Range:	6–10 mos		
Copies or draws circle	33.0[9]	33.0[6]	36.0[8]

[1]VI = Visual impairments
[2]VI/MH = Visual impairments, multiple handicaps
[3]Knobloch, Stevens, & Malone (1980)
[4]Bayley (1969)
[5]Range for children without disabilities is provided when available
[6]Less than 50% of this subgroup had accomplished this skill at the time of the survey
[7]Illingworth (1980)
[8]Less than 25% of this subgroup had accomplished this skill at the time of the survey
[9]Frankenburg, Dodds, & Fandall (1973)
[10]Brigance (1978)

TABLE 11–1

(continued)

Milestone	Infants without Disabilities	Infants with VI[1] (n = 39)	Infants with VI/MH[2] (n = 43)
Communication			
Says first word (mama, baba) Range:	7.9[4] 5–14 mos	10.0	19.0[6]
Uses 2-word sentences Range:	20.6[4] 16–30 mos	18.0	27.0[8]
Uses first person pronouns appropriately	24.0[3]	36.0[6]	38.0[8]
Follows 2-step directions	36.0[7]	24.0[6]	30.0[8]
Social			
Plays interactively with adults Range:	9.7[4] 7–15 mos	11.0	18.0[6]
Cognitive			
Points to 3 of own body parts	18.0[3]	23.0[6]	20.0[6]
Sings a song from memory	40.0[10]	24.0[6]	30.0[8]
Talks about past events	40.0[9]	30.0[6]	27.0[8]
Self-help			
Toilet trained without diapers during day	30.0[7]	25.0[6]	37.0[8]
Removes T-shirt independently	36.0[7]	24.0[6]	24.0[6]

Source: From "The Visually Impaired Infants Research Consortium (VIIRC): First Year Results" by K. A. Ferrell, E. Trief, S. Deitz, M. A. Bonner, D. Cruz, E. Ford, & J. Stratton, in press, *Journal of Visual Impairment and Blindness.* Copyright © 1989 by K. A. Ferrell. Reprinted by permission.

al., in press). Table 11–1 presents the developmental acquisition data from the first year of this study. The consortium has arrived at the following conclusions:

1. Infants with visual impairment and no additional handicapping conditions, in many cases, achieve selected developmental milestones within the range of acquisition demonstrated by sighted infants.
2. Infants with visual impairment who also have additional handicapping conditions, in most cases, acquire these same milestones at a later chronological age.

3. The sequence of acquisition differs in both groups from that demonstrated by sighted infants.
4. The greatest delays in development are in the fine motor domain.

Although this study is limited by its reliance on informants and its lack of specificity on the degree of functional vision, it offers insight into the developmental problems of infants with visual impairment.

Conclusions from Developmental Studies

All of these studies suggest delays in skill acquisition, but they also draw four other conclusions.

1. Visual impairment poses a significant risk to early child development.
2. Handicapping conditions in addition to visual impairment compound the developmental risk.
3. Many skills are not acquired because they have not been introduced. Several authors cite the correspondence between opportunity and acquisition.
4. There is tremendous variability in each sample studied. The interactive nature of development and the range of variables affecting infants with visual impairment make it impossible to establish cause and effect relationships or to predict the developmental course for individual children.

Application of a Sighted Standard

While it is generally thought that infants with visual impairment are delayed in several areas of development, that delay exists only when children are compared to others without the disability. There is little evidence that infants with visual impairment experience the environment and the people around them in the same way as sighted infants. In fact, evidence seems to indicate that their experiences may be totally different (Santin & Simmons, 1977). For example, does the touch and taste of a banana produce the same concept as the sight and taste of a banana? Or does the sound of a mother's voice produce the same concept as the sight of her face? And, little is known about the coordination of the senses. It is not known, for instance, if the sound of a squeeze toy produces the same concept for the visually impaired child when the child holds it or if someone else holds it.

Yet, realistically, infants with visual impairment live in a visual world. Their parents, peers, and teachers are usually sighted. They are evaluated with instruments normed on a sighted population. Even if future research demonstrates that applying a sighted standard to infants with visual impairment is wrong, the fact remains that presently there is no alternative.

Developmental Hurdles

DuBose (1979) identifies 62 curricular concerns for the development of young children with visual impairment. Space does not permit a discussion of each, but some of the principal developmental hurdles for infants and toddlers should be addressed.

Sensory stimulation.   Observing the infant without a visual disability easily demonstrates the role vision plays in early development. Attachment, play, imitation, and motor skills are only a few of the areas that are explicitly related to vision. From the second day of life, infants make eye contact and follow moving objects (Brazelton, 1973). Vision both provides and demonstrates attention, and forms the basis for all future learning. Barraga (1983) suggests that vision integrates all other sensory modalities. For this reason, the loss or distortion of vision necessitates that interventionists carefully guide the visually impaired child so lost sensory information is received in some way.

For infants with visual impairment, the primary mode of obtaining information is limited, unreliable, or missing altogether, so the child must utilize other means to obtain the sensory information that forms concepts. Unfortunately, it is not known how infants do this and there is some evidence that infants with visual impairment experience delays in intersensory coordination (Ferrell, 1984a; 1984b). Consequently, even with intact input from the other senses, there is no guarantee that the information has meaning for the child.

Vision verifies information received through the other modalities for sighted infants. In other words, when the sighted infant hears the sound made by a favorite toy, the child turns to look at it, and then smiles in recognition. The blind infant, however, may hear the sound, may even turn toward it, but requires touch to verify its recognition. The visually impaired child's response is neither immediate nor assured. There is always delay, even assuming that tactile recognition occurs at the same age as visual recognition.

Sensory input that is at times absent, and at other times unbalanced, has a cumulative effect on how the visually impaired child interprets the world. This effect begins in infancy and the child may not catch up until adolescence (Stephens & Grube, 1982; Stephens & Simpkins, 1974).

Imitation.   Visual imitation plays a critical role in early learning (Miller, 1983) and is involved in almost every aspect of the child's development. The infant with visual impairment is unable to observe others in motor activities, in food preparation, in conversations, or in play. It is not uncommon for children with severe visual limitations or blindness to need improvement in some social area because most social skills are learned through visual imitation (Raver & Drash, 1988). Parallel and imitative play are very important to the child's socio-communicative development. Without these experiences, peer-to-peer play and later social skills may be limited in adolescence (Scholl, 1986).

Motor development.   Adelson and Fraiberg (1974) provide an extensive account of motor development in blind infants, which Fraiberg (1977) summarizes. Motor delays tend to be difficulties in locomotion, rather than overall motor development. Visually impaired children tend to acquire gross motor postural milestones within the same range as sighted children. However, items requiring self-initiated mobility and locomotion have a greater chance of presenting delays.

Fraiberg and her colleagues postulate that locomotion delays are attributable to the delay in reaching to sound, which for infants in their study did not occur until

Visual impairment poses a significant risk to early development, so concrete experiences must be arranged to facilitate compensatory skills in young children.

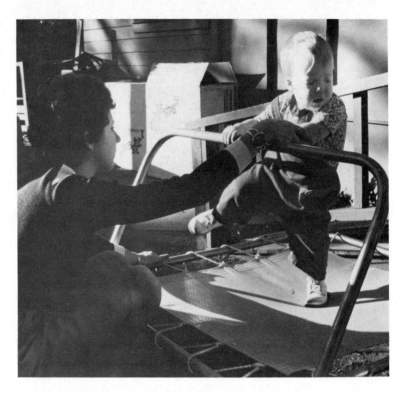

late in the first year. Fraiberg believes that reaching is a significant event in the life of an infant, and that sighted infants who reached at 4 or 5 months of age were actually demonstrating their understanding of objects outside the self. Infants with good vision practice this awareness and develop their knowledge of objects for approximately 5 months before crawling. Blind infants, on the other hand, who are unable physiologically to reach to sound until 9 or 10 months, seem to then need the 5-month practice period before they can crawl.

The theory seems plausible, particularly because later studies seem to support the locomotor delay. However, this hypothesis does not take into account later studies of auditory development which show that reaching to sound can occur earlier than previously thought. The real hurdle may be related to intersensory coordination and the delayed cognitive development of object permanence.

It may also be that locomotor delays are related to inadequate experiences while basic postural skills are acquired. For example, many blind children walk with an unusual gait—feet externally rotated, stiff-legged, center of gravity lowered, almost waddling. It could be that this gait, which is characterized by weight shift without hip and trunk rotation, occurs because the infants' early experiences did not incorporate hip and trunk rotation into daily routines. Sighted infants first practice hip and trunk rotation in the sitting position, by turning to retrieve an object that is picked up by their peripheral vision. This rotation, reach, and retrieve action is the foundation for moving from sitting to crawling.

However, visually impaired infants, because they never see objects in the periphery, may never practice hip and trunk rotation in sitting. For this reason, it is *essential* that visually impaired children have experiences that closely match those their sighted peers spontaneously seek. Interventionists must assist families in establishing *varied* and *continual* prelocomotion experiences (e.g., trunk and hip rotation in reaching, sitting, standing) so that later locomotion skills will be based on adequate early motor preparation. Some of the positioning activities described in Chapter 3 are appropriate for infants with visual impairments before they begin to walk.

In addition, if atypical postures such as head droop, rounding of the lower back, and atypical motor patterns develop, the services of a developmental therapist may be warranted. If these behaviors are not corrected in early childhood, they can negatively affect how people perceive the child's competence and social desirability (Raver, 1987a; 1990). The reader is referred to other sources for specific information for normalizing atypical motor and social patterns (e.g., Raver, 1984; Raver & Dwyer, 1986; Raver, 1987b).

Intersensory coordination.   The ability to use all the sensory modalities simultaneously is critical in early development. Equally important is **cross-modal transfer**, the ability to take information obtained through one sensory modality and apply it to another. Most early intervention strategies assume that intersensory coordination and cross-modal transfer occurs, without evaluating whether it does. If, however, observation indicates that cross-modal transfer is not occurring, then **coactive movements** are needed. Coactive movements occur when the interventionist aids the child through a movement such as crawling, spoon feeding, or completing a puzzle.

Another typical early intervention strategy is the **multisensory approach** in which the interventionist attempts to provide as much simultaneous sensory stimulation as possible for the child. This may assist or compensate for difficulties the child experiences in integrating sensory input. Activities or routines are presented systematically through the remaining four senses of smell, taste, hearing, and touch. (Any vision the child has is also used.) For example, during diapering, the infant is encouraged to smell the difference between fresh cloth and disposable diapers, taste and feel their differences and commonalities, and attend to their different sounds. Parents' comments would guide this type of exploration. It can never be assumed that incidental learning and intersensory coordination spontaneously occur in infants and toddlers with visual impairments.

However, for some visually impaired infants, the multisensory approach leads to sensory bombardment that prompts the child to tune out, instead of integrating the information. Unfortunately, there are few guidelines for deciding which approach, and how much input, is optimal for a child. Generally, if the child appears to withdraw from an activity, it may indicate that input is excessive. Recent research failed to find evidence of cross-modal transfer in 24 children between the ages of 6 and 24 months on a test of tactual-to-visual transfer, even though the infants had all demonstrated residual visual acuity (Ferrell, 1984a; 1984b). Although evidence from interventionists suggests that intersensory coordination is a problem area for many visually impaired children, more information is clearly needed.

Object permanence.   As discussed in Chapter 4, object permanence is the knowledge that an object or person exists when the object or person is not in sensory contact with the individual. For the infant this usually means that a toy played with yesterday is searched for tomorrow. The infant with good visual abilities is able to make this connection easier than the infant with visual impairment because of the immediate feedback and verification provided by vision. Substituting sound or tactual qualities for objects may not provide sufficient information.

Parents of infants with visual impairments must constantly create situations in which play with and explanation of objects is arranged, rewarded, and expected in an effort to compensate for the anticipated delay in this area. Mobiles, playpens, wrist rattles, and toys with short strings aid in keeping toys nearby and retrieving them when they are pushed out of reach.

Fine motor skills.   It is often assumed that tactual development is more highly developed in infants with visual impairment precisely because they are so dependent on it. But this is not the case (Cutsforth, 1951). Fine motor development does not occur in isolation but is interrelated with all aspects of development. Many infants with visual impairment do not receive sufficient opportunities in the prone position and, consequently, miss the experience of weight bearing on the hands and subsequent refinement of grasping. If the child's grasp and object relations do not become refined, self-feeding does not occur (Kitzinger, 1980). If the muscles in the mouth are not exercised through the introduction of new textures, speech does not occur.

Classification.   Abstract thinking, reasoning, and generalization are used in the cognitive process of **classification**. Because of the lack of opportunity to observe objects by size, shape, or color infants who are visually impaired may experience a delay in the first stage of classification: grouping by physical attributes. Gerhardt (1982) found that blind infants between the ages of 14 and 18 months learn to control objects by devising a strategy involving the simultaneous use of two objects, one in each hand. This study reported classification of objects based on their similarities paralleled the development of sighted children, with a slight developmental lag.

Language development.   Visually impaired infants have been described as demonstrating fewer positive vocalizations, making fewer social initiations to the mother, evidencing more negative affect (such as crying and whining), and spending more time ignoring the mothers than sighted infants of the same age (Rogers & Puchalski, 1984; Rowland, 1984). Although language development of blind children generally parallels sighted children's (Bigelow, 1987; Parsons, 1985), deviations and common delays have been identified, such as limited use of object names and requests, heavy reliance on routine phrases and people's names, limited reference to objects and events out of touch, and delayed development of personal pronouns (Urwin, 1984), as well as deviations in some pragmatic aspects of language (Anderson, Dunlea, & Kekelis, 1984).

Attachment. Als, Tronick, and Brazelton (1980) and Fraiberg (1977) have devoted considerable attention to attachment in infants with visual impairment, focusing on the different responses and signal behavior they demonstrate. Infants with visual impairment have a sophisticated repertoire of attachment behaviors that are different from infants with intact vision (Rogers & Puchalski, 1986). Sighted children rely on eye contact for feedback and social engagement. Visually impaired infants, on the other hand, respond with facial expressions, body movements, and autonomic and not easily observable behaviors (e.g., heartbeat, breathing patterns) to communicate.

What is not frequently understood is that infants with visual impairment, because they must rely on their hearing, are unusually quiet—which causes them to be seen as passive. Sudden movements without preparatory cues may frighten the infant, eliciting a startle reflex and extension of body parts. Adults who are unaware of the infant's interaction style may interpret this as emotional rejection when, in fact, it is more likely a response to the adult's insensitive approach. Consequently, it is important for adults to prepare the child before touching, moving, or interacting with the child. Comments such as "Hello, Billy, I am going to give you a hug," signal the child that a change is going to occur. Family members often need to be trained to recognize the unique attachment behaviors and signals of infants with visual impairments. In this way, families can more effectively reward and increase their child's social involvement and reciprocity.

Additionally, visually impaired infants tend to suffer prolonged periods of separation anxiety that seem to be due, in part, to their necessarily greater dependence on caretakers. As infants grow older, visual impairment places other limitations on social interactions. Anyone who was reared by the crook of their mother's eyebrow knows the importance of nonverbal communication and appreciates the amount of information visually impaired infants miss.

The inability to observe the signals of others places them at a disadvantage not only in interpreting and generalizing from the actions of others, but also in monitoring their own behavior. Blind children are often described as manifesting lags in social maturity and as initiating fewer social contacts than their sighted peers (Markovits & Strayer, 1982).

Most people learn social rules from others, such as when it is permissible to scratch, or eat with the fingers. These rules are learned directly through verbal admonishments or indirectly through stares or disapproving facial expressions. The visually handicapped child cannot read the indirect signals, nor can the child change the behavior unless someone tells the child about it. If these behaviors are not changed, relationships with peers and adults will suffer (Ferrell, 1986; Raver, in press; 1987a).

Incidental learning. In normal development, infants acquire new skills almost naturally, with little intervention. However, for the infant with visual impairment, learning can never be left to chance. A good example of this is the skill of dropping objects into containers and then dumping them. No one has to teach an infant without disabilities how to do this. Nonhandicapped children observe the people around them doing this every day as they throw away trash, put money in a purse, take

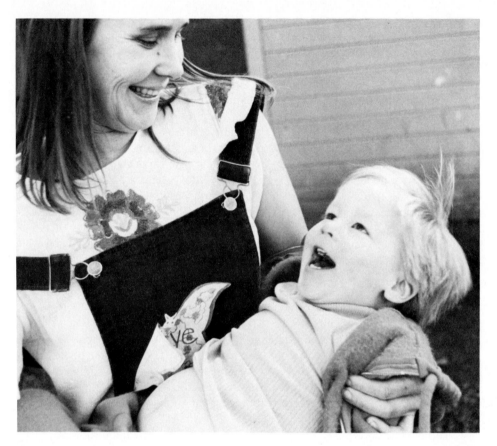

Family members often need to be trained to recognize the unique signals and attachment behaviors of infants with visual impairments so that they may more effectively increase their child's social engagement and reciprocity.

change out of a pocket, pour milk, and take a cookie out of the cookie jar. When an adult introduces a toy that requires the skills of in and out (such as a plastic milk bottle and clothespins), little instruction is needed because the sighted infant has already had a good deal of vicarious experience with the concepts.

The infant with visual impairment cannot profit from vicarious experiences. Consequently, interventionists and families cannot afford to make assumptions about the child's prior experience. Instead, those around the child must take the time to demonstrate and explain, as much as possible, all that is occurring around the child. The child needs to be directly engaged to develop adequate experience with concepts. Experiences must be direct, concrete, and meaningful to the child to expand concept development.

Part to whole.   Most infants learn from global to specific; that is, they observe the totality of an object before they examine the small parts. Infants with visual impairment, however, must learn in the opposite direction. They have to examine the parts and then somehow fit them into a whole concept. This style of learning is clumsy, slow, and easily leads to misinterpretation or the formation of faulty concepts.

The difficulties this learning style imposes are illustrated by the way infants obtain information and concepts about the family pet. The infant with good visual abilities sees a whole cat, simultaneously. When the cat meows, the child sees the mouth open; when it licks or scratches the child's hand, the child sees its tongue or its paw and how these parts fit into the concept of *cat*. In contrast, the infant with visual impairment obtains information about the cat in random pieces. The child can feel only one part of the cat at any time and does not know how all the parts fit together. The child may hear a meow, but does not know where the sound comes from; the tongue and the paw come out of nowhere; and the soft fur may brush against the skin at any time without warning. Giving the infant with visual impairment a stuffed toy and labeling it as a cat adds further confusion to the child's effort to understand the concept of cat. The stuffed toy feels and acts nothing like the real cat. All infants form concepts gradually, utilizing all sensory input; infants with visual impairment do so with disjointed information. Of course, the visually impaired child eventually learns the concept of *cat,* but the concept is based on the child's unique sensory experiences, and the resulting concept may or may not resemble the concept of *cat* held by sighted individuals.

Concrete experiences. As children mature, it is possible to introduce toys or models to illustrate concepts. However, it is important to recognize that visual limitations affect toddlers' abilities to symbolize (to have an object stand for the real object or person), simply because they cannot see it. This is why concrete materials and the child's own body and body movements are preferred for instructional purposes. Concrete materials and direct experiences increase the likelihood of forming both accurate and adequate concepts, because they are genuine and not merely objects that someone with sight, who has already formed the concept, thinks represents reality.

There are many objects that do not lend themselves to concrete experiences: the sun, birds, bumblebees, tigers. Nonetheless, each of these also has sensory qualities such as warmth and brightness, chirping and wing fluttering, buzzing, and roaring. During the first years of life, it is important to focus on concrete, direct experiences that have meaning to the infant, rather than abstract experiences that may have meaning only to sighted adults.

In summary, visual impairment has the potential to affect all aspects of development. Even with early intervention, some of the influences of the loss or reduction of vision, such as delays in locomotive movements, may be difficult to completely compensate for because auditory development does not provide the same advantages as visual development (Adelson & Fraiberg, 1976). Further, the acquisition of visual-perceptual skills and spatial relationship concepts such as body image, body awareness, and space awareness are often not well developed due to visual impairment (Palazesi, 1986). Interventionists must be careful to not be misled. A child can verbally describe a concept and still fail to integrate it intellectually or apply it in life. A critical role of interventionists is to assist visually impaired children in their efforts to integrate developmental domains. Figure 11–1 shows the major skill areas of motor

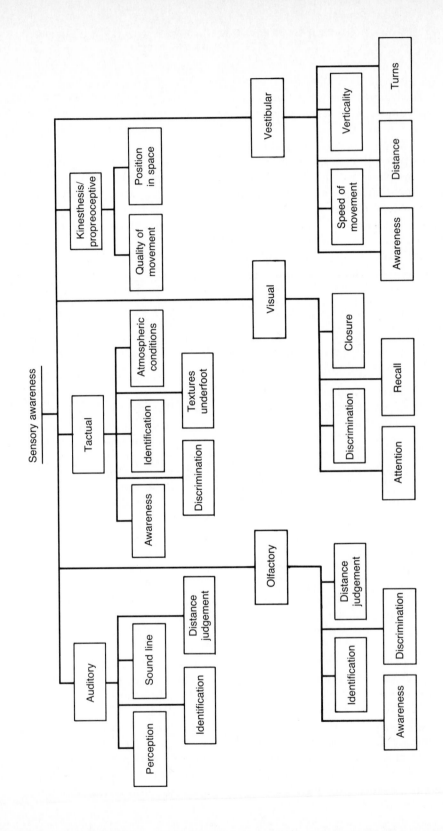

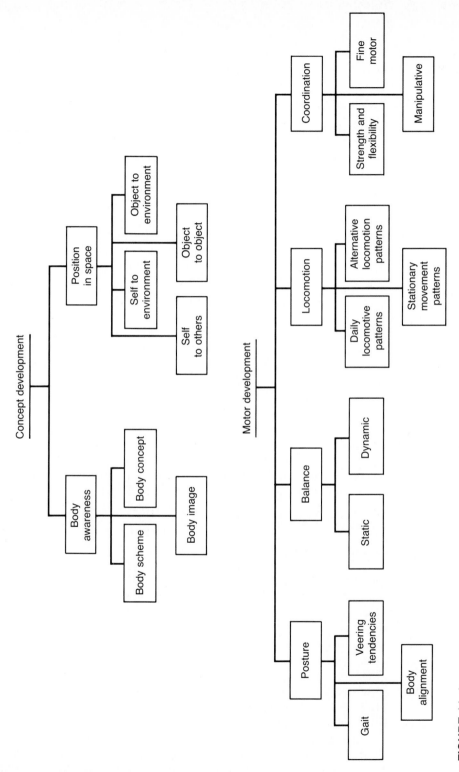

FIGURE 11-1

Major skill areas that must be integrated for optimal learning and locomotion by children with visual impairments. (Source: "The Need for Motor Development Programs for Visually Impaired Preschoolers" by M.A. Palazesi, [Tables 1-3], [*Journal of Visual Impairment & Blindness*, Vol 80, No. 2] is © 1986 by American Foundation for the Blind, Inc., and is reproduced with kind permission of the American Foundation for the Blind, 15 West 16th Street, New York, NY 10011.)

development, sensory awareness, and concept development that visually impaired children need to integrate for optimal learning and independent locomotion.

Good Fairy Syndrome

Lois Harrell from the Blind Babies Foundation in San Francisco speaks frequently of the Good Fairy Syndrome. This phrase describes how visually impaired infants must view a world in which objects and people seem to appear and disappear into a void. From birth, infants who are visually impaired rely on other people to bring them everything, whether it is food, social interaction, or a change of diapers. Although this cannot be avoided completely, the passivity it creates can be reduced if a greater totality of an action, through verbal or tactual feedback, is provided for the child. That is, tell the child where diapers are kept before they are placed on the child and have the child touch the shelves where toys are stored so the child can begin to understand that these things do not just magically appear when the child is ready for them.

The Good Fairy Syndrome may play a large role in the delay in object concepts observed in visually impaired children. Along the same lines, attempts to anticipate every need of infants may delay their understanding that they can have an effect on the world through actions other than crying. Doing too much for the child, and an attitude of over-protection, may work to lower expectations for the child, and ultimately may lower the child's performance.

FAMILY INVOLVEMENT

Because of the unique developmental needs of infants with visual impairment, family involvement is particularly crucial to provide the consistent and sustained intervention needed to facilitate learning. Family involvement is discussed in other chapters and, in general, the strategies and suggestions mentioned also apply to families of infants with visual impairment. However, there are some factors that may be unique to families of infants with visual impairment.

Historical Influence of Visual Impairment

To actively assist families in coping with the demands of the child with visual impairment, interventionists must understand how parents and families may respond to the notion of loss of vision. Lowenfeld (1982) suggests that the way blindness has been treated historically has a continuing impact on families today, particularly in the way family members respond to an infant with visual loss. For example, Judeo-Christian teachings are replete with lessons to look after and take responsibility for the individual who is blind, implying that individuals with visual impairment are unable to care for themselves. These teachings are reflected in diminished expectations and sometimes over-protection of young children with visual impairment. These attitudes may actually contribute to developmental delay because lowered expectations and over-protection become self-fulfilling prophecies. The less infants with visual impairment are expected to do, the less they learn; the less they learn, the more they are in need of protection. As one mother states: "I was so guilt-ridden when my son was born that I did everything in my power to keep him content so I would feel like a good mother. I wouldn't let people outside our family touch him. That probably held him back but I didn't know it then. . . . "

Interventionists can actively assist families in understanding that many blind individuals lead productive lives with families of their own and satisfying careers. Feeling sorry for the child with visual impairment will not facilitate the child's future independence. Rationalizing over-protection with promises of being more strict in the future, when the child is older and bigger, ignores the fact that the greatest opportunity for learning is during the first 3 years; over-protected infants are learning dependence and poor self-concepts (Tuttle, 1984).

In addition, visual impairment has been historically linked to immorality (Cutsforth, 1951; Lowenfeld, 1982). Myths and fairy tales of improper behavior, sexual and otherwise, that are punished by blindness are part of almost every culture. Even modern stories, such as the award-winning late-1980s play, *Into the Woods,* contained a sequence in which three sisters were blinded for their evil ways and then played the part of fools for the rest of the play. It is not surprising that parents frequently blame themselves for their infant's visual impairment, or that blindness carries such a negative stigma in today's society. Visual impairment is more frequently associated with incompetence or secrecy (the umpire is blind; blind carbon copies) than it is with strength and competence.

Family members, and all people coming into contact with infants with visual impairments, are also projecting—they imagine what it would be like if they were visually impaired. Most people perceive a visual loss as devastating and cannot imagine how they would continue a normal life. Again, these attitudes are barriers to effective interaction. A grandfather of a congenitally blind toddler said this: "Everyone would say 'Oh, it could be worse' or 'At least he [my grandson] is healthy.' But one day I couldn't take it anymore. A fella in the bank said 'It could be worse' and I yelled back, 'No it couldn't!' I really lost it."

The best way to overcome these attitudes is to introduce older children or adults who are visually impaired to the young child's family. Parent groups can play a crucial role in helping family members to see the possibilities, rather than the limitations, inherent in the child's visual loss.

Interventionists need to

- ☐ observe parents' attitudes and behavior toward their child
- ☐ teach parents how to respond to their child's pleasure, aggression, and other social signals and reactions
- ☐ teach the parents how to develop object relations in their child (Burlingham, 1975)

Parents also require guidance in identifying critical learning periods so arrangements can be made to nurture the attainment of developmental milestones. Infant transdisciplinary teams are assisted by **intinerant teachers for visually handicapped students,** educators trained in the specific needs of children and adults with visual impairments. Because of the low incidence of visual impairment, itinerant vision teachers most often serve as consultants and train primary service providers and family members as needed.

ASSESSMENT

Assessment of infants with visual impairment follows the same principles of assessment used with any infant with special needs. That is, assessment should be comprehensive, multidisciplinary, unbiased, and conducted by individuals knowledgeable about visual impairment and its effects on development.

Unfortunately, there are several reasons why these principles do not always apply in practice. First, the low prevalence of visual impairment makes it extremely unlikely that early childhood special educators and related service personnel will acquire a great deal of experience working with infants with visual impairment, even in a large city, unless they specifically set out to do so by working in an agency that serves only a visually handicapped population. Second, it is not always possible to avoid bias in test administration, simply because tests used do not meet validity standards for a visually impaired population. It is, therefore, strongly recommended that assessment results only be used to identify the child's strengths and weaknesses in development, rather than to diagnose additional handicapping conditions or to document developmental delay.

Commercial Instruments

Several commercial assessment instruments are currently used with infants with visual impairment. Table 11–2 shows a list of tools used by infant programs responding to the Ferrell (1987) study. It is clear from the table that there is little agreement on what constitutes an adequate and comprehensive assessment, even among programs serving children with visual impairments.

Of these instruments, only five have been developed (though not standardized) on a visually impaired population: the Callier-Azusa (Stillman, 1978), the Maxfield-Buchholz (Maxfield & Buchholz, 1957), the Oregon Project (Brown, Simmons, & Methvin, 1986), the Reynell Zinkin (Reynell, 1983), and the Growing Up (Croft & Robinson, 1984). An additional two, the Adaptive Performance Instrument (Consortium on Adaptive Performance Evaluation, 1982) and the Battelle Developmental Inventory (Newborg, Stock, Wnek, Guidabuldi, & Svinicki, 1984) include adaptations for infants with visual impairment. The Oregon Project and Growing Up are designed as curriculum checklists, rather than assessments. None of these instruments have been developed for the visually impaired child with sufficient methodological soundness to lend confidence to the results.

Informal Assessment

Because formal assessment instruments leave much to be desired, interventionists frequently turn to informal tools to assess infants with visual impairments. Hart (1983) and Ferrell (1985; 1989) use a prerequisite skills approach that examines general themes in development and stresses the interaction of all domains. A sample of this type of informal domain interaction assessment is presented in Figure 11–2.

TABLE 11–2

Instruments used for assessment of young children with visual impairment (listed in order of frequency reported in Ferrell, 1987).

Instrument	Developed for Visually Impaired	Appropriate for Infants
Callier-Azusa Scale	x	x
Brigance Inventory of Early Development		x
Maxfield-Buchholz Social Maturity Scale	x	x
Learning Accomplishment Profile for Infants		x
Bayley Scales of Infant Development		x
Oregon Project Skills Inventory	x	x
Reynell Zinkin Scales	x	x
Adaptive Performance Instrument	*	x
Uzgiris-Hunt Ordinal Scales of Psychological Development		x
Vineland Social Maturity Scale		x
Battelle Developmental Inventory	*	x
Tactile Test of Basic Concepts	x	
Griffiths Scales of Mental Development		x
Growing Up Assessment	x	x
Hawaii Early Learning Profile		x

*Adaptations for infants with visual impairment have been provided, but are not standardized.

Source: Adapted from "State of the Art of Infant and Preschool Services in 1986" by K. A. Ferrell, 1987, *Yearbook of the Association for Education and Rehabilitation of the Blind and Visually Impaired, 4,* p. 30. Copyright © 1987 by K. A. Ferrell. Reprinted by permission.

Functional Vision Assessments

Since Barraga (1964) first demonstrated that children could be taught to use their **residual vision,** any vision or light perception the child may possess, specialists working with infants with visual impairment include in their assessments procedures to evaluate how infants use their vision. These components are usually included in functional vision assessments.

□ **pupillary response**: to determine how the pupils respond to light and how much control the infant has over the environment
□ **muscle balance**: to determine whether or not the eyes work together
□ **visual fields**: to determine if the infant has a full field of vision
□ **fixation**: to determine if the infant can attend in all parts of the visual field
□ **tracking**: to determine the eyes' ability to move together in various directions and to sustain fixation on a moving target
□ **unusual head posture and eye movement**: to record atypical behaviors that might suggest visual field losses or muscle imbalance

These components must be evaluated together for an accurate diagnostic assessment of the child's vision. For example, a head tilt down and to the right does

Child: _____ Birthdate_____

Today's date_____

Does child exhibit skill?

	Yes	Not Yet
Motor development		
Absence of atypical reflexes: _____ ATNR	___	___
_____ STNR	___	___
_____ Landau	___	___
_____ Moro	___	___
Tone (describe): _____	___	___
_____		
_____		
Balance: _____ Head	___	___
_____ Shoulders	___	___
_____ Trunk	___	___
_____ Hip	___	___
_____ Legs & feet	___	___
_____ Standing	___	___
_____ Moving	___	___
Rotation: _____ Head	___	___
_____ Shoulders	___	___
_____ Trunk	___	___
_____ Hip	___	___
Protective reactions: _____ Front	___	___
_____ Side	___	___
_____ Back	___	___
Fine motor/Self-help development		
Grasp: _____ Reflexive	___	___
_____ Palmar	___	___
_____ Raking	___	___
_____ Scissors	___	___
_____ Inferior pincer	___	___
_____ Superior pincer	___	___
Reach: _____ One-hand	___	___
_____ Two-hand	___	___
_____ Front	___	___
_____ Right	___	___
_____ Left	___	___
Voluntary release: _____ Against surface	___	___
_____ Free space	___	___
Wrist rotation: _____ Forward	___	___
_____ Back	___	___

FIGURE 11–2

Corequisite skills assessment of infants. (From *Corequisite Skills Assessment of Infants* by K. A. Ferrell, 1989, unpublished instrument. New York: Columbia University. Copyright © 1989 by K. A. Ferrell. Reprinted by permission.)

	Does child exhibit skill?	
	Yes	Not Yet
Cognitive development		
Object permanence:	___	___
Object constancy:	___	___
Means-end behavior:	___	___
Categorization: Physical	___	___
Groups	___	___
Function	___	___
Association	___	___
Communication/Social development		
Eye contact:	___	___
Imitation: Vocal	___	___
Verbal	___	___
Physical	___	___
Imagination:	___	___
Interaction:	___	___

FIGURE 11–2
(continued)

not necessarily indicate a left field loss. This posture may indicate that the left eye is **amblyopic** (a dimness or loss of vision), perhaps due to a muscle imbalance. However, if the evaluator relied only on the information from the unusual head posture, conclusions from the assessment would be inaccurate and misleading.

A full discussion of procedures used in a functional vision assessment of infants is beyond the scope of this chapter. Fortunately, several excellent functional vision assessments are available that provide guidelines for both the novice and the experienced vision specialist. Three of these warrant discussion.

The *Functional Vision Inventory* (Langley, 1980) provides considerable detail about how to administer and interpret procedures to evaluate functional vision. The instrument is written by an experienced teacher of infants and young children.

The book, *Look at Me* (Smith & Cote, 1982), offers a good introduction to functional vision assessment. This book also covers eye anatomy, common eye disorders, and outlines a suggested vision stimulation sequence with stimulation activities. The book is appropriate for young children, particularly those who are multi-handicapped, but it does not address the specific needs of infants.

The *Program to Develop Efficiency in Visual Functioning* (Barraga & Morris, 1980) is a set of materials including the Diagnostic Assessment Procedure as well as a curriculum for training individuals with low vision to use their residual vision. Although the materials are appropriate for children with a cognitive level of at least 3 years, the sourcebook and other materials give useful information for professionals and families of visually handicapped children of all ages.

PROGRAMMING

Many of the issues involved in instructional programming for infants with visual impairments were discussed earlier in this chapter. Essentially, the basic issues are the same as they are for any infant with a significant sensory loss or limitation:

- ☐ programming should be based on assessment
- ☐ the strengths of the child must be used to address the weaknesses
- ☐ a perspective which focuses on the child's competence tends to facilitate developmental gains

Although it is true that visually impaired infants and toddlers are like other children, it is also true that they are different. Visually impaired children must receive the right type of attention early so they may develop a framework for effectively interacting with the world around them. When one sense is absent or limited, the other senses *do not* suddenly improve. The other senses must be developed. That is, each time the infant who is visually impaired is assisted in substituting touch and listening for sight, the remaining senses are enhanced.

These recommendations, largely drawn from *Get a Wiggle On* (Raynor & Drouillard, 1975), are additional practical suggestions for optimizing the development of visually impaired infants and toddlers.

Tie together all the separate pieces of information children receive. Describe what children are touching, smelling, tasting, hearing, and seeing. This helps children understand and integrate information about what objects are, what they do, and how they feel.

Touch and kiss children often. Touching children is more powerful than just talking lovingly, because children with visual impairments cannot see the loving smiles. Consequently, families must communicate affection through pats, hugs, and affectionate words. Also, individuals outside families should be encouraged to openly express affection to children so they learn to trust others.

Keep children engaged. Although visually impaired children may be content to stay in the crib for long periods of time, the stimulation received there is very limited. Encourage families to carry their child with them as they do household tasks, talk about what they're doing, and explain the sounds they make. Sharing with children and keeping them involved will discourage children from tuning out the world.

Change children's position and objects of interest often. Although a child may prefer one position to another, it is critical that all positions are experienced frequently. Lying on the stomach is necessary for strengthening neck muscles to lift the head, and for learning weightbearing on the hands. Change the objects placed near children often so they have a reason to reach out. Family members need to be reminded that their child can only keep track of them by touch or sound.

Create situations that lead to the next developmental milestone.   To encourage reaching, for example, put toys just within children's reach, demonstrate where they are, and talk about the objects. Sighted infants see objects and are motivated to touch them, but visually impaired infants must be taught that there are things just beyond their reach.

To encourage sitting, frequently let the child sit facing in or out on a parent's lap. To facilitate walking, regularly walk with the child before independent walking occurs. Push toys such as shopping carts, lawn mowers, and some wagons encourage walking and exploration. (They also run into things before children do.) As with the child with sight, installing gates on stairways and covers on sockets just before the child is mobile may be necessary for safety.

While children are learning to move around the home, it is best to keep furniture in the same place. However, after children are walking, it is appropriate to move furniture—as long as the child is told and shown where items have been placed.

After children are walking, encourage them to follow the walls with their hands to learn the way around.   Instead of walking in open spaces, following the walls, which is called **trailing**, permits children to map an area more efficiently. Concepts for later independent travel, such as spatial orientation, are most successfully taught during the first years of life (Ferrell, 1979). Leading the child around communicates that independent travel is something the child cannot do safely. Additionally, encourage children to practice walking up and down steps and climbing. With supervision, visually impaired children should experience everything sighted children experience.

Use playpens sparingly.   Playpens are helpful for children who reach out because toys are in a controlled space, and consequently, are easier to find. However, the whole house offers a wider range of experiences and should be viewed as a child's first playground. Toys should be placed around the house to be discovered during the child's travels. Leave some low cupboards open slightly so the child is encouraged to explore. Remember to remove all unsafe items.

Increase children's sensory input.   The child needs to learn all the different textures inside (e.g., carpet, hardwood, tile) and outside (grass, mud puddles, cement, dirt) the home. Encouraging children to go barefoot maximizes sensory information. As much as possible, let children directly experience climate changes (e.g., walk in the rain, feel snow, blow against the wind).

Describe everything children cannot see.   Descriptions keep children's curiosity about the world alive and help them to be less timid of the unfamiliar. Families should be reminded to use words to describe the world they are able to see (e.g., traffic jams, disappointed expressions, someone waving from down the block, the faucet leaking). Identifying sounds and describing the world helps children make sense of apparently random sounds. Eventually, children will be able to use sounds to map their house, yard, and neighborhood (e.g., toilet running, car door slamming, brother's bike being thrown on the walkway).

Control situations in which rocking is permitted.   Due to limited sensory input, some visually impaired children may repeatedly rock, spin, or flap their hands. Rocking horses or rocking chairs can offer opportunities to experience these sensations in more appropriate ways. If children engage in these movements at other times, it is essential that their behavior be interrupted and they be directed to another activity. Atypical movements can be altered in early childhood, but only if they are consistently replaced by appealing alternatives.

All objects in the home are potential toys for learning.   Visually impaired children, like all children, often prefer household objects (e.g., shoes, pans, cups) to conventional toys. Selecting educational toys for visually impaired children can be difficult, because the toy that seems appropriate to parents or professionals may have limited appeal to the child. Appropriate toys should fulfill the child's developmental needs, have enough sensory information to stimulate the child's interest, and have the ability to be adapted to fulfill other purposes or functions. It is important to gradually and consistently introduce new toys, objects, and experiences even if the child seems frightened by them at first.

Insist that children run, climb, play with other children, and experience something new every day.   Visually impaired children often exercise less than other children their age. Yet the reality is that they need as many, or more, physical experiences to form good spatial relationships and body image. Interventionists should encourage parents to promote independence in play and movement. A fenced yard allows the child to move freely and safely. Placing a radio on the back porch allows the child to learn the way back to the house easily. Because other children may be unpredictable in their interaction and play, the visually impaired child may prefer the company of familiar adults. However, the child needs to learn how to take turns, share materials, and enjoy other children. In most cases, social skills may need to be taught systematically.

Commercial Curricula

With certain adaptations, nearly all early childhood curricula may be used as long as the particular limitations of the child's visual impairment are considered. Three curricula developed for young children with visual impairment provide specific suggestions for interventionists.

The Oregon Project (Brown, Simmons, & Methvin, 1986).   These materials were developed by asking experienced teachers of young visually impaired children to identify the skills in the Portage Project Curriculum that they found blind and low vision children to be delayed in acquiring. Teachers' responses were then organized into a new checklist and field tested. The final product became the Oregon Project Skills Inventory that was supported by a grant from the Handicapped Children's Early Education Program (HCEEP). The manual includes suggested activities and a good selection of finger plays appropriate for young children with visual impairments. The inventory is appropriate for instructional assessment only and should not be used to document developmental levels.

Growing Up (Croft & Robinson, 1984).   This curriculum was also an HCEEP Project and was known as Vision Up. It provides teaching strategies for approximately 600 criterion-referenced skills. The materials are color-coded by domain and include a "card sort" assessment for parents. Parents sort the cards into piles of yes, no, and don't know according to whether or not their child performs a behavior. *Growing Up* is available in both English and Spanish.

Reach Out and Teach (Ferrell, 1985).   These materials are the result of a research and development project sponsored by the U. S. Department of Education and are designed specifically for families to use at home, in conjunction with an early interventionist or a correspondence vision educator. The materials are sold as a two-volume set, including a handbook and an interactive workbook in which parents practice and apply the information to their child. A set of eight slide-tapes and a Teacher's Manual are also available.

Mainstreaming Issues

Although children with visual impairments have been mainstreamed into regular education classes since the 1950s (Roberts, 1986), little research is available either to refute or support the practice. Most of the issues relating to the mainstreaming of infants focuses on adapting the environment and adapting teaching methodology to meet the specialized needs of the child. Successful mainstreamed arrangements place special demands on the case manager and require continual communication and training of all professionals working with the child and the child's family. When these parameters are met, there is often little reason why the child with a visual impairment cannot be successfully integrated into a community setting.

SUMMARY OF PROCEDURES

Bearing in mind that the needs of the visually limited child are different from those of the blind child, a few general statements about working with visually impaired children can be made. Some of the key concepts from this chapter follow:

1. Introduce skills to visually impaired children with no additional handicapping conditions at roughly the same time as other children their age because a correspondence exists between the opportunity to learn and the acquisition of skills.
2. Create situations in which play with objects and object relations are arranged, rewarded, and expected in an effort to compensate for the anticipated delay in this developmental area.
3. Make special efforts to present sensory activities designed to compensate for difficulties in sensory integration. Never assume incidental learning or intersensory coordination is spontaneously occurring.

TRANSDISCIPLINARY CASES

The following case studies demonstrate the different demands placed on families and professionals in serving low vision and blind children.

THE GARCIA FAMILY

Ramona is a happy 20-month-old with Charge Syndrome, which involves multiple congenital anomalies including myopia (nearsightedness), colobomas (malformation of the iris), microcephaly (a small head), growth failure, monoarticular arthritis, congenital hip dysplasia, and anemia. Ramona is the youngest of three children, with a fourth on the way. Mr. and Mrs. Garcia are in their early 30s. Mr. Garcia is a military officer and Mrs. Garcia is a homemaker. They are both actively involved in Ramona's intervention activities.

Ramona has had surgery for a hiatal hernia, has been hospitalized three times for recurrent pneumonia, and currently has a gastrostomy tube. She exhibits significant developmental delay, but she is doing well considering her extensive medical problems. Ramona is enrolled in an early intervention program sponsored by a school district that offers weekly home visits. She attends a center-based program once a week to receive occupational and physical therapy, and participates in a small Mommy-and-Me group. Because of her repeated hospitalizations and susceptibility to infection, Ramona's participation has been sporadic.

An itinerant teacher of the visually handicapped also serves on Ramona's team and visits the center monthly to consult, provide information and materials, and train team members in techniques to encourage Ramona to use her limited vision. The staff is highly motivated because Ramona is the first infant with a visual impairment enrolled in the program. Initially, the itinerant vision teacher gave inservice training for the team on the effects of visual impairment on development and useful strategies to facilitate early development. The itinerant teacher also conducted a functional vision assessment with Ramona as team members observed, explaining what she was doing and why, as each item was completed. Based on this assessment, the team discovered that Ramona's central vision was extremely poor and that she relied on her peripheral vision most of the time. This explained why she turned her head slightly to the side whenever her attention was drawn to people or toys (some team members felt she was trying to avoid them and the activity) and why she brought objects close to her eyes. Team members quickly found out that presenting food and materials off-center engaged Ramona's attention, and permitted her to better manipulate them.

In addition, the itinerant vision teacher registered Ramona with the American Printing House for the Blind (APH) so she could obtain instructional materials developed specifically for young visually handicapped children. Although it is not yet known if Ramona is legally blind (and, consequently, eligible for APH materials on quota), her ophthalmologist has certified her as severely visually limited. Currently, interventionists are using a set of vision stimulation materials from APH, Bright

4. Establish varied and continual pre-locomotion experiences (e.g., trunk and hip rotation in reaching, sitting, standing) so later locomotion skills are based on adequate early motor preparation.

5. Train family members to recognize the unique attachment behaviors and signals so they may more effectively increase their child's social engagement and reciprocity.

6. Use concrete experiences that are meaningful to the child to expand concept development.

7. Assist parents in their efforts to avoid anticipating their child's every need (the Good Fairy Syndrome) so their child may learn to influence the environment as well as be influenced by it. Also, help family members to control

Lights—Learning To See, and other materials have been ordered. The low vision materials are also being used with several other children in the program, which facilitates Ramona's social involvement in the group.

THE BLAKE FAMILY

Jesse Blake, born at 26 weeks' gestational age, was hospitalized for almost 4 months with bronchiopulmonary dysplasia, apnea, and jaundice. About 1 week prior to discharge from the hospital, a routine ophthalmological examination diagnosed retinopathy of prematurity (ROP), stage 3 (ridge with extraretinal proliferation). Mr. Blake is an attorney and Mrs. Blake is a financial consultant. Jesse is their first child, born after a difficult pregnancy. The Blakes and the maternal grandmother are very involved in Jesse's treatments. Mrs. Blake works part-time now, but plans to return to fulltime work once suitable child care can be located.

Jesse's mother visited the pediatric ophthalmologist biweekly after Jesse came home from the hospital. The family recently learned that the ROP had progressed to bilateral retinal detachment, meaning that Jesse is totally blind. His glaucoma (a disease caused by increased intraocular pressure) is now being controlled by medication. There is no evidence of intracranial bleeds or brain damage.

The family physician recommended an early intervention program for Jesse when he was 8 months old. At that time, Jesse was not functioning as well as his 5-month-old cousin, even when corrections were made for his prematurity. His parents expressed concern because he was not sitting up or playing with toys. In the prone position, he kept his head lowered and did not push up on his hands. Mrs. Blake described Jesse as a very good, almost passive baby.

The early interventionist explained to the family that Jesse's behavior was not unusual for a totally blind child who had spent so much time in the hospital. Motor problems are always a concern with infants with visual impairment, so a physical therapist participates on the team to provide additional suggestions for facilitating Jesse's motor development. An itinerant teacher of the visually handicapped participates on the team, too, providing the primary service provider (an educator from the infant program) and other team members specific strategies for working with Jesse and other visually impaired infants in the program. This teacher registered Jesse with the American Printing House for the Blind and asked a colleague who is an **orientation and mobility specialist,** a professional trained to teach visually impaired children and adults independent travel, to assist the physical therapist with Jesse's motor development. Although Jesse's progress seems to be slow, the support the family receives from the transdisciplinary team seems to have increased the family's confidence in their ability to effectively parent their visually impaired son.

feelings of guilt and an attitude of over-protection which lead to lowered expectations, and ultimately lowered performances in their child.
8. Encourage families to actively engage the child, to explain all that is happening, and to provide varied sensory experiences to facilitate development.

SUMMARY

Early developmental experiences and expectations are very important for later successful adjustment in visually impaired infants and toddlers. At the very least, visual impairment means imperfect sensations and inaccurate feedback that may slow the child's concept development and learning. Appropriate early intervention experiences may mitigate some of the limitations imposed by visual loss and may appropriately guide the child's family in its efforts to realize the child's fullest developmental potential.

DISCUSSION QUESTIONS

1. Discuss three domains that are significantly affected by visual impairment. What strategies might be used to assist the low vision child and the blind child in compensating for these influences?
2. What are three of the limitations of assessment tools used with visually impaired infants and toddlers? How can interventionists minimize these limitations?
3. What are team members' responsibilities to the visually impaired child and the family when an itinerant teacher of the visually handicapped is not available in their community? If you were director of an infant program, what would be your plan of action?

APPLIED ACTIVITIES/PROJECTS

1. Interview a visually impaired adolescent or adult who received early intervention services. Ask this individual and the family to identify the most valuable supports and services early intervention provided.
2. Observe comprehensive assessments of a low vision and a blind child. Identify critical developmental needs for each child and develop an Individualized Family Service Plan (IFSP). Analyze differences and similarities in the children.

SUGGESTED READING

Drouillard, R., & Raynor, S. (1977). *Move it.* Lanham, MD: American Alliance Publications.

Freeman, P. (1975). *Understanding the deaf-blind child.* London: Heinemann Health Books.

Kastein, S., Spaulding, I., & Scharf, B. (1980). *Raising the young blind child: A guide for parents and educators.* New York: Human Sciences Press. (Chapters 6, 11, and 16 discuss learning through play.)

Picture books for the blind. New York: Philomel Publishing. (Offers braille and inkprint books with textured pictures.)

Raynor, S., & Drouillard, R. (1975). *Get a wiggle on.* Lanham, MD: American Alliance Publications.

Some children are more special than others . . . A guide to Mattel toys for parents of the visually handicapped child. Toys for special children, Mattel Toys, Hawthorne, CA 90250 (catalog of selected toys for visually impaired children).

Webster, R. (1977). *The road to freedom: A parent's guide to prepare the blind child to travel independently.* Jacksonville, IL: Katan Publications.

REFERENCES

Adelson, E., & Fraiberg, S. (1976). Sensory deficit and motor development in infants blind from birth. In Z. S. Jastrzembska (Ed.), *The effects of blindness and other impairments on early development* (pp. 103–121). New York: American Foundation for the Blind.

Als, H., Tronick, E., & Brazelton, T. B. (1980). Affective reciprocity and the development of autonomy. *Journal of the American Academy of Child Psychiatry, 19,* 22–40.

Anderson, E., Dunlea, A., & Kekelis, L. (1984). Blind children's language: Resolving some differences. *Journal of Child Language, 11,* 645–664.

Barraga, N. (1964). *Increased visual behavior in low vision children* (Research Series No. 13). New York: American Foundation for the Blind.

Barraga, N. (1977, March). *Development of low vision.* Paper presented at Staff Meeting of the Virginia Commission for the Visually Handicapped, Virginia Beach, VA.

Barraga, N. (1983). *Visual handicaps and learning* (rev. ed.). Austin, TX: Exceptional Resources.

Barraga, N., & Morris, J. (1980). *Program to develop efficiency in visual functioning.* Louisville, KY: American Printing House for the Blind.

Bayley, N. (1969). *Bayley Scales of Infant Development.* New York: The Psychological Corporation.

Bigelow, A. (1987). Early words of blind children. *Journal of Child Language, 14,* 47–56.

Brazelton, T. B. (1973). Neonatal Behavioral Assessment Scale. *Clinics in Developmental Medicine* (No. 50). Philadelphia: Lippincott.

Brigance, A. (1978). *Diagnostic Inventory of Early Development.* North Billerica, MA: Curriculum Associates.

Brown, D., Simmons, V., & Methvin, J. (1986). *The Oregon Project for visually impaired and blind preschool children* (3rd ed.). Medford, OR: Jackson County Education Service District.

Burlingham, D. (1975). Special problems of blind infants: Blind baby profile. *Psychoanalytic Study of the Child, 30,* 3–13.

Cattell, P. (1940). *The measurement of intelligence of infants and young children.* New York: Johnson Reprint Corporation.

Consortium on Adaptive Performance Evaluation (1982). *Adaptive Performance Instrument* (experimental ed.). Moscow: University of Idaho, Department of Special Education.

Croft, N. B., & Robinson, L. W. (1984). *Growing Up: A developmental curriculum.* Austin, TX: Parent Consultants.

Cutsforth, T. (1951). *The blind in school and society.* New York: American Foundation for the Blind.

Doll, E. A. (1953). *A measurement of social competence: A manual for the Vineland Social Maturity Scale.* Edison, NJ: Educational Test Bureau.

DuBose, R. F. (1979). Working with sensorily impaired children. Part I: Visual impairments. In S. G. Garwood (Ed.), *Educating young handicapped children: A developmental approach* (pp. 323–359). Germantown, MD: Aspen.

Education of the Handicapped Act of 1975, Part B (P.L. 94–142), Title XX, U.S.C. §1400–1420.

Ferrell, K. A. (1979). Comment—Orientation and mobility for preschool children: What we have and what we need. *Journal of Visual Impairment and Blindness, 73*(4), 147–150.

Ferrell, K. A. (1984a). A second look at sensory aids in early childhood. *Education of the Visually Handicapped, 16,* 83–101.

Ferrell, K. A. (1984b). Visual perceptual performance of visually handicapped infants with and without the use of binaural sensory aids (Doctoral dissertation, University of Pittsburgh,

1983). *Dissertation Abstracts International, 44,* 2437A. (University Microfilms No. 83–27,684).

Ferrell, K. A. (1985). *Reach out and teach.* New York: American Foundation for the Blind.

Ferrell, K. A. (1986). Infancy and early childhood. In G. T. Scholl (Ed.), *Foundations of education for blind and visually handicapped children and youth* (pp. 265–273). New York: American Foundation for the Blind.

Ferrell, K. A. (1987). State of the art of infant and preschool services in 1986. *Yearbook of the Association for Education and Rehabilitation of the Blind and Visually Impaired, 4,* 22–39.

Ferrell, K. A. (1989). *Corequisite Skills Assessment of Infants,* Unpublished instrument. New York: Columbia University.

Ferrell, K. A., Trief, E., Deitz, S., Bonner, M. A., Cruz, D., Ford, E., & Stratton, J. (in press). The Visually Impaired Infants Research Consortium (VIIRC): First year results. *Journal of Visual Impairment and Blindness.*

Flynn, J. T. (1987). Retinopathy of prematurity. *Pediatric Clinics of North America, 34,* 1487–1510.

Fraiberg, S. (1977). *Insights from the blind: Comparative studies of blind and sighted infants.* New York: Basic Books.

Frankenburg, W. K., Dodds, J. B., & Fandall, A. W. (1973). *Denver Developmental Screening Test.* Denver: University of Colorado Medical Center.

Gerhardt, J. B. (1982). The development of object play and classification skills in a blind child. *Journal of Visual Impairment and Blindness, 76,* 219–223.

Glass, P., Avery, G., Subramondan, K., Keys, M., Fostek, A., & Friendly, D. (1985). Effects of bright light in the hospital nursery on the incidence of retinopathy of prematurity. *New England Journal of Medicine, 313,* 401–404.

Hammer, M. E., Mullen, P. W., Ferguson, J. G., Pai, S., Cosby, C., & Jackson, K. L. (1986). Logistic analysis of risk factors in acute retinopathy of prematurity. *American Journal of Ophthalmology, 93,* 574–579.

Hart, V. (1983). Motor development in blind children. In M. Wurster & M. E. Mulholland (Eds.), *Help me become everything I can be. Proceedings of the North American Conference on Visually Handicapped Infants and Young Children* (pp. 74–79). New York: American Foundation for the Blind.

Hatfield, E. M. (1975). Why are they blind? *The Sight-Saving Review, 45,* 3–22.

Huebner, K. M., & Ferrell, K. A. (1986). Ethical practice in the provision of services to blind and visually impaired infants, children, and youth. In M. E. Mulholland (Ed.), *Ethical issues in the field of blindness* (pp. 9–19). New York: American Foundation for the Blind.

Illingworth, R. S. (1980). *The development of the infant and young child: Normal and abnormal* (7th ed.). Edinburgh: Churchill Livingstone.

Kirchner, C. (1989). National estimates of prevalence and demographics of children with visual impairments. In M. C. Wang, M. C. Reynolds, & H. J. Walberg, (Eds.), *Handbook of special education: Research and practice. Volume 3, Low incidence conditions* (pp. 135–153). Oxford: Pergamon Press.

Kitzinger, M. (1980). Planning management of feeding in the visually handicapped child. *Child Care, Health & Development, 6,* 291–299.

Knobloch, H., Stevens, F., & Malone, A. F. (1980). *Manual of developmental diagnosis: The administration and interpretation of the revised Gesell and Amatruda Developmental and Neurologic Examination,* Hagerstown, MD: Harper & Row.

Koestler, F. A. (1976). *The unseen minority: A social history of blindness in America.* New York: David McKay.

Langley, M. B. (1980). *Functional Vision Inventory for the multiply and severely handicapped.* Chicago: Stoelting.

Lowenfeld, B. (1982). *Berthold Lowenfeld on blindness and blind people.* New York: American Foundation for the Blind.

Markovits, H., & Strayer, F. (1982). Toward an applied social ethology: A case study of social skills among blind children. In K. H. Rubin & H. Ross (Eds.), *Peer relationships and social skills in childhood* (pp. 274–301). New York: Springer-Verlag.

Maxfield, K. E., & Buchholz, S. (1957). *A Social Maturity Scale for Blind Preschool Children: A guide to its use.* New York: American Foundation for the Blind.

Miller, P. H. (1983). *Theories of developmental psychology.* San Francisco: W. H. Freeman.

Newborg, J., Stock, J. R., Wnek, L., Guidubaldi, J., & Svinicki, J. (1984). *The Battelle Developmental Inventory.* Allen, TX: DLM Teaching Resources.

Norris, M., Spaulding, P. J., & Brodie, F. H. (1957) *Blindness in children.* Chicago: University of Chicago Press.

Packer, J., & Kirchner, C. (1985). State level counts on blind and visually handicapped school children. *Journal of Visual Impairment and Blindness, 79,* 357–361.

Palazesi, M. (1986). The need for motor development programs for visually impaired preschoolers. *Journal of Visual Impairment and Blindness, 80*(2), 573–576.

Parsons, S. (1985). The performancce of low vision children on the Preschool Language Scale. *Education of the Visually Handicapped, 17,* 117–125.

Phelps, D. L. (1981). Retinopathy of prematurity: An estimate of vision loss in the United States—1979. *Pediatrics, 67,* 924–926.

Raver, S. (1984). Modification of head droop during conversation in a 3-year-old visually impaired child: A case study. *Journal of Visual Impairment and Blindness, 78,* 307–310.

Raver, S. (1987a). Training gaze direction in blind children: Attitude effects on the sighted. *Remedial and Special Education, 8*(5), 40–45.

Raver, S. (1987b). Training blind children to employ appropriate gaze direction and sitting behavior during conversation. *Education and Treatment of Children, 10*(3), 237–246.

Raver, S. (1990). Effect of gaze direction on evaluation of visually impaired children by informed respondents. *Journal of Visual Impairments and Blindness, 84*(1), 67–70.

Raver, S., & Drash, P. (1988). Increasing social skills training for visually impaired children. *Education of the Visually Handicapped, 19*(4), 147–155.

Raver, S., & Dwyer, R. (1986). Using a substitute activity to eliminate eye poking in a 3-year-old visually impaired child in the classroom. *The Exceptional Child, 33*(1), 65–72.

Raynor, S., & Drouillard, R. (1975). *Get a wiggle on: A guide for helping visually impaired children grow.* Lanham, MD: American Alliance Publications.

Reynell, J. (1983). *Manual for the Reynell-Zinkin Scales.* Windsor, Berks, UK: NFER-NELSON Publishing Co.

Roberts, F. K. (1986). Education for the visually handicapped: A social and educational history. In G. T. Scholl (Ed.), *Foundations of education for blind and visually handicapped children and youth: Theory and practice* (pp. 1–18). New York: American Foundation for the Blind.

Rogers, S., & Puchalski, C. (1984). Social characteristics of visually impaired infants' play. *Topics in Early Childhood Special Education, 3,* 52–56.

Rogers, S., & Puchalski, C. (1986). Social smiles of visually impaired infants. *Journal of Visual Impairment and Blindness, 80,* 863–865.

Rowland, C. (1984). Preverbal communication of blind infants and their mothers. *Journal of Visual Impairments and Blindness, 78,* 297–302.

Santin, S., & Simmons, J. (1977). Problems in the construction of reality in congenitally blind children. *Journal of Visual Impairments and Blindness, 71,* 425–459.

Scholl, G. T. (1986). What does it mean to be blind? In G. T. Scholl (Ed.), *Foundations of education for blind and visually handicapped children and youth: Theory and practice* (pp. 23–33). New York: American Foundation for the Blind.

Silverman, W. A. (1982). Retinopathy of prematurity: Oxygen dogma challenged. *Archives of Disease in Childhood, 57,* 731–733.

Smith, A. J., & Cote, K. S. (1982). *Look at me: A resource manual for the development of residual vision in multiply impaired children.* Philadelphia: Pennsylvania College of Optometry Press.

Stephens, B., & Grube, C. (1982). Development of Piagetian reasoning in congenitally blind children. *Journal of Visual Impairment and Blindness, 76,* 133–143.

Stephens, B., & Simpkins, K. (1974). *The reasoning, moral judgment, and moral conduct of the congenitally blind* (Report No. H23–3197). Washington, DC: U. S. Office of Education, Bureau of Education for the Handicapped.

Stillman, R. (1978). *Callier-Azusa Scale.* Dallas, TX: Callier Center for Communication Disorders.

Tuttle, D. W. (1984). *Self-esteem and adjusting with blindness.* Springfield, IL: Charles C. Thomas.

Urwin, C. (1984). Language for absent things: Learning from visually handicapped children. *Topics in Language Disorders, 4,* 24–37.

Vaughn, M., & Scholl, G. (1980). Where have all the children gone? *DVH Newsletter, 25*(2), 6–7.

Warren, D. H. (1989). Implications of visual impairments for child development. In M. C. Wang, M. C. Reynolds, & H. J. Walberg (Eds.), *Handbook of special education, research and practice: Volume 3, low incidence conditions* (pp. 155–172). Oxford: Pergamon Press.

PART V

WORKING WITH FAMILIES

12

Working with Parents and Families

Jennifer Kilgo and Sharon A. Raver

OVERVIEW

This chapter discusses issues relating to serving families, including:

- parental reactions to the birth of a child who is at risk or handicapped
- effects of the child on the immediate and extended family
- guidelines for serving culturally diverse families
- family systems theory
- factors affecting family adaptation
- techniques for effective communication
- guidelines for a family-centered approach to early intervention
- parental rights

As has been indicated throughout this book, the family-centered approach is the cornerstone of exemplary practice in early intervention. Rather than asking families to adjust to programs' policies and needs, programs now adjust services to families' needs. Parents are seen as full partners, decision makers, and evaluators of services. A family-centered approach is based on family systems theory. That is, infants and toddlers with special needs are viewed as part of their family system, which in turn is viewed as part of a larger network of informal and formal systems. What happens to one member of the family affects all members, and each family member has their own needs and skills. Thus, interventionists must devise an individualized approach for each family served. To do this, professionals need an understanding of the effects the birth of a child with a handicap, or the diagnosis of an exceptionality, may have on how families function.

PARENTAL REACTIONS TO AT-RISK AND HANDICAPPING CONDITIONS

The birth of an atypical infant or the diagnosis of the child's handicap often comes as a shock to families and creates a deep sense of loss of the expected child (Solnit & Stark, 1961). The arrival or diagnosis of an atypical infant destroys parents' expectations of a perfect child and requires parents to adjust to the actual infant (Perske, 1973).

There is much discussion and debate in the literature over parental responses to the birth of an infant who is at risk or handicapped. Some families experience increased stress following the birth of a handicapped child, but this experience is not necessarily universal. Some researchers suggest parents appear to experience a series of emotional reactions similar to those of mourning the death of a loved one or the death of the normal child they were expecting. However, Featherstone (1980) points out that important differences exist between mourning the birth of a handicapped child and the bereavement process associated with death. Death is final and the significance is clear. The implications of a child's handicap are ambiguous because of the uncertainty about how it will influence the child's development.

Parents report variations in their initial or early reactions to the birth of a handicapped child: confusion or shock, refusal or denial, anger, ambivalence, bitterness, guilt, depression, envy, rejection, helplessness, and finally acceptance and understanding (Blacher, 1984). It has been suggested that parents move through these stages of acceptance: shock; denial; sadness, anger, or anxiety; adaptation; and reorganization (Drotar, Baskiewicz, Irvin, Kennell, & Klaus, 1975). Still Featherstone (1980) cautions that stage theories are an oversimplification of a complex process. Parents may not pass through these stages or they may progress through them in different orders, or at varying rates or intensities. Even within the same family, mothers and fathers often experience different levels of acceptance and grief. Consequently, stage theories should only be used as a reference for the range of parental reactions. Some parents feel chronic sorrow and may never achieve complete acceptance (Olshansky, 1962).

Variations in parental reactions appear to be related to the nature and severity of the infant's condition, the parents' overall personalities and coping styles, the family's composition and dynamics, the availability of support systems, the availability of early intervention services, and the family's culture (Gabel, McDowell, & Cerreto, 1983). These elements seem to combine in unique ways for families, resulting in a variety of parental reactions. As one father remembers, "I felt mostly disbelief. I just couldn't believe the doctors could be right. My wife was angry. She went into a rage. She stayed angry a long time. I got angry about 3 years later."

The age at which the child is diagnosed and the severity of the condition can make a difference in parents' reactions. A family's response to an infant with a congenital birth defect or obvious abnormality may be much different than their reaction to an infant with a milder, less obvious condition that is recognized gradually.

Yet, not all parental reactions and influences on the family may be characterized as negative. Turnbull and Turnbull (1990) found that the professional literature has a tendency to discount the positive influences of a child with special needs on the family. Despite the potential negative effects, many parents and families make successful adjustments to their situation. The guidance of appropriate early intervention seems to help by fostering coping strategies, reducing stress, reducing feelings of inadequacy and guilt, and increasing self-esteem (Vadasy, Fewell, Meyer, Schell, & Greenberg, 1984).

Each parent with an infant or toddler who is handicapped faces a personal combination of situations and factors that result in individual reactions and special needs. Individualization, used traditionally with children, has to be used to appropriately serve families as well.

IMPACT OF HANDICAPS ON IMMEDIATE AND EXTENDED FAMILY

The birth of an atypical infant can have profound effects on **intrafamilial** individuals, immediate family members, and **extrafamilial** individuals, extended family members. Because of the transactional nature of human relationships, each family member and extended family member operates both as an agent for change in the family system and as a target of influence from others.

Siblings

It is often not recognized how strongly a handicapped brother or sister can affect sibling reactions and interactions. The dynamics of the family can be a significant factor in how siblings adjust. The climate in some families may be so unstable that the adjustment of siblings may be unfavorable even if the handicapped child were not considered (Seligman, 1983). In some cases, the able-bodied sibling's needs may be neglected due to disproportionate parental time and energy devoted to the child with the disability. The desired goal in early intervention is a *balanced* family life in which parents include the handicapped child and, at the same time, focus on the needs of all other family members.

Parents' attitudes and adjustment are reflected in their interactions with their handicapped child. Waisbren (1980) found that parents of very young developmentally delayed children describe themselves negatively after the birth of a handicapped child and express more negative feelings than parents of nonhandicapped children. Clearly, such negative feelings shape siblings' reactions.

Besides positive parental adjustment, the encouragement of open communication regarding feelings toward the handicapped sibling can have an influence on sibling adjustment (Seligman, 1983). Open communication implies acceptance of both positive and negative feelings. In addition, siblings need accurate information about their brother's or sister's handicapping condition and its implications (Wasserman, 1983). Siblings often harbor fears stemming from misunderstandings about the handicapping condition.

The responsibilities that normal siblings assume for their handicapped brother or sister are a pervasive element in short- and long-term reactions to their handicapped sibling. Sometimes older children, especially daughters, are given increased caregiving responsibilities. Stoneman and Brody (1982) caution that siblings should not be given extended responsibilities beyond their level of maturity.

Many siblings make successful adjustments to their handicapped brother or sister, and in fact, cite positive results from their relationship, such as an increased appreciation of their own good health and a greater understanding and compassion for others (Grossman, 1972). After an extensive review of the literature, Gallagher and Powell (1989) conclude that the effects of a child with a handicap on siblings are not static; they suggest that siblings may express positive feelings toward the handicapped child at certain times and negative reactions at others. One teenage sibling remarked: "I was always mad at Nicky because I could tell he made Mom tired. After he was born we just never had as much fun. Mom was always too tired for fun. I never thought it was fair. But I was real happy when he learned something new at school."

Extended Family Members

Extended family is a term used to identify family members outside the immediate family such as grandparents, aunts, uncles, cousins, or other close relatives. These people may experience strong reactions to the birth of an atypical family member.

Grandparents tend to experience sorrow for their grandchild and tend to have concerns about their own child's burdens and responsibilities in caring for the child (Gabel & Kotsch, 1981). Extended family members, particularly grandparents, can provide resources of support, comfort, and understanding (Schell, 1981). But some extended family members may experience difficulty with acceptance, and may, consequently, be of limited assistance. To help extended family members work toward acceptance so they may be more involved, more early intervention programs are offering support groups, information sessions, and program open houses that highlight the needs of these family members.

Significant Others

The family's community and the nature of the family's relationships within that community are critical factors in family adjustment. As a group, families of handicapped children appear to be susceptible to increased stress (Gallagher, Beckman, & Cross, 1983), report feelings of loneliness or social isolation from friends, neighbors, and the community (Darling, 1979), and have smaller and less supportive networks than families with nonhandicapped children (Kazak & Marvin, 1984). Due to caregiving demands and emotional distress, and the uncomfortable feelings of friends and neighbors, families may have fewer informal contacts in their community after the birth of an atypical infant. Feelings of isolation may be related to changes in neighborhood friendships. Contact with neighbors may be limited to quick exchanges on weekends. Today, other systems such as co-workers may take the place of neighbors. Although co-workers are an important support network, they may not live close by and may be unable to fulfill the same roles as neighbors (e.g., emergency caregiving, car pooling).

The amount of stress experienced seems to be closely related to the family's social supports. Some families receive tremendous support from family, friends, and neighbors. These families appear to be less likely to become dependent on formal service systems (Trivette, Deal, & Dunst, 1986). Others may not be as fortunate. Rural or small urban communities still offer limited professional services, so families are forced to rely more heavily on their informal supports within the community. Providing activities for individuals outside the immediate family may expand families' social support, even when families are not directly involved. At times, the amount of social support families enjoy may be associated with their cultural background.

SERVING CULTURALLY DIVERSE FAMILIES

As stated in Chapter 8, infant interventionists must be sensitive to cultural nuances which may influence interactions with families when the cultural backgrounds of interventionists and caregivers differ. Culture is probably best thought of as a set of possibilities from which the family may choose (Anderson & Fenichel, 1989). However, a family's cultural identity does not dictate how the family will respond to the many circumstances families face in their efforts to receive early intervention services. Professionals must be careful to avoid assuming that all individuals within a cultural group react in a predetermined manner. Such assumptions lead to stereotyping, which limits understanding, and are difficult to overcome.

Interventionists must accept that there is no entity such as *the* Native American family, or *the* African American family. (The preferred terminology for cultural groups changes with time and among individuals. Professionals should use the terminology considered most appropriate in their community). Any generalizations made about different cultural groups are only valid when they are considered in the broadest sense of the term.

Infant interventionists are often advised to be culturally sensitive in serving children and their families. Being culturally sensitive does not mean that interventionists must know everything about the cultures they serve. Yet, at the most fundamental level, cultural sensitivity does imply a refusal to assign values such as better or worse, more or less intelligent, right or wrong, to cultural differences and similarities (Anderson & Fenichel, 1989). All children are raised in a way that socializes them "for optimal adjustment and success in their home culture" (Westby, in press). The most effective infant interventionists tend to acknowledge and respect the diverse practices of families. The most effective professionals acknowledge the cultures represented in their region, learn the general characteristics of those cultures, and realize that cultural diversity will affect families' participation in intervention programs.

Cultural knowledge permits professionals to be aware of potential interactional differences and to respond appropriately. Practices that may seem incomprehensible to uninformed professionals may seem logical in the context of the family's culture. For example, professionals aware that some cultural groups may avoid eye contact out of respect (e.g., Asian, Native American) will interpret minimal eye contact appropriately, rather than attach negative assumptions drawn by the mainstream culture such as uncooperativeness or embarrassment. Culturally knowledgeable professionals would not expect all individuals from the same cultural group to avoid eye contact, but would be aware that this is a possible behavior.

Interpreting behavior from the perspective of the family's culture allows more positive family-professional interaction. For example, contrary to the impression given by some studies of low-income African Americans, Stack (1974) suggests that the system of shared child care and parenting is not indicative of disorganization or broken family life. Stack suggests that this kinship system is a creative adaptation to poverty, maximizing the exchange of goods and services. Although this exchange lessens somewhat as families climb the socioeconomic ladder, McAdoo (1979) has found that mutually supporting family and kin networks persist in middle-class African American families and concludes that it is a cultural tendency rather than a strict adaptation to poverty.

Effective interventionists tend to allow families to take the lead in expressing how their culture is managed in their family. This is helpful because within each cultural group there may be numerous cultures represented and families may not traditionally follow all the aspects of their cultural group.

Examples of Diversity

Culture shapes beliefs, family practices, childrearing practices, and communication. Variations in beliefs and behaviors, of course, are found both within and between cultural groups. Some of the general cultural tendencies outlined by Anderson and Fenichel (1989) in *Serving Culturally Diverse Families of Infants and Toddlers with Disabilities* may serve as a guide for interventionists' initial inquiry into major cultural groups in the United States.

For instance, an *Asian American family* may function with a strict gender, sibling, and age hierarchy. Traditional Asian families tend to be extended, with many generations living under one roof. Parents may take active roles in their children's learning activities, but may be reluctant to participate in situations in which language and cultural barriers are present, such as intervention program functions. Infants born with disabilities may be viewed, to some extent, as punishment for sins of parents and ancestors (Nguyen, 1987). Many Southeast Asian families expect older family members to be treated with respect, so interventionists should address the oldest family member first. This individual may be the principal decision maker for the family. Family members may be reluctant to ask questions and make direct eye contact because this may be considered disrespectful. Additionally, families may see dress as reflecting the degree of respect between people, so a casually dressed home visitor may be viewed as showing disrespect.

An *African American family* may be extended with the mother and grandmother taking strong roles in the rearing of young children. Inappropriate behavior may be disciplined regularly. Family bonding, the importance of spirituality, and sharing may be important issues for families (E. Bailey, 1987). African American families have repeatedly experienced discrimination and disrespect, which may influence their communication with professionals. Professionals may also unconsciously alter their style of interaction. Jenkins (1981) reports that mainstream professionals may have inappropriately low expectations for African Americans as clients or students.

A *Hispanic American family* may have strong extended family connections. In patriarchal Hispanic families, the father/husband may be viewed as having ultimate responsibility for the care and well-being of the family. Any disability may be seen as intertwined with religion and perceived as punishment for some wrongdoing. Children with disabilities may be indulged and not expected to share in their own care. Family members may be more present-oriented, rather than future-oriented as the professionals are (Kunce, 1983). Hispanic families may place a value on developing a personal relationship with interventionists and require time to establish a climate of trust. Until trust is developed, it is important to use formal titles (e.g., Mr., Mrs.) to communicate respect for family members.

A *Native American family* may also find the extended family a source of support and identity. In a number of tribal cultures, grandparents and elders have significant control over adult children and control the raising of grandchildren. Parental behavior may be considered causally linked to birth defects and disease. Native American parents may be slow to judge professionals and may require time to develop trust. Out of respect for professionals, some Native Americans may not discuss their concerns if they feel the professional (e.g., doctor, infant interventionist, educator) is in a hurry.

Working within the family's cultural network may mean the difference between successful and unsuccessful early intervention efforts. At times this may involve learning the family's language or actively becoming more knowledgeable about the family's customs. Such efforts are made to establish trust. The following factors must be determined when serving multicultural families (Anderson & Fenichel, 1989):

- □ *Position on cultural continuum.* Where does the family lie along its cultural continuum? For example, how is the family organized? What is the pattern of decision making? What is the language spoken at home?
- □ *Values.* What values are shared with the Anglo mainstream? What values differ from the Anglo mainstream?
- □ *Comfortable interaction.* What is the most comfortable way for the family to work with the service system?
- □ *Additional information.* Is there other information that may be important for professionals to know to most effectively work with this family or individual family members?

Interventionists must rely upon sensitivity and understanding to demonstrate respect for cultural, familial, and individual diversity. Cultural awareness and sensitivity must be stated as a priority at the onset if family-centered intervention is to be achieved. Good intentions will not produce appropriate services for culturally diverse young children and their families.

FAMILY SYSTEMS APPROACH

The family systems approach to working with families is the anchor of Part H of P.L. 99–457. A major premise of family systems theory is that the child is an integral member of the larger family unit. All family members interact with one another, influencing the entire family unit. The family unit is defined by each family, and definitions vary greatly. For example, a single mother and an infant may constitute a family unit; a two-parent family with several children and a grandmother may comprise another family unit.

Family system theory suggests that there are interrelated subsystems in each family, so the handicapped child, the parents, and other family members are all changed by the process of living together and childrearing.

Turnbull and Turnbull (1990) organize family system concepts into these four elements:

- □ family characteristics
- □ family interactions
- □ family functions
- □ family life cycle

These four elements are interrelated so it is the interventionist's task to foster positive interactions in each toward good family health. The main elements of this framework of intervention are illustrated in Figure 12–1.

FIGURE 12–1

Family systems conceptual framework. (From *Working with Families with Disabled Members: A Family Systems Approach* [p. 60] by A. P. Turnbull, J. A. Summers, and M. J. Brotherson, 1984, Lawrence, KS: The University of Kansas, Kansas University Affiliated Facility. Adapted by permission.)

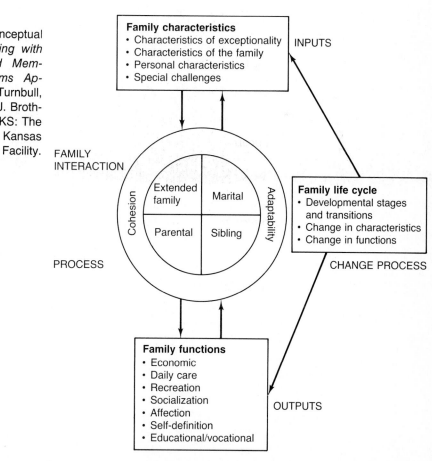

Characteristics

Family characteristics are descriptive attributes of the family such as features of the child's exceptionality, family characteristics, personal traits of individuals, as well as the family's means of addressing the needs of family members. Features of the exceptionality include dimensions such as the severity of the child's disability, physical appearance, and behavior. A young child diagnosed as deaf/blind with spastic quadriplegic cerebral palsy would obviously present different challenges than a child who has a language delay but has a normal physical appearance and mental abilities.

Family characteristics are family size and constellation, cultural background, socioeconomic status, and geographic location. An unemployed, drug-addicted single mother living with her only child in a low-income inner-city neighborhood has different resources than a middle-income family living in the suburbs with three children and a housekeeper.

Personal traits, too, vary greatly. Research indicates that chronic depression in parents is associated with impaired parenting behaviors and deficits in child emotional development (Paterson, 1982), but parents who receive early intervention services tend to have more positive attitudes about their lives than parents who do not receive services (Burden, 1980). Clearly, a family whose members display physical and mental well-being will have more resources to draw upon during periods of stress.

Interaction

Family interaction represents the relationships between individual family members and **family subsystems**, or subgroups. Relationships within the family can be discussed within four subsystems:

- □ marital (husband-wife)
- □ parental (parent-child)
- □ sibling (child-child)
- □ extra-familial (family, friends, neighbors, larger community including professionals) (Turnbull & Turnbull, 1990)

When family conditions change, as with the birth of an atypical infant, dramatic changes may occur in the roles within the family, as well as the family's overall functioning. An illustration of this is revealed in this mother's remarks: "Before our child I was always the one who took care of the details and keep us going as a family. But after we adopted Mark, and then found out he was handicapped, I fell to pieces. Since Mark, our responsibilities have switched. ... Now he [the husband] does the big stuff because I just can't seem to remember anything or get myself organized."

Functions

The third element of the family systems theory, **family functions**, are the needs that families are responsible for regularly addressing such as economic, domestic/health care, recreation, socialization, affection, self-definition, and educational/vocational tasks (Turnbull & Turnbull, 1990). The tasks involved in family functions are provided in Table 12–1. Often family goals on Individualized Family Service Plans (IFSP) address the needs required for family functioning.

The handicapped infant introduces changes in family routines; schedules and resources often must be altered to accommodate the needs of the newest member. The family may be forced to prioritize needs, emphasizing certain family functions required for survival (e.g., economics) while deemphasizing others either temporarily or longterm (e.g., recreation or socialization).

The functions of individual subsystems are also affected by the arrival of a handicapped infant. The demands of the handicapped child often use energy that was previously available for siblings, the parents' relationship, or family friends and extended family. Often interventionists assist families in creating a balance between the needs of individual family members and the family unit as a whole. How a balance is achieved is each family's decision, and as such, must be respected by professionals. In some cases, families may chose noninvolvement or minimal involvement to establish a balance. Although generally viewed unfavorably by professionals, this decision may result in more time for the parents to be involved with their handicapped child and other family members (MacMillan & Turnbull, 1983) producing positive effects on the family as a unit.

TABLE 12–1
Tasks associated with family functions.

Economic	**Recreation**	**Affection**
Generating income	Participating in individual and family-oriented recreation	Nurturing and loving
Paying bills and banking		Sharing companionship
Handling investments	Setting aside demands	Enjoying intimacy
Overseeing insurance benefit programs	Developing and enjoying hobbies	Expressing emotions
Earning allowance	Building skills and talents	**Educational/Vocational**
Dispensing allowance	**Socialization**	Continuing education for parents
Saving for the future	Building relationships	Completing homework
Daily Care	Developing social skills	Developing cultural appreciation
Purchasing and preparing food	Engaging in social activities	Building social responsibility
Purchasing and preparing clothing	**Self-Identity**	Making career choices
Maintaining health care	Establishing self-identity and self-image	Developing work skills and attitudes
Providing safety and protection	Recognizing strengths and weaknesses	Supporting career interests and problems
Transporting family members	Belonging to groups	Developing family values
Maintaining and cleaning home	Developing self-confidence	

Source: From *Working with Families with Disabled Members: A Family System Perspective* (p. 36) by A. P. Turnbull, J. A. Summers, and M. J. Brotherson, 1984, Lawrence, KS: The University of Kansas. Adapted by permission.

Life Cycle

The effects on the family of a member who is handicapped are never static. The **family life cycle** is a way of conceptualizing the sequence of changes that occur in families at different times. Effects on family members change as they move through major life stages: birth and early childhood, elementary school years, adolescence, young adulthood, empty nest, and elderly years (Turnbull & Turnbull, 1990). In the beginning of the family life cycle, during the birth and early childhood stage, adjustments to the birth of a new family member are compounded by the challenge of obtaining a diagnosis, seeking information regarding the condition, and securing services for the child. Each successive life stage has stresses that affect the family's interactions and functions.

FAMILY ADAPTATIONS

The way in which a family adapts to life with an exceptional child is influenced by

- □ the availability of support systems
- □ the coordination of family services
- □ the temperament of the child

One of the best ways to foster adaptation in families is to use anticipatory guidance in an attempt to minimize the effects of stress-related circumstances on the family.

Support Systems

Any support is helpful for a family, but the type and amount of support tends to be the significant factor in family adaptation. For example, if a child needs physical therapy, but only speech therapy services are available, the family has access to support, but it does not help the family. Many families indicate informal supports (relatives, friends, neighbors) are as necessary as formal supports (professionals, services) in meeting their ever-changing needs. Guiding families in ways to build their own support systems is one way to strengthen family adaptation (Dunst, Trivette, & Deal, 1988). The type of supports likely to mediate stress varies with the characteristics of the family and child, and the family's placement in the life cycle.

Coordination of Services

An important factor related to family adaptation is the coordination of early intervention services. Because multiple agencies are usually involved, families may experience the frustration of fragmented services. The coordination of services dictated in Part H of P.L. 99–457 is an enormous task requiring linkage between multiple public and private agencies and professionals from a number of disciplines.

Infant intervention consists of a number of potential service settings such as the Neonatal Intensive Care Unit, follow-up clinics, public and/or private child care, infant programs, and public school services. Each setting means transitions, with accompanying stress, for families. Offering a regular, carefully orchestrated multiagency transition process may ease family stress (Noonan & Kilgo, 1987).

Temperament of the Child

Infants are born with a set of personality characteristics that can be referred to as **temperament**. Temperament characteristics have been described as individual differences in the behavioral style of the child to which a family must adjust (Thomas & Chess, 1977). Parental perceptions of their child's temperament can influence their interactions with the child (Huntington, Simeonsson, Bailey, & Comfort, 1987), and ultimately, the child's development. An infant who is responsive to adults, adaptable, and playful is usually perceived by parents as a child with an easy temperament and attracts a lot of parent attention. In contrast, an infant who is fussy, hard to soothe, and exhibits irregular sleeping and eating patterns is routinely referred to as a difficult child and usually receives less attention from parents. Children who are described as slow to warm up frequently take longer to adapt to others. To increase family adaptation, relationship-oriented interventions may be necessary to modify the infant's contribution to interactions.

Considerable individual differences in temperament characteristics exist among infants with various handicapping conditions. Parents are strongly influenced by their infant's contribution to interactions. Handicapped infants may have more difficulty contributing. The interplay of parenting style, parents' ages, the number of children in the family, cultural and ethnic values, family functions, communication patterns, supports, and socioeconomic status can affect family relationships and adaptation. Specific child characteristics associated with different handicapping conditions that differentially affect parent-child relationships, and consequently family adaptations, are displayed in Table 12–2.

FAMILY-PROFESSIONAL COMMUNICATION TECHNIQUES

In order to support families, positive relationships must be established between parents and professionals. Positive relationships involve effective communication (Winton & Bailey, 1988). **Communication** is a process by which information and feelings are received and sent between individuals. Recently, attention has been placed on the importance of quality communication skills in early intervention.

Strategies for Effective Communication

Successful communication skills tend to be related to certain characteristics of communication, the physical surroundings, the needs of those communicating, and aspects of verbal and nonverbal communication.

Communication characteristics.   Effective communicators are usually associated with particular characteristics that affect the direction and outcome of interaction with others. Two of the most important characteristics of quality family-professional communication, and the most difficult to quantify, are respect and trust. To communicate respect, professionals acknowledge the family's decisions, lifestyle, values, beliefs, and efforts to care for their child, even when these conflict with those held by interventionists (Horejsi, 1979). As discussed earlier, within some cultural groups this might involve addressing the most elderly family member, using titles of respect (Mr.,

TABLE 12–2
Effects of specific handicaps on children's interactional skills.

Handicap	Reported Findings
Mental retardation	Reduced responsivity to others Decreased vocalization Lack of smiling or delayed smiling More solitary play Fewer initiations to others More likely to resist or not respond to cuddling
Hearing impairment	Impaired communication Inconsistent responses to communicative attempts Fewer social initiations
Visual impairment	Irregular smiling Smiling in response to auditory cues only Child must "maintain contact" by tactile and auditory (rather than visual) cues
Physical and motor impairments	Limp or physically unresponsive Difficulty in relaxing Decreased ability to laugh or smile Smile may look like a grimace Impaired communication skills Impaired locomotion skills prevent child from independently seeking out parent

Source: From *Teaching Infants and Preschoolers with Handicaps* (p. 148) by D. B. Bailey and M. Wolery, 1984, Columbus, OH: Merrill. Copyright © 1984 by Merrill, an imprint of Macmillan Publishing Company. Reprinted by permission.

Mrs.), and dressing to communicate respect for the family (avoiding casual clothing). To communicate trust, professionals must follow through with commitments, offer unhurried contact time, communicate empathy, and admit, when appropriate, if answers are not available.

Physical surroundings.   Attending to another person, either visually or auditorially, can be extremely difficult when there are distractions. Minor physical barriers to quality communication can often be controlled. For instance, slight distractions such as a television playing during a home visit, can be eliminated by scheduling visits when they do not interfere with favorite programs. Sibling interferences can be handled by bringing a distractor toy or activity for the sibling or giving the sibling some role in intervention activities. Notetaking during meetings may inhibit the flow of conversation with some parents, while others do not appear affected. The decision to take notes should be the prerogative of each family.

Jargon-free communication.   Communication is only effective when everyone involved understands the message. Professional jargon interferes with clarity and may serve as a barrier to developing quality relationships with families. Occasionally it may be appropriate for professionals to use an unfamiliar term because it is the most effective and accurate descriptor. In this case, the new term and its purpose needs to be clarified so it becomes a part of professionals' and parents' shared language. A mother with a newly diagnosed infant offers this perspective: "I feel like I need a medical dictionary to just talk to the doctors and school people I see. After awhile, I ask them to write things down and I look it up when I get home. But half the time, I nod and act like I'm not stupid and completely lost. Sometimes, I leave with knots in my stomach."

Unfortunately, some professionals are unaware that their communication skills make it difficult to form warm relationships with families. Effective communication skills demand practice and experience. Because communication skills are the platform for all effective early intervention, interventionists are wise to develop these skills with the same professional dedication that they develop other skills related to serving children and families.

Nonverbal Communication

Eighty-five percent of all information conveyed is communicated nonverbally. **Nonverbal communication** is the use of body language including gestures, facial expressions, posture, and body movements that convey information. It is important to learn to monitor one's body language, to respond to others' body language, to become familiar with culturally diverse nonverbal signals (e.g., avoiding eye contact, avoiding asking questions), and to note discrepancies in nonverbal and verbal messages. Table 12–3 provides a list of desirable and undesirable nonverbal communication behaviors appropriate for the mainstreamed Anglo culture.

Paralanguage. **Paralanguage** refers to the manner of speech or vocal effects, such as voice tone, volume, or intonation, that accompany or modify an utterance and communicate meaning. A monotone voice, for example, conveys boredom, while a high-pitched voice signifies disbelief. The way in which one speaks is often more important than what is actually said.

Listening. The importance of active and purposeful **listening** for effective communication cannot be overemphasized. A common complaint of parents is that professionals do not listen to them (Johnson, McGonigel, & Kauffman, 1989). Quality listening is an *active* process requiring conscious attending skills. The active listener leans slightly forward and maintains more than the usual amount of eye contact during a conversation (Knapp, 1972). A face-to-face position with an open posture (i.e., arms not crossed in front), remaining relaxed and alert, establishing proximity within a comfort zone, and using natural gestures are nonverbal behaviors that demonstrate attentive listening. (Readers are reminded that these behaviors may communicate disrespect in some cultural groups and should be used in situations only in which they are appropriate.) Fatigue and strong feelings about what is being discussed, however, can operate as deterrents to listening (Kroth, 1985).

Verbal Communication Skills

Verbal communication skills of following, reflecting, questioning, and structuring combine with nonverbal skills to form the foundation of quality communication.

TABLE 12–3
Inventory of Practitioner's Nonverbal Communication.

Desirable	Undesirable
Facial expressions	
Direct eye contact (except when culturally proscribed)	Avoidance of eye contact
	Eye level higher or lower than client's
Warmth and concern reflected in facial expression	Staring or fixating on person or object
	Lifting eyebrow critically
Eyes at same level as client's	Nodding head excessively
Appropriately varied and animated facial expressions	Yawning
	Frozen or rigid facial expressions
Mouth relaxed; occasional smiles	Inappropriate slight smile
	Pursing or biting lips
Posture	
Arms and hands moderately expressive; appropriate gestures	Rigid body position; arms tightly folded
	Body turned at an angle to client
Body leaning slightly forward; attentive but relaxed	Fidgeting with hands (including clipping nails or cleaning pipe)
	Squirming or rocking in chair
	Slouching or placing feet on desk
	Hand or fingers over mouth
	Pointing finger for emphasis
Voice	
Clearly audible but not loud	Mumbling or speaking inaudibly
Warmth in tone of voice	Monotonic voice
Voice modulated to reflect nuances of feeling and emotional tone of client messages	Halting speech
	Frequent grammatical errors
	Prolonged silences
Moderate speech tempo	Excessively animated speech
	Slow, rapid, or staccato speech
	Nervous laughter
	Consistent clearing of throat
	Speaking loudly
Physical proximity	
Three to five feet between chairs	Excessive closeness or distance
	Talking across desk or other barrier

Source: From *Social Work Practice: Theory and Skills* by Dean H. Hepworth and J. Ann Larsen © 1982 by The Dorsey Press. Reprinted by permission of Wadsworth, Inc.

Following skills. A number of responses, referred to as **following skills,** facilitate dialogue by encouraging the speaker to continue speaking. **Door-opener statements** such as "I'd like to know more about.... " or "What do you see Leslie doing in 6 months' time ... ?" encourage parents to share and seek information. **Minimal encouragers** are brief responses by the listener such as "uh-huh," "yes," a slight head nod, or a smile that invite parents to continue to offer information (Winton, 1988). These techniques convey that the listener is interested and wants to hear more.

Although some professionals find it difficult, it is best to avoid communication behaviors with evaluative components, such as judging the parent or offering explanations or solutions. Such behaviors may block communication. For instance, instead of saying "Well, she does that because...." and beginning to offer solutions, it is usually better to ask something such as "Why do you think she is doing that?" In this way, solutions are not handed to the family but they are generated collaboratively.

Reflecting content and feelings.   **Reflecting** is a method of checking with the speaker to determine if what was said was understood correctly by the listener. **Paraphrasing** is used to restate important or complex statements in a concise manner while emphasizing the main idea of the message (Winton, 1988). Statements such as "I understood you to say...." test the listener's perceptions, so inaccuracies in interpretation of the original message may be corrected. Comments may then be made to expand on what was said (e.g., "Tell me more about...." or "Anything else?"). Another method of reflecting content involves summarizing lengthy comments or recapitulating what has been said (Winton & Bailey, 1988).

Reflecting feelings refers to the ability to identify how a person really feels, even if the speaker may not verbally express those feelings. This process involves listening for feeling words, listening for the content of the message, observing body language, and asking one's self "What would I feel?" One might say, "You felt angry when he said that?" or "It hurt?" to demonstrate that the listener is listening empathically.

Effective questioning.   Johnson and colleagues (1989) describe **effective questioning** as the ability to ask questions in a manner in which information is shared. These authors urge interventionists to have a rationale for all questions asked of families, so that intrusive questions or questions that cause discomfort are avoided.

There are two types of questions: open-ended and close-ended. A **close-ended question** can usually be answered with a "yes," "no," or other brief response. Close-ended questions request specific information such as "Does Anna have seizures?" or "Does Anna eat breakfast?" When more extensive information is desired, open-ended questions are used. **Open-ended questions**, such as "How are mealtimes with Anna?" elicit more complete responses to a question.

All questions should be asked straightforwardly, while maintaining eye contact. Questions that inhibit freedom of response (e.g., "You don't have difficulty feeding Anna, do you?") should be avoided. This type of questioning can make parents feel that their behavior is incorrect or unacceptable.

Effective questioning assists family members in generating goals and solutions to their own problems (Tomm, 1987). For example, "What do you see Anna doing at mealtimes in 6 months?" or "How can we help Anna develop self-feeding skills?" clearly communicate *shared* problem solving. Readers are referred to Winton and Bailey (1988) and Johnson, McGonigel, & Kaufmann (1989) for more examples of interview and interactional questions for families.

Structuring.   Having a structure for formal meetings with parents ensures more effective communication. The purpose of the meeting and the time allotted should be stated before the meeting. At the onset of the meeting, the objectives for the meeting and activities or tasks to be accomplished need to be stated. At the end of the meeting, a summary of the meeting or the objectives accomplished and a re-statement of the agreed plan of action should be given.

Handling Confrontations and Negotiations

Especially in the beginning of the early intervention process, many parents experience feelings of powerlessness. In some individuals, intense emotions trigger anger or hostility toward a system or an individual who seems unable to "fix" their child.

Also, certain words may elicit powerful emotional reactions. Statements to parents such as "Your child is retarded," or statements from parents to professionals such as "You are the worst teacher I have ever seen," interfere with one's ability to listen. Professionals need to be sensitive to the potential hurtful impact of even casual comments to family members.

When conflicts do develop, they should be resolved swiftly. If the family member is confrontational or hostile, it is best to remain calm, soften one's voice, and permit the family member to express the point of view with little interruption except to ask for elaborations or clarifications when needed. The key ingredient to resolving confrontations is listening empathetically (e.g., "How would I feel if I were this parent?"), rather than blaming.

Most people say they listen, but in actuality, a good listener is a rare find. Many individuals use the time the other person is speaking to plan their own points, and outline their own agenda. By following families' priorities and engaging in quality communication and negotiation, professionals design partnerships in which parents feel valued and respected.

To diffuse a confrontation, professionals must make sincere efforts to come to a joint, mutually acceptable solution or resolution. This may involve gaining the family member's permission to write down the issues so that each may be systematically handled. However, some family members may not feel comfortable with notetaking and their preference should be honored.

Although there is never one way to handle any situation interventionists may encounter, confrontational interactions in which the legitimacy of the family member's strong feelings are acknowledged tend to promote prompt negotiations, and work to expand the family member's trust in the professional.

Practicing communication strategies under supervised role-play situations seems to be most effective in changing behavior. Because nonverbal and verbal communication skills are essential for effective communication, activities designed to improve these skills are included at the end of this chapter.

ASSESSMENT INVOLVING FAMILIES

The family-centered approach to early intervention has a number of implications for the assessment process with families. Like most types of assessment, family assessment is best if information is gathered using a number of sources and modes. Family assessment may involve assessing parent-child interaction, responsivity, and/or family strengths and needs. Refer to Bailey and Simeonsson (1988) for an extensive review of family assessment tools.

Parent-child Interaction Scales

Research demonstrates that parent-infant interaction is related to later child development and associated with other dimensions of the family system (Comfort, 1988). Consequently, one principal purpose of early intervention is to foster quality parent-child relationships. To help parents adjust their interactional style, Hedlund (1989) recommends professionals take these actions:

- □ educate parents about their child's unique communication/body language
- □ assist parents in becoming attuned to their own interactional style and how that style affects their child
- □ provide parents with guided practice and encouragement to adapt their styles as their child develops
- □ highlight the child's developmental progress so parents can see the results of their efforts

When children are handicapped, their abilities and responsiveness in play interactions can influence reciprocal parent-child play. Parents may experience frustration if the child's ability to play is significantly impaired. Assessment information helps to determine parent-child interactional strengths, in addition to needs, so rewarding aspects of the relationship may be increased. The interventionists can build on strengths (e.g., mother is devoted to child), and select for intervention those areas in which assistance may be needed (e.g., mother gives mostly noncontingent attention).

Formal assessment of parent-child interactions should never be considered routine. Instead, families should determine if this is a desired area of attention for intervention efforts (Fewell & Kaminski, 1988). In addition to the instruments listed in Chapter 13, Table 13.2, the Social Interaction Assessment/Intervention (McCollum & Stayton, 1985), the Teaching Skills Inventory (Rosenberg, Robinson, & Beckman, 1984), the Nursing Child Assessment—Teaching and Feeding Scales (Barnard, 1978), and the Maternal Behavior Rating Scale (Mahoney, 1985) are available.

Responsivity Scales

Infants and toddlers who are at risk and handicapped demonstrate behaviors that are indicators of their readability, predictability, and responsiveness. The Neonatal Behavioral Assessment Scale (Brazelton, 1984) and the Assessment of Preterm Infant Behavior (Als, Lester, Tronick, & Brazelton, 1982) are tools used for determining the cues and interpretability of young children's behaviors.

Determination of Family Strengths and Needs

Determining the family's unique strengths and needs as they relate to the child's development is a complex undertaking that requires many professionals to develop

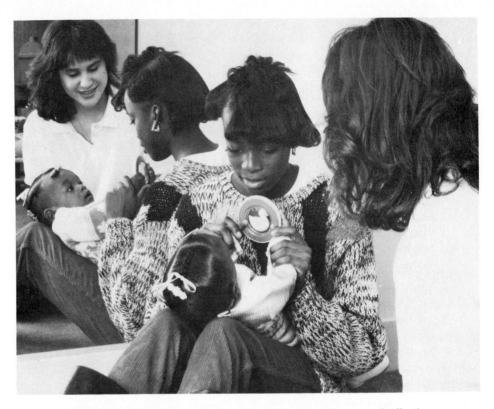

Serving families with a family-centered approach involves the use of effective communication skills and responding to the needs of the family so that they may better facilitate the child's development.

an entirely new set of skills. Any survey and questionnaire selected to determine families' strengths and needs must

□ meet the family's individual needs (e.g., language of household)
□ be easy for parents to read
□ be nonintrusive
□ offer space for parents to add concerns
□ be reasonable in length
□ assist in determining family strengths

A list of commonly used family needs assessment instruments is included in Chapter 13, Table 13.2.

FAMILY-CENTERED APPROACH TO PROGRAMMING

The child with special needs may introduce stressors or add to existing family stress, which may lead to a dysfunctional family. By addressing the family's most pressing needs, the effects of intervention on family members may improve family functioning, and this may contribute to positive outcomes in the child (Odom, Yoder, & Hill, 1988). As professionals have become convinced of the wisdom of family-centered services in theory, however, a number of questions have emerged regarding how to implement family-centered practices.

Professional-family Partnerships in Planning

Professional-family partnerships mean actively involving families in assessing their own and their child's needs. It means accepting families' expectations and limits on the degree to which they desire to be involved as parents, not professionals (Garland & Linder, 1988). As Barnard (1985) states: "We need to begin to view our work with families as a partnership in which we are consultants, but the family is in charge" (p. 4).

Kovach (1986) found that when the staff contributes more goals and strategies to the service plan, parents followed through with only half of the strategies. But when parents contribute at least equally to the service plan, parents' implementation was 80% to 100%. Not surprisingly, parents and professionals often differ in their priorities for goals or services. D. B. Bailey (1987) offers reasons that may account for these differences.

> Parent motivation may be lacking if they do not see the relevance of recommended activities. Other parents may be motivated, but lack the time, resources, energy or skill to follow through. Professionals may have limited insight into family needs and priorities. Furthermore, professionals may have limited ability to motivate and challenge parents. (p. 61)

When differences occur, it is important that interventionists do not attempt to force their values on families. Rather, differences should be discussed openly with families so a range of alternatives can be generated. By using a collaborative approach to selecting goals, interventionists objectively demonstrate that they recognize the value of the family's perspective and its cultural value system.

Family-professional Partnerships in Intervention

Working with families as partners does not necessarily mean making parents therapists or teachers. It does mean supporting families in their efforts to cope with the problems and stresses associated with raising a handicapped child and helping them to encourage the development of that child. A partnership means that families may choose the way and extent to which they desire to be involved in the intervention process with their child. This sounds simple, but many professionals are more comfortable going into a home and doing their "thing" with the child and then leaving. Truly sharing the intervention role with families changes the dynamics of intervention for everyone involved. Vincent (1985) issued this challenge to early interventionists:

> If we are to be successful with families, we are going to have to reorient as professionals. We are going to need to look to parents as the leaders, parents as the experts, parents as the bosses. We are going to need to ask them to join us cooperatively as equals in this partnership so that we create a reality out there that matches what all of us want to see. (p. 1)

Certainly families vary in their abilities and desire for services and this changes as the children and families change. Despite the fact that some professionals claim that families are equal partners and that they are nonjudgmental about families' decisions about how much participation they desire, some professionals still communicate dissatisfaction with families who desire less involvement. A single father reported: "I didn't want to, but with my jobs and never seeing my son, I had to cut back on home visits and never get to meetings no more. I feel guilty about it and even though [my home visitor] don't say so, I know she isn't happy about it. What can I do about it?"

At other times, professionals may try to assume too much responsibility or send a message to families that they are not really sufficiently competent to cope without the professional. Turnbull and Turnbull (1990) and Dunst and his colleagues (1988) have discussed this notion of **noncontingent help**, and suggest that the long-term effects of providing assistance and information that is neither requested nor needed may foster dependency rather than growth in family members.

Enablement and **empowerment** are terms at the heart of the family-centered approach. Enabling is a concept defined by Deal, Dunst, and Trivette (1989) as "creating opportunities for family members to become more competent and self-sustaining with respect to their abilities to get needs met and attain desired goals" (p. 33). The term *empowerment* is described as "carrying out interventions in a manner in which family members acquire a sense of control over their own developmental course as a result of their efforts to meet needs" (Deal et al., 1989, p. 33).

Attempting to find a balance between independence and emotional support forces professionals to be flexible in their transactions with families. What may be an enabling approach with one family may be viewed as an unwillingness to help to another. Families' needs must be met in ways that are respectful of their cultural preferences and the many other factors that vary considerably across families.

Parental Rights

Professionals who advocate partnerships with families must be willing to offer a range of liberties to families. Some liberties might mean that parents are not perfectly compliant with the desires of professionals. Exercising their rights might be part of the acceptance process for some families; for other families, it might be part of becoming less dependent on professionals for support and decision making. Ferrell (1985) has outlined these 12 fundamental parental rights:

The right to feel angry. Little in life prepares someone for parenting a handicapped child. The anger parents feel often comes from not being able to control, or change, the situation. Professionals can help parents to direct their anger toward getting the best possible services for their child.

The right to seek another opinion. It is considered good practice to seek a second opinion with major medical decisions such as surgery. Parents may desire the same prerogative with early intervention if they do not believe or like the diagnosis or intervention plans. It is unwise for professionals to take this search for information personally, and be hurt by it. The process of searching can afford parents a small sense of control over their lives and often facilitates their acceptance in the long run.

The right to keep trying.   Sometimes parents are convinced that a particular goal, such as walking, is what their child needs. Even when the therapist indicates that walking isn't feasible at that time in the child's life, some parents are still determined to realize their goal. By continuing to pursue the goal, parents may feel more involved and purposeful.

The right to stop trying.   Parents need to learn to protect their time and energy. Even though from a professional's point of view, what has been asked only takes 10 minutes a day or can be incorporated into daily routines, for some exhausted parents, it may still be impossible that day. Truly respecting the dignity of the family means that professionals allow families to decide how their time with their family will be used. Parents must balance all members of the family, not just the handicapped child, and at times this means that parents make decisions about their time that differ from professionals' priorities.

The right to privacy.   Dealing with a parade of professionals, no matter how well intentioned, can be very difficult for some parents. Because of their handicapped or at-risk child, aspects of their family are of interest to people they may not know very well. It is every family's right to set limits on how intrusive professionals can be in their lives.

The right to be a parent.   It is unrealistic to expect parents to "work with" their children all the time. Families need time to relax, to play without a goal, and to simply enjoy one another's company. Some activities professionals ask parents to do are unnatural for parents and make them feel like teachers, not parents. For parents who desire it, separating the roles of teacher and parent may allow the family to find new joy in their handicapped family member.

The right to be unenthusiastic.   Some days with a child who is handicapped can be thrilling because the child learned something new or smiled. Other days the child may be less responsive and the parent may feel less enthusiastic. Communicating to parents that having "up" and "down" days is all part of the adaptation process will help them to better understand ebbs in their emotional energy. It may be easier for professionals to be enthusiastic because they only enter a family's life for short periods of time, but parents must ration their physical and emotional energy for a lifetime of challenges.

The right to be annoyed with their child.   No fine quality relationship is without its difficult times. Parents of handicapped children may feel guilty for feeling disappointed or irritated by their child. To handle stress for long periods of time, parents need to be able to express and understand that their feelings will not always be all good or all bad toward their child. Their child is a child first, and a handicapped child second. All children are annoying sometimes.

The right to time off.   Parents have aspects of their lives that do not involve their handicapped child, such as their marital relationship and personal hobbies. Parents who allow themselves time off and have interests outside their families tend to express the strongest feelings of personal well-being. Parents of handicapped children often struggle for this balance in their personal lives.

The right to be the expert.   The reality is that the family knows the child better than anyone—even the professionals. Respecting parents' points of view about their child is at the very heart of the family-centered approach.

The right to set limits.   Often parents get contradictory messages from professionals. On one hand, they are told to just relax and enjoy their child. On the other, they are told not to relax too much because they can make significant changes in their child's development if they "work with the child." Parents have the right to be a family— not a family that revolves around the needs of the handicapped child. Parents are the best judges of what limits are best for their family, in their unique circumstances.

The right to dignity.   Professionals receive and expect respect and dignity, and parents should receive and expect the same. Talking to parents as peers, respecting their time and perspectives, and really listening all communicate to parents that professionals are their advocates, not their adversaries.

Few will say parenting is an easy task, but most will agree that the majority of parents do the best job they can. By giving families a central role in early intervention, professionals work toward fostering the family's autonomy for the good of the child. Certain dimensions of family life have emerged as important in the development of children's competencies during the first years of life:

- the presence of a responsive, warm, and attentive attachment figure
- parental use of consistent disciplinary standards that involve explanation and appropriate positive affect
- a well organized and stimulating environment
- parental encouragement of learning by use of questioning and graduated cues that are responsive to feedback from the child
- parental expectations for child competence
- harmonious relations within the family
- a positive relationship with the environment outside the family including extended family, friends, and community (Silber, 1989)

Families may need to be alerted to the signs of stress: tiredness or fatigue, lack of interest, boredom, no desire to go out, never inviting friends over, and lack of sexual intimacy. The exact way stress is played out in families varies as much as the individual members in a family. A mother of a mildly handicapped toddler put it this way: "Sometimes I feel that I can't go on. [begins to cry softly] I am so tired and so sick of being pleasant and brave. Sometimes I just want to lock myself in my room and send everyone away—my husband, the kids, the therapists, and all those doctors we see every year, even when we don't want to. I want sympathy . . . and I get mad when I get it. But I really want Stephanie to be normal. Who is going to do that for me?"

TRANSDISCIPLINARY CASES

The following case studies and the Applied Activities/Projects provide opportunities to practice skills discussed throughout this book and in this chapter.

THE HUNTER FAMILY

Desiree, 24 months old, has no verbal expressive language, and primarily uses gestures or grunts to communicate. She has been diagnosed as oral-motor apraxic. Desiree lives with her mother, Lena (17); her maternal grandmother, Lillian (39); her maternal aunt, (19); and two cousins (2 and 4). Her father has not seen her since she was 2 months old. The Hunters are an African American family who live in a rural area in the house in which all the adults were raised and the family has resided for four generations.

Desiree's mother and aunt work as waitresses in the nearby small town. Desiree and the other children are cared for by their maternal grandmother. Because the grandmother has primary responsibility for care of the children, she makes all of the decisions regarding them. She feels that Desiree is slow and does not need the medical and therapy attention that the infant transdisciplinary team has recommended. Desiree's grandmother states that the family should be able to care for itself, not rely on others for help. Desiree's mother feels differently, especially regarding her daughter's therapy needs, but is fearful of contradicting her mother.

Although the Hunters live in a rural community, they have many friends and extended family members in the area. These friends and family have little economic means, but they have many skills, talents, and personal resources they willingly share with the Hunters.

THE MARTIN FAMILY

Shelly, 18 months old, functions at approximately a 9-month level according to a recent transdisciplinary assessment. She has seizures, is hypotonic, and experiences repeated infections due to her diagnosed congenital disorder, **Wolf's Syndrome**. Shelly lives with her mother, Joan (32); her father, Stuart (39); and her sisters, Debra (4), Susan (8), and Jayne (10). Although the Martins moved to their rural community 6 years ago, they have few friends in the area. No extended family members live nearby.

Shelly's mother cares for her family. She was a nurse for a brief period prior to the birth of her first child. Shelly's father works as an electrical engineer for a communications company 60 miles away. He works 50- to 60-hour weeks and is away from home at least 3 nights a week. The family's income is stable and provides enough for a comfortable home, good medical care, and an occasional vacation.

Shelly's sisters are all active in school and extracurricular activities. Debra is taking dance lessons. Susan participates in a drama program and takes piano lessons. Jayne is in a 4-H club and attends a girls' group sponsored by the family's church. Shelly's sisters help in her care but are also frustrated at times by the amount of time their sister requires. While Shelly's mother and three sisters attend church on Sundays, her father stays home with her. He occasionally assists with household chores on weekends.

SUMMARY OF PROCEDURES

There is no doubt that the diversity of family needs, the complex nature of family functioning, and the multicultural identities of families pose special challenges to professionals. The most successful programs are those that respond to the individualized strengths and needs of families. When strengths and needs are respected and used in the intervention plan, there is a greater chance of a positive family impact. A summary of key strategies of this chapter follows:

1. Use direct teaching, modeling, and communication to demonstrate to families the importance of their role in facilitating, guiding, and supporting their child's development.
2. Support family members as they move through their own sequences of acceptance. All individual family members, as well as extended family members, experience adjustment differently. Some individuals may never completely accept their situation.
3. Ask parents to encourage siblings to discuss their handicapped sibling's condition. Remind parents that their attitudes and adjustments set the stage for their children's adjustment.
4. Provide support services (e.g., groups, information sessions, program open houses) to extended family members and significant others, in addition to families. This may extend the support network of some families which may facilitate their adaptation.
5. Learn as much as possible about the family structure, childrearing practices, beliefs, and communication styles of different cultural groups. Cultural knowledge and sensitivity must be stated priorities of early intervention programs serving culturally diverse young children and their families.
6. Learn and practice effective communication skills—controlling paralanguage factors, listening, following skills, reflecting content and feelings, questioning—with the same professional dedication that other areas of early intervention have been learned. Effective communication, which may be defined differently by various cultural groups, is a learned skill that can be improved and refined.
7. Actively demonstrate and communicate trust and respect in all transactions with families to implement a family-centered approach to early intervention. Use nonjudgmental listening and negotiation when differences in priorities and values arise with families.
8. Actively nurture and encourage parental self-assurance in all interactions with families. Parents have problem-solving and coping skills that interventionists need to respect, promote, and encourage.
9. Promote family autonomy by acknowledging parental rights: to feel angry, to seek another opinion, to keep trying, to stop trying, to privacy, to parent, to be unenthusiastic, to be annoyed with their child, to take time off, to be the expert, to set limits, and to be treated with dignity.

SUMMARY

The idea of a partnership between professionals and families appears to be a natural, and perhaps even logical approach to early intervention. However, the changes in professional and family interactions necessary for such a partnership to be successful are far from simple. Parental emotional distress and anxiety, a lack of parental knowledge of child development, the zeal of interventionists, interventionists' lack of cultural knowledge, and conflicts in values between professionals and families often mitigate against real partnerships. Nonetheless, working with families to find joy in small developmental gains, modeling encouragement and interactional patterns, and organizing parents as resources for one another can go a long way toward building partnerships.

Interventionists must remain sensitive to the idiosyncracies and multicultural considerations of families. To do this, a flexible approach and appropriate communication skills are necessary. Professionals should encourage families to decide in what way, and to what degree, early intervention will be included in their lives. The ability to feel competent in their handling of their child and in making decisions for their family are critical skills for families who are just beginning what may be many long years of special services directed by professionals.

DISCUSSION QUESTIONS

1. Today more is understood about the impact of a handicapped child on family members. What resources and assistance may infant interventionists offer families to facilitate their interaction? How might the effectiveness of such efforts be evaluated?
2. Explain what it means to work within the family's cultural network. Name five ways in which interventionists may become more knowledgeable about a family's culture. What effect may this knowledge have on the effectiveness of serving the family?
3. This chapter discussed parental rights. What are interventionists' rights and how do professionals balance parental and professional rights when they conflict?

APPLIED ACTIVITIES/PROJECTS

1. **Case study exercise**. After reading the Hunter and Martin case studies, discuss the following questions:
   □ Compare and contrast the families in terms of the four elements of the Family Systems Framework (e.g., characteristics, interactions, functions, life cycle).
   □ Identify major strengths and needs apparent in these brief descriptions of each family.
   □ List any obstacles there might be to meeting child and family needs. For each obstacle, generate a possible strategy or solution.
2. **Jargon-free communication exercise**.
   □ Make a list of the 10 most frequently used jargon words in early intervention.
   □ Select a partner from a different discipline (or assume different discipline roles). Define each jargon word to your partner without using other jargon words.
   □ Role-play a conference with the Hunter and Martin families, discussing this information without using jargon.
3. **Interpersonal communication exercise**. Divide into groups of three. Each student will assume the roles of speaker, listener, and observer at least once. The speaker talks for 2 to 3 minutes on a topic of interest to the Hunters or Martins using effective communication skills. The listener should demonstrate good listening behaviors. At the end of each 2- to 3-minute exchange, the observer provides feedback on speaker and listener communication behaviors (e.g., eye contact, attending, hand gestures, facial expressions, voice tone). Switch roles until everyone has had an opportunity to play each role. Then, repeat the previous

steps with a confrontational situation you create from the case studies. Practice negotiation skills and collaborative goal setting.

4. **Values assessment and clarification exercise**. Divide into groups of three and select a leader. Each person reads the following list of value statements. Then as a group, go through each statement and discuss whether to keep, eliminate, or revise the statement so that it is acceptable to *all* group members. If time allows, additional statements should be added to the following:

□ The family is the primary decision maker regarding early intervention service needs and child and family program priorities.

□ When services needed are not available, the early intervention program should provide them.

□ Parents should be encouraged to be case managers.

□ Dependence is encouraged when professionals provide services which could more appropriately be provided or arranged for by families.

□ Parents should be co-equal members of the early intervention team.

□ Parents should be captains of the early transdisciplinary intervention team. (Activity used with permission from a working document from Child Development Resources [CDR], Lightfoot, Virginia).

SUGGESTED READINGS

A number of parents have written personal accounts of raising a child who is handicapped, with particular emphasis placed on the impact of their early interactions with professionals. The following are recommended:

Featherstone, H. (1980). *A difference in the family: Life with a disabled child*. New York: Basic Books.

Kupfer, F. (1982). *Before and after Zachariah*. New York: Delacorte Press.

Simons, R. (1987). *After the tears: Parents talk about raising a child with a disability*. San Diego: Harcourt Brace Jovanovich.

Turnbull, A. P., & Turnbull, H. R. (1985). *Parents speak out: Then and now*. Columbus, OH: Merrill.

Other books and resources of interest:

Anderson, P. P., & Fenichel, E. S. (1989). *Serving culturally diverse families of infants and toddlers with disabilities*. Washington, DC: National Center for Clinical Infant Programs.

Especially grandparents: A newsletter for and about grandparents of children with special needs. (For information about this newsletter write: *Especially Grandparents*, 2230 Eighth Ave., Seattle, WA 98121).

Fewell, R. R., & Vadasy, P. F. (1986). *Families of handicapped children: Needs and supports across the life span*. Austin, TX: PRO-ED.

Meyer, D., Vadasy, P., & Fewell, R. (1985). *Living with a brother or sister with special needs: A book for sibs*. Seattle: University of Washington Press.

Parks, S., Furuno, S., O'Reilly, K., Inatsuka, T., Hosaka, C., & Zeisloft-Falbey, B. (1989). *HELP ... at Home*. Palo Alto, CA: VORT.

Randall-David, E. (1989). *Strategies for working with culturally diverse communities and clients*. Washington, DC: American Association for the Care of Children's Health.

Tingey-Michaelis, C. (1983). *Handicapped infants and children: A handbook for parents and professionals*. Austin, TX: PRO-ED.

Turnbull, A. P., & Turnbull, H. R. (1990). *Families, professionals, and exceptionality: A special partnership*. Columbus, OH: Merrill.

Workshops and handbooks of interest:

Ivey, A. (1971). *Microteaching: Innovations in interview training*. Springfield, IL: Charles C. Thomas.

Kirkham, M., Norelius, K., Meltzer, N., Schilling, R., & Schinke, S. (1988). *Reducing stress in mothers of children with special needs*. Seattle: University of Washington Press.

Meyer, D. J., & Vadasy, P. (1987). *Grandparent workshops: How to organize workshops for grandparents of children with handicaps*. Seattle: University of Washington Press.

Meyer, D. J., Vadasy, P., & Fewell, R. R. (1986). *Sibshops: A handbook for implementing workshops for siblings of children with special needs*. Seattle: University of Washington Press.

Meyer, D. J., Vadasy, P., Fewell, R. R., & Schell, G. (1985). *A handbook for the Fathers Program: How to organize a program for fathers and their handicapped children*. Seattle: University of Washington Press.

REFERENCES

Als, H., Lester, B. M., Tronick, E. Z., & Brazelton, T. B. (1982). Towards a research instrument for the assessment of preterm infants' behavior (APIB). In H. E. Fitzgerald, B. M. Lester, & M. W. Yogman (Eds.), *Theory and research in behavioral pediatrics* (pp. 35–132). New York: Plenum.

Anderson, P. P., & Fenichel, E. S. (1989). *Serving culturally diverse families of infants and toddlers with disabilities*. Washington, DC: National Center for Clinical Infant Programs.

Bailey, D. B. (1987). Collaborative goal-setting with families: Resolving differences in values and priorities for services. *Topics in Early Childhood Special Education, 7,* 59–71.

Bailey, D. B., & Simeonsson, R. J. (1988). *Family assessment in early intervention*. Columbus, OH: Merrill.

Bailey, D. B., & Wolery, M. (1984), *Teaching infants and preschoolers with handicaps*. Columbus, OH: Merrill.

Bailey, D. B., & Wolery, M. (1989). *Assessing infants and preschoolers with handicaps*. Columbus, OH: Merrill.

Bailey, E. (1987). Sociocultural factors and health care-seeking behavior among Black Americans. *Journal of the National Medical Association, 4,* 389–392.

Barnard, K. (1978). *Nursing Child Assessment—Teaching and Feeding Scales*. Seattle: University of Washington School of Nursing.

Barnard, K. (1985). Toward an era of family partnership. In *Equals in this partnership: Parents of disabled and at-risk infants and toddlers speak to professionals* (pp. 4–5). Washington, DC: National Center for Clinical Infant Programs.

Blacher, J. (1984). Sequential stages of parental adjustment to the birth of a child with handicaps. *Mental Retardation, 22,* 55–68.

Brazelton, T. B. (1984). *Neonatal Behavioral Assessment Scale* (2nd ed.) (Clinics in Developmental Medicine, No. 50). Philadelphia: Lippincott.

Burden, R. (1980). Measuring the effect of stress on the mothers of handicapped infants: Must depression always follow? *Child Care, Health, & Development, 6,* 111–125.

Comfort, M. L. (1988). Assessing parent-child interactions. In D. B. Bailey & R. J. Simeonsson (Eds.), *Family assessment in early intervention* (pp. 65–94). Columbus, OH: Merrill.

Darling, R. (1979). *Families against society: A study of reactions of children with birth defects*. Beverly Hills, CA: Sage Publications.

Deal, A. G., Dunst, C. J., & Trivette, C. M. (1989). A flexible and functional approach to developing individualized family support plans. *Infants and Young Children, 1,* 32–43.

Drotar, D., Baskiewicz, A., Irvin, N., Kennell, J., & Klaus, M. (1975). The adaptation of parents to the birth of an infant with a congenital malformation: A hypothetical model. *Pediatrics, 56,* 710–717.

Dunst, C. J., Trivette, C. M., & Deal, A. (1988). *Enabling and empowering families: Principles and guidelines for practice.* Cambridge, MA: Brookline Books.

Featherstone, H. (1980). *A difference in the family: Life with a disabled child.* New York: Basic Books.

Ferrell, K. A. (1985). *Reach out and teach.* New York: American Foundation for the Blind.

Fewell, R. R., & Kaminski, R. R. (1988). Play skill development and instruction for young children with handicaps. In S. Odom & M. Karnes (Eds.), *Early intervention for infants and children with handicaps: An empirical base* (pp. 145–158). Baltimore: Paul H. Brookes.

Gabel, H., & Kotsch, L. S. (1981). Extended families and young handicapped children. *Topics in Early Childhood Special Education, 1,* 29–35.

Gabel, H., McDowell, J., & Cerreto, M. C. (1983). Family adaptation to the handicapped infant. In R. Fewell & G. Garwood (Eds.), *Educating handicapped infants: Issues in development and intervention* (pp. 299–322). Rockville, MD: Aspen.

Gallagher, J. J., Beckman, P., & Cross, A. H. (1983). Families of handicapped children: Sources of stress and its amelioration. *Exceptional Children, 50,* 10–19.

Gallagher, P. A., & Powell, T. H. (1989). Brothers and sisters: Meeting special needs. *Topics in Early Childhood Special Education, 8,* 24–37.

Garland, C., & Linder, T. (1988). Administrative challenges in early intervention. In J. B. Jordan, J. J. Gallagher, P. L. Hutinger, & M. B. Karnes (Eds.), *Early childhood special education: Birth to three* (pp. 5–28). Reston, VA: The Council for Exceptional Children.

Grossman, F. K. (1972). *Brothers and sisters of retarded children: An exploratory study.* Syracuse, NY: Syracuse University Press.

Hedlund, R. (1989). Fostering positive social interactions between parents and infants. *Teaching Exceptional Children, 21,* 45–48.

Horejsi, C. R. (1979). Social and psychological factors in family care. In R. H. Bruininks & G. C. Krantz, (Eds.), *Family care of developmentally disabled members* (pp. 13–24). Minneapolis: University of Minnesota.

Huntington, G. S., Simeonsson, R. J., Bailey, D. B., & Comfort, M. L. (1987). Handicapped child characteristics and maternal involvement. *Journal of Reproductive and Infant Psychology, 5,* 105–118.

Jenkins, S. (1981). *The ethnic dilemma in social services.* New York: The Free Press.

Johnson, B. H., McGonigel, M. J., & Kauffman, R. K. (1989). *Guidelines and recommended practices for the Individualized Family Service Plan.* Washington, DC: National Early Childhood Technical Assistance System and American Association for the Care of Children's Health.

Kazak, A. E., & Marvin, R. S. (1984). Differences, difficulties, and adaptations: Stress and social networks in families with a handicapped child. *Family Relations, 33,* 67–77.

Knapp, M. L. (1972). *Nonverbal communication in human interaction.* New York: Holt, Rinehart & Winston.

Kovach, J. (1986). *Project Dakota Final Report (1983–1986).* Eagan, MN: Project Dakota Outreach.

Kroth, R. (1985). *Communicating with parents of exceptional children.* Denver, CO: Love Publishing.

Kunce, J. (1983). *The Mexican-American: Cross-cultural rehabilitation counseling implications.* Final Report of World Rehabilitation Fund Grant No. G008 103982.

MacMillan, D., & Turnbull, A. (1983). Parent involvement with special education: Respecting individual differences. *Education and Training of the Mentally Retarded, 18,* 5–9.

Mahoney, G. A. (1985). *Maternal Behavior Rating Scale.* Unpublished rating scale. Available from Gerald Mahoney, Pediatric Research and Training Center, Department of Pediatrics, University of Connecticut, School of Medicine, Farmington, CT.

McAdoo, H. (1979). Black kinship. *Psychology Today, 5,* 67–110.

McCollum, J. A., & Stayton, V. D. (1985). Infant/parent interactions: Studies and intervention guidelines based on the SIAI Model. *Journal of the Division of Early Childhood, 9,* 125–145.

Nguyen, D. (1987, December). *Multicultural issues.* Presentation at Topical Conference of the Technical Assistance for Parent Programs (TAPP) Project, Boston, MA.

Noonan, M. J., & Kilgo, J. L. (1987). Transition services for early age individuals with severe mental retardation. In R. N. Ianacone & R. A. Stodden (Eds.), *Transition issues and directions* (pp. 25–37). Reston, VA: The Council for Exceptional Children.

Odom, S., Yoder, P., & Hill, G. (1988). Developmental intervention for infants with handicaps: Purposes and programs. *The Journal of Special Education, 22*(1), 11–24.

Olshansky, S. (1962). Chronic sorrow: A response to having a mentally defective child. *Social Casework, 43,* 190–194.

Paterson, R. (1982). *Cohesive family process.* Eugene, OR: Cartalia Publishing.

Perske, R. (1973). *New directions for parents of persons who are retarded.* Nashville, TN: Abingdon Press.

Rosenberg, S., Robinson, C., & Beckman, P. (1984). Teaching skills inventory: A measure of parent performance. *Journal of the Division for Early Childhood, 8,* 107–114.

Schell, G. C. (1981). The young handicapped child: A family perspective. *Topics in Early Childhood Special Education, 1,* 21–27.

Seligman, M. (1983). Sources of psychological disturbances among siblings of handicapped children. *The Personnel and Guidance Journal, 61,* 529–531.

Silber, S. (1989). Family influences on early development. *Topics in Early Childhood Special Education, 4,* 1–23.

Solnit, A. J., & Stark, M. H. (1961). Mourning the birth of a defective child. *Psychoanalytic Study of the Child, 16,* 523–537.

Stack, C. (1974). *All our kin: Strategies for survival in a Black community.* New York: Harper & Row.

Stoneman, Z., & Brody, G. H. (1982). Strengths inherent in sibling interactions involving a retarded child: A functional role theory approach. In N. Stinnett, B. Chesser, J. DeFrain, & P. Knaub (Eds.), *Family strengths: Positive models for family life.* Lincoln: University of Nebraska.

Thomas, A., & Chess, S. (1977). *Temperament and development.* New York: Brunner/Mazel.

Tomm, K. (1987). Interventive interviewing. Part II. Reflexive questioning as a means to enable self-healing. *Family Process, 26,* 167–184.

Trivette, C., Deal, A., & Dunst, C. (1986). Family needs, sources of support, and professional roles: Critical elements of family systems assessment and intervention. *Diagnostique, 11,* 246–267.

Turnbull, A. P., & Turnbull, H. R. (1990). *Families, professionals, and exceptionality: A special partnership.* Columbus, OH: Merrill.

Vadasy, P., Fewell, R., Meyer, D., Schell, G., & Greenberg, M. (1984). Involved parents: Characteristics and resources of fathers and mothers of young handicapped children. *Journal of the Division for Early Childhood, 9,* 13–25.

Verderber, R. F. (1981). *Communicate*. Belmont, CA: Wadsworth.

Vincent, L. J. (1985). Family relationships. In *Equals in this partnership: Parents of disabled and at-risk infants and toddlers speak to professionals* (pp. 34–41). Washington, DC: National Center for Clinical Infant Programs.

Waisbren, S. (1980). Parents' reactions after the birth of a developmentally disabled child. *American Journal of Mental Deficiency, 84,* 345–351.

Wasserman, R. (1983). Identifying the counseling needs of the siblings of mentally retarded children. *The Personnel and Guidance Journal, 61,* 622–627.

Westby, C. E. (in press). Cultural differences in caregiver-child interaction: Implications for assessment and intervention. In L. Cole and V. Deal (Eds.) *Communication disorders in multicultural populations*. Rockville, MD: American Speech-Language-Hearing Association.

Winton, P. J. (1988). Effective communication between parents and professionals. In D. B. Bailey & R. J. Simeonsson (Eds.), *Family assessment in early intervention* (pp. 207–228). Columbus, OH: Merrill.

Winton, P. J., & Bailey, D. B. (1988). The family-focused interview: A collaborative mechanism for family assessment and goal-setting. *Journal of Division for Early Childhood, 12,* 195–207.

13

The Individualized Family Service Plan Process

Sharon A. Raver

_____ **OVERVIEW** _____

This chapter discusses how to write Individualized Family Service Plans (IFSPs) and issues relating to successful implementation and evaluation of plans, including:

- □ principles underlying the IFSP process
- □ issues relating to IFSP development
- □ major components of the IFSP
- □ interagency collaboration

One of the most discussed components of P.L. 99–457, Part H, is the IFSP. Prior to passage of this law, most infant programs approached the development of service plans from the IEP model; Individualized Educational Programs (IEP) written for preschool through school-aged children. Although some of the information included in both plans is similar, their orientations are different. The purpose of the IEP is primarily to specify resources and services directed toward satisfying child-oriented goals. The purpose of the IFSP is to identify and organize formal and informal resources to facilitate *the family's goals* for the children and themselves. The IFSP is designed to accomplish this by building on the family's strengths.

The IFSP reflects a change in the field's conception of teamwork and family involvement as a result of Part H of P.L. 99–457. Early interventionists used to make efforts to involve parents at all costs (McGonigel & Garland, 1988). After parents were involved, however, their roles were often limited to rubber stamping the professionals' recommendations, and attending parent meetings.

The process of the IFSP forces professionals to view intervention from an ecological perspective. Services are conceived as family focused—assisting the family, not just the mother or the parents, and assisting the family in ways the family recommends. The success of family-focused interventions seems to be related to the goodness-of-fit concept (Thomas & Chess, 1977). That is, the better the fit between the characteristics of the child and the family's expectations, the better the outcome. Successful family-focused interventions are also associated with the family's agenda (Johnson, McGonigel, & Kaufmann, 1989). The IFSP outlines the family's priorities for how early intervention will be incorporated into their family life. If family and professional agendas do not coincide, successful family-focused activities are difficult.

PRINCIPLES UNDERLYING THE IFSP PROCESS

Dunst and colleagues (1988) identify eight roles for infant interventionists: empathetic listener, teacher-therapist, consultant, resource, enabler, mobilizer, mediator, and advocate. All of these roles are evident in the way in which IFSPs are written and implemented. The IFSP process is designed to reduce family stress and build family competence by strengthening coping techniques that assist the family in satisfying their own unmet needs.

The sequence of the IFSP process, from identification to service delivery for families of handicapped and at-risk children younger than 3 years of age as outlined in Part H of P.L. 99–457 is presented in Figure 13.1. The sequence is motivated by the goal of establishing a satisfying relationship between caregivers and the child that leads to increased stimulation, attention, and support. The activities of the IFSP process are

- initial contact between the family and early intervention services
- planning of assessments
- child assessment
- identification of family strengths and needs
- development of outcomes to meet child and family needs
- implementation of the IFSP
- formal and informal evaluation of the plan

The IFSP process mirrors how infant intervention is now conceptualized. Johnson, McGonigel, and Kaufmann (1989) identify these principles as guiding the IFSP process:

1. The dependence infants and toddlers have on their families necessitates a family-centered approach to early intervention.
2. States and programs should define *family* to reflect the diversity of family patterns and structures.
3. Respect for and acceptance of the diversity of each family's structure, roles, values, beliefs, and coping styles is a cornerstone of family-centered early intervention.
4. Early intervention systems and strategies must reflect a respect for the racial, ethnic, and cultural diversity of the family.

FIGURE 13–1

A system of identification processes and services for families of handicapped and at-risk children under 3 eligible for early intervention services. (From *Early Childhood Special Education: Birth to Three* [p. 31] by J. B. Jordan, J. J. Gallagher, P. L. Hutinger, & M. B. Karnes [Eds.], 1988, Reston, VA: The Council for Exceptional Children. This material is in the public domain.)

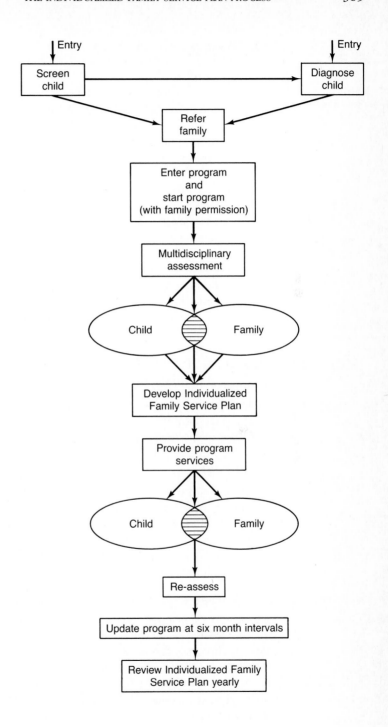

5. Respect for family autonomy and independence means the family must be able to choose the level and nature of early intervention involvement in their life.

6. Family-professional collaboration and partnership are the keys to family-centered early intervention and to successful implementation of the IFSP process.

7. An enabling approach to working with the family requires that professionals re-examine their traditional roles and practices and develop new practices when necessary—practices that promote mutual respect and partnership.

8. Early intervention services should be flexible, accessible, and responsive to family needs.

9. Early intervention services should be provided according to the normalization principle, which means that the family should have access to services in as normal a fashion and environment as possible and that services should promote the integration of the child and family within their community.

10. Because no one agency or discipline can meet the diverse needs of infants and toddlers with special needs and their families, a team approach to assessing, planning, and implementing the IFSP is necessary.

ISSUES RELATING TO IFSP DEVELOPMENT

P.L. 99–457, Part H, requires the redefinition of some practices, and in other cases, the introduction of new service delivery practices. Child Find, family assessment, and case management are issues involved in the IFSP process that will be clarified by each state in the next decade.

Child Find

Child Find is a type of affirmative action campaign designed to aggressively search for eligible handicapped children and to provide services to those children. Part H of P.L. 99–457 states that a comprehensive Child Find system include a process for referrals to service providers. According to Garwood and Sheehan (1989), the authors of P.L. 99–457 did not necessarily envision the development of new programs, but believed that existing systems must be modified or expanded to reach appropriate children.

Child Find responsibilities are shared by hospitals, parents, child care programs, pediatricians and other physicians, diagnostic clinics, and other professionals who may not work directly with infants and toddlers but make referrals to services (Smith, 1988a). The exact nature of Child Find activities varies from state to state. Generally, high-risk children such as medically fragile and/or premature children are tracked or monitored by states to ensure appropriate health and developmental services are referred when needed. Child Find activities often involve offering free screenings in shopping malls and child care centers. Common screening instruments used in early intervention, with ordering information, age range, and areas screened are presented in Table 13.1.

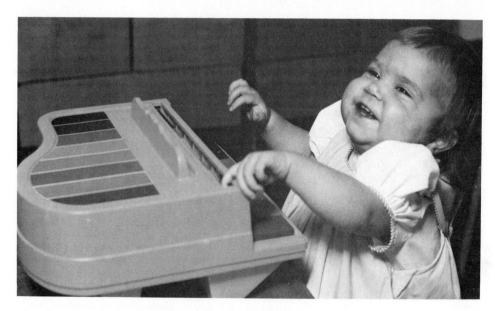

Respect for and acceptance of the diversity of each family's structure, roles, values, beliefs, and coping styles are the cornerstones of family-centered early intervention.

Family Assessment

Part H of P.L. 99–457 does *not* mandate an assessment of the family. The law states only that information about family strengths and needs that relates to its ability to enhance the child's development be gathered. As a rule, this includes information needed to identify the family's strengths, resources, needs, and concerns. The premise behind this approach is that with the right kind of resources, *every* family can support the development of a child with special needs, and services should assist, not supplant, the family (Smith, 1988a). This type of assessment is not designed to give professionals permission to further intrude into the family's life. In fact, the family decides what is relevant for each of these areas. Because of the potentially sensitive nature of family assessment, Johnson and colleagues (1989) suggest that family assessment occur *after* the child has been assessed. In this way, if the child does not require services, the family does not have to be assessed.

In the past, assessment for service plans centered on evaluating the child's needs. Now assessment considers the needs of the child as well as the child-family unit. For instance, if the child needs adaptive equipment but the family cannot afford it, obtaining the equipment is a family goal that is necessary for desired changes in the child. Because family assessment addresses potentially sensitive issues, they must be handled in a highly professional manner. The only reason to assess family functions is to better instill in the family a sense of competence about their ability to nurture and facilitate their child's development.

TABLE 13–1
Screening instruments for early intervention.

Instrument Name	Ordering Information	Age Range	Area(s) Screened
Basic Developmental Screening 0–4	Blackwell Mosby Books 11830 Westline Dr. St. Louis, MO 63141	Birth–4 yrs	All
Communicative Evaluation Chart	Educators Publishing Svc. 75 Maulton St. Cambridge, MA 01238	Birth–5 yrs	Language
Comprehensive Early Education Profile (CEEP)	Comprehensive Early Education Program 1720 7th Ave. S. Birmingham, AL 35294	Birth–7 yrs	All
Comprehensive Identification Process (CIP)	Scholastic Testing Svc. 480 Meyer Rd. Bensenville, IL 60106	2.5–5.5 yrs	All
Denver Developmental Screening Test (DDST)	LADOCA E. 51st & Lincoln St. Denver, CO 80216	Birth–6 yrs	All
Denver Prescreening Developmental Questionnaire	LADOCA E. 51st & Lincoln St. Denver, CO 80216	Birth–6 yrs	All
Developmental Activities Screening Inventory Revised (DASI-R)	DLM/Teaching Resources Corporation 50 Pond Park Rd. Hingman, MA 02043	6–60 mos	Cognitive Fine motor
Developmental Assessment Schema	Special Education Infant/Preschool Prog. Minneapolis Public Schools Minneapolis, MN	Birth–5 yrs	All
Developmental Indicators for the Assessment of Learning (DIAL-R)	Childcraft 20 Kilmer Rd. Edison, NJ 08817	2–6 yrs	All

Family functioning is assessed on three dimensions (Bailey et al., 1986). First, certain child variables are related to family functioning. For example, family stress tends to increase as a function of a child's diagnosis, responsiveness, temperament, and caregiving demands. Second, the family's need for support, information, or training influences how the family functions. And third, parent-child interactions affect how the family operates. Family functioning may be assessed with formally administered instruments, self-report scales, or naturalistic assessments (Odom & Schuster, 1986). Table 13–2 lists parent/family assessment instruments by tool, ordering infor-

TABLE 13–1
(continued)

Instrument Name	Ordering Information	Age Range	Area(s) Screened
Developmental Profile	Psychological Developmental Publications Indianapolis, IN	6 mos– 12 yrs	All
Developmental Screening Inventory 1980 (Revised)	Gesell Developmental Test Materials, Inc. P.O. Box 272391 Houston, TX 77277–2391	4 wks– 36 mos	All
EMI Assessment Scale	EMI Dept. of Pediatrics UVA Medical Center Box 232 Charlottesville, VA 22098	Birth–24 mos	All
Infant Monitoring Questionnaire	Center on Human Development University of Oregon 901 E. 18th Ave. Eugene, OR 97403	4–24 mos	All
McCarthy Scales	Psychological Corporation 304 E. 45th St. New York, NY 10017	2.5–8.5 yrs	All
Milani-Comparetti Motor Development Screening Test	Meyer Children's Rehab. University of Nebraska Medical Center Omaha, NE 68131	Birth–2 yrs	Neuromotor
Minnesota Child Development Inventory	Behavior Science Systems Box 1108 Minneapolis, MN 55440	1–6 yrs	All
Preschool Inventory	Addison-Wesley Reading, MA	2–6.5 yrs	Cognitive
Screening for Motor Delay	Children's Hospital 2924 Brook Rd. Richmond, VA 23220	Birth–6 mos	Motor

mation, age range, and areas evaluated. Readers are also referred to Bailey and Simeonsson (1988) and Johnson, McGonigel, and Kaufmann (1989) for detailed discussions of tools and family assessment issues.

Family resources and strengths. **Family strengths** are individual or family resources that can be used in the intervention process with the family's child. Part H of P.L. 99–457 only indicates an assessment of family strengths. Family strengths and resources tend to be related to the family's personal coping systems. Strengths in

TABLE 13–2
Parent/family assessment instruments.

Tool	Ordering Information	Areas Evaluated
FACES II and Family Satisfaction Scale	Family Stress & Coping Project Dept. of Family Social Science Univ. of Minnesota St. Paul, MN 58108	Family cohesion Family adaptability
Home Observation for Measurement of the Environment (HOME)	Robert H. Bradley Center for Child Development and Education University of AR at Little Rock 33rd & University Ave. Little Rock, AR 72204	Child's environment
Needs Assessment Inventory	Family-Centered Resource Project Antietam Valley Center Reading, PA 19606	Family needs
Parent Attitude Assessment	ECE-SMH Center Dept. of Special Education Arizona State University Tempe, AZ 85281	Parent(s) attitudes toward services, staff, their child, themselves, and their parenting abilities
Parent Behavior Profile	The ME TOO Program 655 Washington St. Fairfield, CA 94533	Parent(s) behavior toward their handicapped child
Parent Behavior Progression	Center for Research Development and Services Dept. of Educational Psychology California State University Northridge, CA 91330	Parenting behavior

families tend to fall into three resource categories (Bailey & Simeonsson, 1988). **Personal resources** are characteristics that give meaning to life and allow individuals to address problems constructively. Resources might be personality types; a strong sense of control over life; and religious, cultural, or philosophical beliefs. **Within-family resources** are drawn from the nuclear or extended family members. These resources might be help with child care or housekeeping, and family members who are good listeners and can provide emotional support. **Extra-family resources** are resources that come from outside the family and extended family, such as support from neighbors, church, professionals, and friends. Generally, the more access to these resources the family has, the wider an array of coping mechanisms the family has to assist them through difficulties.

Family strengths were included in the IFSP process to ensure that the family, as well as service providers, focus on the family's strengths, not merely their needs. At times, strengths may be difficult to quantify or articulate in the IFSP. As one father

TABLE 13–2
(continued)

Tool	Ordering Information	Areas Evaluated
Parent Questionnaire Preschool Handicapped Program	Preschool Program Director Board of Cooperative Educational Services Yorktown Heights, NY 10598	Parent(s) involvement in program; attitude toward services; perception of change in child; program strengths and weaknesses
Parent Scales	Project RHISE Outreach Children's Development Center 650 N. Main St. Rockford, IL 61103	Parent(s) attitudes and feelings
Parenting Stress Index	Pediatric Psychology Press 2915 Idlewood Dr. Charlottesville, VA 22091	Identifies parent/child systems under stress
The Professional Assessment of Parent Needs and Progress	Project RHISE Outreach Children's Development Center 650 N. Main St. Rockford, IL 61103	Parent(s) needs
Readiness Levels of Parents	Project RHISE Outreach Children's Development Center 650 N. Main St. Rockford, IL 61103	Parenting skills and abilities, primarily in relationship to educational environment

states, "When I was asked what our strengths as a family were, I had to pause and think. I could only think of stupid things like we have fun together and we argue a lot. My wife is calm and I'm not. We balance each other out. We make sure the other is out of the bed in the morning. And our other kids are a great help in keeping us from going crazy."

The lack of appropriate instruments, the lack of appropriate training, and institutional and family resistance can serve as barriers to family assessment (Bailey & Simeonsson, 1988). Yet the best way to find out how a family would like to identify their strengths and needs is to ask them (Johnson et al., 1989). The way questions are asked can greatly enhance or hinder communication. Interventionists must explain fully why they ask certain questions and remain sensitive to parents' reactions as questions are asked and answered (Shelton, Jeppson, & Johnson, 1987). The family's cultural background may also affect how, or if, questions are asked directly.

Interventionists cannot be too careful when they deal with the complex, and at times, fragile family system. Unless specifically trained, it is inappropriate for interventionists to act as counselors to families in the areas of marital relationships, family conflict, and family stress. In general, substantial needs in these areas warrant a referral to specialized services.

Family needs.   The term **family needs** is not clarified by Part H of P.L. 99–457, but in general, it refers to the process of identifying concerns, desires, or areas needing development in family members so that they may more fully participate in the intervention activities of their child. Needs refer to such things as information about the child's condition, knowledge about typical child development, time away from the child (respite care), job training, or perhaps information about child care facilities. Any of these needs may influence the success of intervention with children at risk or who have disabilities (Garwood & Sheehan, 1989).

Families are often capable of identifying their own coping strategies and unmet needs. An assumption of family-focused intervention is that both the family's and the interventionist's perceptions are valid sources of information to assess family needs. Therefore, assessment of needs often includes self-report and self-ratings by parents in addition to ratings by interventionists when necessary or appropriate (Bailey et al., 1986). And as with information about the family's strengths, one of the best ways to get information about the family's needs is to ask them in a family-focused interview (Winton & Bailey, 1988). The use of open-ended questions, such as "What are your greatest problems as a family?" in which parents either write or verbally indicate pressing concerns for their family is usually less threatening.

Parents and professionals collaborate to identify the family's needs and generate potential outcomes. This process inevitably involves value-loaded decision making (Kaiser & Hemmeter, 1989). Nonetheless, as much as possible, professionals have a responsibility in family-centered intervention to follow the family's value system, if it does not place the child in jeopardy. Interventionists must keep in mind that P.L. 99–457, Part H does *not* state that all the family's needs must be met. In fact, such a goal is far beyond the scope of most early intervention programs.

Formal tools such as the Family Needs Survey (Bailey & Simeonsson, 1985) assist in identifying general areas of concern for families. All items of this self-rating survey begin with "I need...," or "Our family needs..." to encourage personal responses. To allow for the diversity of families, many programs choose self-report family needs assessments so the IFSPs more accurately reflect family goals. Ideally, the needs assessment process should function as a learning process, assisting everyone involved to have a better understanding of the other's perspectives. Frequently, family needs are related to critical times and events, parent-child interactions, and community access.

Critical times and events. Critical events influence the type of needs the family may have at particular times. Nondevelopmental events, such as the birth of another child, program transitions, and critical illnesses, can affect what the family needs. As the time approaches for children's major developmental achievements such as walking, talking, and self-feeding—and the family recognizes the child cannot perform these tasks, disappointments arise that call for additional coping skills from the family.

Three specific periods bring about increased stress for families with handicapped young children:

☐ the initial diagnosis of the handicapping condition
☐ the first efforts at seeking help or intervention
☐ the transition from infant to preschool programs (Bernheimer, Young, & Winton, 1983).

Professionals are aware that such critical events and times create greater needs and increased vulnerability in the family, so support must be adjusted accordingly. Instruments, such as Hanline's (1988) self-report needs checklist for families enrolling their toddlers in preschool programs, allow interventionists to better support families and their children during critical times in the family's life.

Parent-child interactions. The IFSP demonstrates the transition in infant intervention from an infant-centered model to a transactional model that focuses on the child as well as the broader context of the parent-child relationship. Studies comparing mother-child interactional patterns in normal and atypical families suggest that mothers of at-risk and developmentally delayed children as a group need extra support. Early strains on parent-child relationships (such as health concerns and an unexpected diagnosis) can have long-term consequences.

Information gained from parent-child assessments is used to foster positive interactions between parents and their infants by helping parents become more sensitive to their infant's communication system. Parent-child interactions may be evaluated using behavioral observation systems (molar rating, molecular coding) and interaction assessment systems (molar rating scales, molecular coding systems, checklists) (Rosenberg, Robinson, & Beckman, 1986). **Molar** units are broad classes of behaviors such as responsivity or directiveness. **Molecular** categories are narrow behavioral events such as smiles, hugs, or vocalizations. The type of instrument used depends on the type of information desired.

Access to the community. Being a part of the community is a valued goal for individuals with disabilities, even young children. Often the child with disabilities is restricted to specialized settings such as clinics, hospitals, special classes, and therapy centers. Social experiences may be restricted to relatives, therapists, and other children with special needs. The broader community offers other opportunities for the child and family to learn. However, access to the community may be limited by physical inaccessibility, lack of appropriate adaptive equipment, and parental reluctance. As one father stated, "Everyone stares at us and I find I want to leave every place we go as soon as we get there. The bigger Jason gets, the harder it is. He acts like a baby but he looks even older than he is. I'm not ashamed exactly, but I can't relax."

The discomfort this parent reports is not uncommon. Some families need support to minimize the stress attached to outings in order to more fully participate in their community. Calhoun, Rose, and Armstrong (1989) suggest families use these strategies to broaden their community involvement

☐ take a support person along on first outings
☐ investigate possible architectural barriers ahead of time

□ start slowly
□ brainstorm solutions with other families
□ share successes with other families

After the family's needs are assessed by the transdisciplinary team, the next step is to translate those needs into goals for the IFSP. Negotiation between team members and the family is required to do this successfully. By encouraging the family to select the direction of their IFSP, professionals acknowledge that a person's perception of what is the most important need at a particular time is most likely to dominate that person's energy. Interventionists must be careful about the way in which family goals are written on IFSPs. For example, McGonigel and Garland (1988) caution against using family goals to increase family compliance with program policies and procedures. An example of that is: "When the home visitor arrives at the home, Mrs. Smith will be up and dressed and will have Travis dressed and fed at least 90% of the time" (p. 10). Although this goal focuses on the mother rather than the child, it does not capture the purpose of family goals. A more appropriate goal might be: "Mrs. Smith would like to continue home visits and would like them changed to late afternoons

Child and family strengths are included in the IFSP process to ensure that the family and service providers focus on strengths, not merely needs.

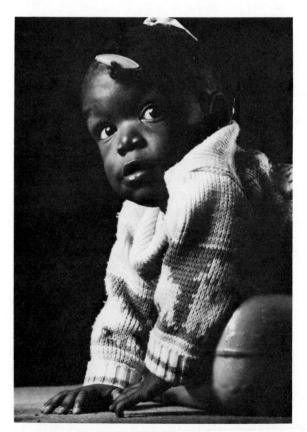

if possible by June 1." Table 13–3 lists common family-needs assessment and parent-infant interaction tools with author and addresses to write for information.

Case Management

The case manager confirms that services are offered at a time and location suitable for the family, avoid scheduling conflicts, and eliminate wasteful or duplicative efforts (Itagliata, 1982). The case manager serves as family advocate by ensuring that collaboration in assessment and intervention processes occurs.

The case manager needs a thorough awareness of available services and means of securing those services for families. This individual needs to be skilled in bargaining, negotiating, and mediating. Case managers need the ability and willingness to share skills and information and learn from team members. The case manager should increase the family's confidence in its own abilities, and contribute skills, encouragement, support, and feedback (Garland, Woodruff, & Buck, 1988). Part H of P.L. 99–457 states that the case manager must be from the profession most closely associated with the infant's or toddler's developmental needs.

Ideally, case managers are assigned early in the early intervention process, preferably at intake. The size of a caseload is designated by each state. Case management responsibilities can be transferred from one staff member or agency to another as the child's or family's needs change. For instance, if a child is language delayed and later motor delay becomes the critical developmental issue, it may be useful in this case to switch case managers. Or if a child's health care necessitates, it may be possible, with the request of parents, to provide co-case management. A child with severe respiratory disorder, for example, may be handled by an infant program and a pediatric pulmonary center in a hospital. The hospital staff may handle the family's medical management issues and the infant program may deal with other developmental needs and transitions to community programs.

As mentioned in Chapter 9, Dunst, Trivette, and Deal (1988) suggest an enabling model of case management based on promoting family competence and using family empowerment as the major desired outcome of case management practices. They define **empowerment** as family identification and recognition of needs and the process of acquiring resources in a way that increases self-sufficiency, self-esteem, and the family's sense of control over life events. They state that "enabling case managers" do not mobilize resources for families, but rather promote the behavior needed by families to actively seek their own resources.

The original intent of case management was to use the early intervention system to help parents take charge of the issues that affect them and their child, thus ensuring that parental empowerment is seen as a primary function of case management services (Garwood & Sheehan, 1989). Professionals must make whatever special efforts are required so that case management practices do not cause additional burden or strain on the families. When appropriate, it may be necessary for professionals to seek training in case management skills so that interactions with families and professionals from other disciplines and agencies are facilitated.

TABLE 13–3
Family needs assessment and parent-infant interaction instruments.

Instrument/Author	Address
Self-rated	
The Coping Inventory Shirley Zeitlin	Scholastic Testing Service, Inc. 480 Meyer Rd. P.O. Box 1056 Bensenville, IL 60106–8056
Family Resource Scale Hope E. Leet and Carl J. Dunst.	Family, Infant & Preschool Program Western Carolina Center Morganton, NC 28655
Mother's Perceptions of Their Needs and Resources Lisbeth J. Vincent and Sherry Laten	Lisbeth J. Vincent University of Wisconsin 432 N. Murray Madison, WI 53706
The Nisonger Questionnaire for Parents William Loadman, F. Arthur Benson, and Douglas McElwain	Nisonger Center Ohio State University Publications Department McCampbell Hall 1581 Dodd Dr. Columbus, OH 43219
Parent Appraisal of Needs Wendy Numata	Preschool Training Coordinator Educational Service District 101 1025 Indiana Ave. Spokane, WA 99205
Parent Stress Index (PSI) R. R. Abidin	Pediatric Psychology Press 320 W. Terrell Rd. Charlottesville, VA 22901
Family Needs Survey Don Bailey and Rune Simeonsson	FAMILIES Project Frank Porter Graham Child Development Center 301 NCNB Plaza, Room 322–A Chapel Hill, NC 27514

The outcomes of case management are difficult to measure. However, Smith (1988a) suggests these questions for evaluating the accountability of case management:

1. Are all possible resources being considered to meet the needs of the infant and family as specified in the IFSP?
2. Has there been duplication of referral efforts or services; or have agencies been working at cross purposes?
3. Have family members and service providers been aware of who was doing what, where, when, and why?
4. Has the family been satisfied with the way in which its needs were met? Was family participation encouraged?

TABLE 13–3
(continued)

Instrument/Author	Address
Staff-rated	
Needs Assessment Inventory Gilbert Foley, Luzviminda Parco, and Thomas Evaul	Family-Centered Resource Project Albright College P.O. Box 15234 Reading, PA 19606
Parent Behavior Profile Esther Anderson and Sharon Jobson	The ME TOO Program 655 Washington St. Fairfield, CA 94533
Parent/Family Involvement Index John D. Cone, David DeLawyer, and Vicky Wolfe	The West Virginia System 311 Oglebay Hall West Virginia University Morgantwon, WV 26506–6040
Readiness Levels of Parents Dick Rundall	Project RHISE Outreach Children's Development Center 650 N. Main St. Rockford, IL 61103
Parent-infant interaction instruments	
Home Observation for Measurement of the Environment (HOME) Bettye Caldwell and Robert Bradley	Robert H. Bradley Center for Child Development and Education University of Arkansas at Little Rock 2801 S. University Ave. Little Rock, AR 72204
Parent/Caregiver Involvement Scale (PCIS) D. C. Kasari, M. Comfort, and S. Jay	Center for Development of Early Education Kamehameha Schools Kapalama Heights Honolulu, HI 96817

Under Part H of P.L. 99–457, the family is provided due process and an appeal process for resolving conflicts. It is very important that case management practices do not cause additional burdens or strains on the families they were designed to serve (Johnson, McGonigel, & Kaufmann, 1989).

WRITING IFSPs

Some states provide general guidelines to ensure that all necessary components of the IFSP are met; others provide preprinted forms. Some may use computer technology to formulate IFSP goals and objectives (Hochman et al., 1987). Each state determines the specific guidelines and style of its IFSP. Section 677 of P.L. 99–457

TABLE 13–4
How the infant intervention process has changed as a result of P.L. 99–457.

Infant Intervention Process	
Prior to P.L. 99–457	**With P.L. 99–457**
1. Each staff plans his/her own assessment by developmental area.	1. Planning the assessment: ☐ The facilitator asks the parents for priorities/questions they wish to have addressed. ☐ The facilitator then shares this with other team members who help plan a comprehensive assessment that focuses on issues raised by parents.
2. Each staff conducts his/her own assessments, if possible at a time when a parent can be present so that each assessment can be discussed with the parent. This usually means 3 to 5 assessment sessions.	2. An assessment is scheduled when parents can be present. Only the facilitator and parent interact with the child; other staff on the team observe and record.
3. Each staff summarizes his/her assessment findings and recommends goals and treatment settings at a meeting of staff. These staff recommendations are shared with parents at the planning conference.	3. Immediately after the assessment, the parents share what they have seen during the assessment—the child's strengths, interests, motivators, problems, and frustrations. Staff supplement these observations as needed to produce a complete description of the child.
4. Parents are asked if they agree with the recommended goals or have other goals. Staff share their recommended setting(s).	4. Next, parents draw conclusions or state what seems most important to them regarding the child and define major goals. Again, staff supplement as needed.
5. To carry out the goals, a primary service setting is chosen by the team. (Generally either home or center.)	5. To carry out the goals, strategies are created that draw upon adults and other children the child encounters throughout the day. Contact with non-delayed peers is a priority.

requires that the IFSP be developed promptly following assessment. The authors of the law believed that infant development is relatively rapid, so administrative concerns should not delay the initiation of services (Garwood & Sheehan, 1989). Consequently, with parental permission, services may begin before the IFSP process is completed.

The plan must be evaluated once a year, and reviewed with the family at 6-month intervals or more frequently as appropriate. Each state determines if changes can be included without requiring the development of a new IFSP and for what period of time the goals should be written. Interventionists needing specific guidelines are referred to Johnson, McGonigel and Kaufmann (1989).

Each component of an IFSP has specific information for the family and service providers relating to services and expected outcomes so all those involved are clear on how the family will be served. A summary of how the infant intervention process

TABLE 13–4
(continued)

Infant Intervention Process

Prior to P.L. 99–457	With P.L. 99–457
6. Each staff provides direct service or consults in his/her area of development as needed and plans the center-based services. Parents reinforce goals in activities at home.	6. The facilitator consults with family and community resources to carry out the plan and provides direct service only when it cannot be accomplished through consultation. The other staff remain accountable for their area of expertise through active consultation with the facilitator.
7. The IFSP is reviewed and revised semiannually; reassessment occurs annually.	7. The IFSP is reviewed and revised monthly; reassessment and planning occur every 4 to 6 months.
8. Success is measured by: ☐ child progress	8. Success is measured by: ☐ child progress ☐ parent satisfaction ☐ integrated versus segregated service settings and contact with non-delayed peers ☐ parents' gains in knowledge, skill and confidence in describing their child, setting goals, carrying out strategies, and getting others to carry out strategies

Source: Adapted from *Early Intervention Tailor Made* (pp. D1–D2) by L. Kjerland, 1986, Eagan, MN: Project Dakota Outreach. Copyright © 1986 by L. Kjerland, Project Dakota Outreach. Adapted and reprinted by permission.

has changed largely as a result of P.L. 99–457 is presented in Table 13–4. A discussion of each major component of the IFSP, as shown in the sample IFSP in Figure 13–2 follows.

Statement of Developmental Levels

This is the part of the service plan in which developmental, health, and medical information is listed and summarized as child strengths and needs. The instruments used to assess the child's functioning level for this section are determined by the family's priorities and information needs, the characteristics of the child and diagnostic concerns, and the professional judgement of team members. In some cases, child assessments may be conducted at child diagnostic clinics when appropriate and available, especially the initial assessment. Child diagnostic clinics tend to use a multidisciplinary or transdisciplinary model, with the family interacting with a number of professionals. A medical evaluation may be also needed. (However, even with current technologies, physicians are still unable to make a specific diagnosis on at least 50% of children with significant developmental delays.)

Interventionists are wise to use families as a resource to determine the level of the child's functioning. One way to facilitate this is to invite family input first in team

Individualized Family Service Plan (IFSP)

Child's Name: _____Jesse Webster_____

Birthdate: _____10/5/87_____ **Age** _____18 months_____

Developmental Levels:

_10–14_ months Fine motor   _5–9_ months Gross motor

_8–16_ months Cognitive   _6–12_ months Language

_10–12_ months Self-help   _8–14_ months Social-emotional

Health and Medical Information:

Other Information:

FIGURE 13–2
Individualized Family Service Plan (IFSP) (pp. 380–389).

Child's Name: _____ J.W.

Child Strengths and Needs:

Jesse's developmental strengths are his social, cognitive, and fine motor skills. Jesse is very pleasant and outgoing. He enjoys, and actively seeks, adult and child attention. He vocalizes frequently and is playing independently for longer periods of time. He is healthy, but a prolonged ear infection this winter has the family concerned about his hearing. Jesse is beginning to crawl, and is reluctant to stand, even with support.

FIGURE 13–2
(continued)

Child's Name: _____J.W._____

Family Strengths and Needs:

The Websters continue to be very involved in the area Down Syndrome support group and the infant program support group. Michael was elected secretary of the Down Syndrome group this year. The parents report they are enjoying Jesse more now that he is getting older and is more responsive. They indicated they are pleased with the home visits they receive. Jenny indicates that although financial burdens are created by her working only part-time, both she and Michael believe the benefits for Jesse and their family make it worthwhile. Jenny's parents now pay for Walton's (Jenny's older son) tennis lessons. Jenny states this makes her feel that now Walton does not have to make unfair sacrifices because of Jesse. Both parents continue to praise the support they receive from Walton in their care of Jesse.

Both parents indicate that they continue to be concerned about Jesse's future, what they might be able to expect from him, and what services might be available. Jenny said she continues to have feelings of guilt about her age possibly being a contributing factor to Jesse's condition. She requested help finding short-term counseling to "work it out."

Gross motor development continues to be an area of need for Jesse, so the family asked that physical therapy be increased. Because of a serious ear infection last winter, the parents requested a hearing assessment for Jesse.

FIGURE 13–2
(continued)

Child's Name: _____J.W._____

Outcomes:

1. The Websters want more information about future services for Jesse, particularly when he is a young adult.

2. Jenny Webster wants more written information about Down Syndrome and wants to participate in personal counseling to discuss her adjustment to Jesse's handicapping condition.

3. The Websters want more physical therapy for Jesse.

4. The Websters want a hearing assessment conducted.

FIGURE 13–2
(continued)

Child's Name: _____ J.W. _____

Outcome: #1

The Websters want more information about future services for Jesse, particularly when he is a young adult.

Strategies/Activities:

1. The Websters will meet with representatives of the area Association for Retarded Citizens (ARC) to discuss and visit supported employment sites and adult homes in the community. Michael Webster will set this up.

2. The Websters will get information about waiting lists for these services.

3. The Websters will meet some workers with Down Syndrome at the local sheltered workshop to try to get more understanding of the quality of their lives.

4. The Websters will visit the public schools to observe their programs.

Criteria/Timelines:

The Websters will make these visits by September. If more information is needed, the Websters will call their case manager.

FIGURE 13–2
(continued)

Outcome: #2

Jenny Webster wants more written information about Down Syndrome and wants to participate in personal counseling to discuss her adjustment to Jesse's handicapping condition.

Strategies/Activities:

1. Marie (the case manager) will give Jenny a list of counselors and counseling centers by June 15th.

2. Marie will give Jenny information about financial assistance for counseling services by June 15th.

3. By September, Jenny will ask the Down Syndrome support group to have a counselor as a speaker at one of their meetings to discuss family adjustments.

4. Jenny will discuss her feelings and concerns with her family, and her neighbor, Mrs. Brooke, in the next two weeks.

5. Marie will loan Jenny a book and some pamphlets on Down Syndrome by June 15.

Criteria/Timelines:

The timelines are listed next to each activity. Jenny will reevaluate the need for counseling in 6 months.

FIGURE 13–2
(continued)

Child's Name: _____ J.W. _____

Outcome: #3

The Websters want more physical therapy for Jesse.

Strategies/Activities:

1. Marie (case manager) will arrange for another physical therapy evaluation for Jesse to occur by July 1st.

2. The physical therapist will be asked to determine if additional physical therapy time is appropriate for Jesse at this time, and if enrollment in the physical therapy play group is appropriate. The evaluation with recommendations is due August 1st.

3. The physical therapist will give more activities for Bella (home visitor) to share with the Websters. Walton (older brother) will be at the next home visit so he can learn the procedures from Bella too.

4. The once-a-week home visits will continue focusing on Jesse's total development.

Criteria/Timelines:

Timeline for the physical therapy evaluation and recommendation is indicated. Additional physical therapy home activities will be provided at the next home visit, May 15.

FIGURE 13–2
(continued)

Outcome: #4

The Websters want a hearing assessment conducted.

Strategies/Activities:

1. Marie (case manager) will call the Websters' pediatrician to get more information about Jesse's hearing infection and treatment within the next 2 weeks.

2. Marie will notify the Websters after she has spoken to the pediatrician, and let them know if a hearing assessment is warranted. If one is appropriate, Marie will arrange for the Child Diagnostic Clinic to contact the Websters with their earliest appointment in August, as the family has requested.

3. The Websters will continue to monitor Jesse's hearing reactions and notify Bella if new infections develop.

Criteria/Timelines:

Timelines are indicated next to strategies/activities.

FIGURE 13–2
(continued)

Child's Name: _____ J.W. _____

Notes on the IFSP Process:

The Websters are articulate, friendly people who are comfortable discussing, in detail, their family's concerns. They are able to identify the types of support they want, and are good at seeking social and professional support when needed. Although Jenny Webster said a goal was not appropriate for the family at this time, she was concerned that Michael may be overworking, and trying to be a "superparent."

FIGURE 13–2
(continued)

388

Child's Name: Jesse Webster   **Birthdate:** 10/5/87

Address: Urban City, USA

Phone: 431-0051

Service Coordinator (Case Manager): Marie Brown, M.S.W.

IFSP Team Members and Signatures:

Jenny & Michael Webster, parents _Jenny & Michael Webster_

Harriet Cole, grandmother _Harriet Cole_

Bella Green, Speech Pathologist _Bella Green_

Margo Young, L.P.T. _Margo Young_

Marie Eldridge, M.A. _Marie Eldridge_

Jon Frontlin, B.A. _Jon Frontlin_

Frequency, Intensity, and Duration of Services:

Services will begin immediately and continue until the September after Jesse's third birthday when he is eligible for public school preschool. Frequency and intensity will vary; see individual outcomes.

IFSP Review Dates: 12/15/87   Intake   6/20/88

                        1/10/89   4/3/89

Transition Plan: ___X___ **Not Applicable** _____ **Yes, (see outcomes)**

Parent Signature(s):

This plan represents our wishes. I (we) understand and agree with it, and I (we) authorize Urban Infant Services to carry out this plan with me (us).

Michael Webster _Jenny Webster_   4-3-89

Parent(s)   Date

FIGURE 13–2

(continued)

meetings, before professionals give their observations. Another is to use open-ended statements such as "I would describe my child this way . . . ;" "A typical day with my child includes . . . ;" "My child is really interested in . . . ." These offer families opportunities to think and talk about their child's strengths and weaknesses.

It is usually preferred to discuss information with families soon after the child's special needs are suspected or formally identified. Honor family preferences for the amount of information they can absorb in one meeting. ("We have discussed so much today. We can discuss these findings any other time you like.") Interventionists should be prepared to discuss assessment results a number of times, if family members seem to need it and/or if they have difficulty remembering information from previous meetings. The inability or difficulty to recall or retain information is a predictable reaction to stress. As one parent relates: "I probably asked the same three questions of every person I saw that first 6 months. 'What is wrong with my son?' 'Will it go away?' 'Will he ever be able to take care of himself?' I always felt they knew more than they would tell me. I still feel that. I wanted to see if they had the same answers. And of course, they didn't."

Statement of Family Needs and Strengths

A significant challenge of the transdisciplinary team during the IFSP process is to avoid making the family feel that they are being evaluated. Parents are more likely to be supportive of their child's service plan if they are active participants in the development of the IFSP, and if they are satisfied with the process by which it is developed (Cooper & Ward, 1974).

It is not desirable, or necessary, to examine all areas of family functioning. If information does not lead *directly* to more appropriate services for the child and family, there is no reason to collect it. The type of assessment tool(s) used must relate directly to the purpose of the assessment. That is, if team members want knowledge of parental attitudes toward services, they would select a different tool than if they want information about the family's level of stress.

Further, whenever possible, needs and strengths need to be stated in measurable terms. When a family receives an unexpected medical diagnosis, the family might say their goal is to "get used to the new equipment." This goal is difficult to evaluate. However, specific variables involved in "getting used to" can be evaluated. The family's goal might be stated as: "(The family) wants to learn to independently hook up, operate, and maintain (the child's) monitor by the end of August."

Expected Outcomes, Strategies, Activities, and Services

The major expected outcomes for the child and family are stated clearly in the IFSP. The family-focused orientation of selecting objectives may mean that, at times, professionals may need to sacrifice personal beliefs about intervention priorities in favor of collaborative goal setting with the family. If parents do not agree or are not interested in the goals professionals desire, treatment will not be successful. Along the same line, the language of the IFSP should include family preferences as much as possible, and avoid jargon to encourage full participation from the family. Any medical or technical jargon must be translated each time it is used so all members of the team are comfortable and have a shared understanding.

Criteria, Procedures for Evaluation

The goal of evaluation is to determine if services are meeting the needs of the child and family. Again, how specifically criteria and procedures are stated in the IFSP depends on state and local policy. Evaluation of outcomes may be as simple as checking to ensure the existence of mandated components of the IFSP, or as complex as an analysis of treatment programs across an entire early education agency. Garwood & Sheehan (1989) have developed a form to analyze the components of an IFSP. See Appendix D.

All team members should be involved in decisions about evaluation of services before data collection begins. Chaos results when data are collected without thinking of how they will be used or analyzed (Sheehan, 1989). In general, evaluation of program effectiveness includes changes in child functioning, evaluation of expected outcomes, and effects on families and community.

Changes in child functioning. The first step in evaluating changes in the child's developmental level would seem to be to re-administer tools used in the initial or previous assessment. However, few infant assessment tools contain sufficient number of items to be very useful for educational assessment and program planning. The major difficulty in program evaluation stems from the need to demonstrate that advances in child performance are the result of educational services rather than maturation. For example, the Bayley Scales contain only 20 items on the motor scale between the developmental ages of 6 and 12 months. Little information regarding child progress is demonstrated when such an instrument is used (Sheehan, 1989). Nonetheless, the Bayley Scales is the most frequently used instrument for measuring child growth in surveyed infant programs (Karnes & Stayton, 1988).

Rosenberg, Robinson, Finkler, and Rose (1987) thoroughly compare major formulas used to evaluate changes in child functioning. Nevertheless Fewell and Sandall (1986) suggest that the results of intervention may vary depending on the analysis used and consequently, different interpretations of program effectiveness may be made. In some states, arena assessments with criterion-referenced tools may be appropriate for determining changes in child functioning. When child assessment is approached as an evolving and continuous process, rather than a discrete activity with a prescribed beginning and end, program changes and modifications can be made at any point. Clearly, whatever choice is made, evaluation of child functioning must be approached with caution.

Evaluation of outcomes. Programs must devise evaluation strategies that measure actual program work and that provide information for program improvement. Deal, Dunst, and Trivette (in press) suggest a rating scale for evaluating the extent to which an outcome goal has been achieved. The scale ranges from a rating of 1 (situation changed or worsened; no longer a need, goal, or project) to a rating of 7 (outcome completely accomplished or attained to the family's satisfaction).

Effects on family and community.   Before the team can evaluate the effects of a program on the family and community, it is essential that desired changes are clear to everyone involved, and that indicators of those changes can be identified. If the expected changes are in the areas of family cohesion and family adaptability, the FACES II Scale and the Family Satisfaction Scale (Olson et al., 1982) may be particularly useful evaluation tools. As a rule, tests with several subtests generally give a more accurate picture of family progress.

Bear in mind that it was not the goal of P.L. 99–457, Part H, to meet all the family's needs. Emphasis should be directed only to family goals or outcomes that can be changed so that the child's functioning is maximized. Addressing all the needs of any family is beyond the scope of infant intervention.

Some programs for infants and toddlers with disabilities evaluate the quality of parent-child interactions and parent satisfaction as indices of program effectiveness. To ensure parent perceptions of satisfaction, team members can

- □ allow sufficient time for meetings
- □ collect input from a variety of professionals to formulate plans
- □ place blame or dissatisfaction on sources besides the parents
- □ increase parent participation in meetings/staffings (Witt, Miller, McIntyre, & Smith, 1984)

Clearly, evaluation procedures vary; most programs evaluate goals and objectives achieved. Nonetheless, Karnes and Stayton (1988) found that the assessment tools infant programs use are not always consistent with the program's stated philosophical model, and in some programs, assessment instruments are used for purposes other than those for which they were designed (e.g., diagnostic instruments were being used to measure the child's progress).

Service Plan

This section of the IFSP lists the specific services needed to meet the family and child's needs, including a statement of frequency, intensity, and method of delivering these services. This may include home visits, therapies, and/or outside consultations and collaborations. General services such as respite care are also listed.

The transdisciplinary approach applies to the assessment process, the development of the IFSP, and the implementation of the IFSP. Although one team member is designated to carry out the plan with the family (the primary service provider or the case manager), this team member relies on regular consultations with and support from other team members to carry out the IFSP successfully (Woodruff & McGonigel, 1988).

Despite frequent support voiced for the transdisciplinary model, McCollum and Hughes (1988) found the interdisciplinary model (team members share their separate plans with one another and implement their section separately) was the most common team model used at the intervention stage in the programs they surveyed. This may be because programs have misunderstood the differences between team approaches, and because prior to P.L. 99–457 there was limited access to training in the transdisciplinary model. Whatever the team approach, services to families need to be integrated, coordinated, and continuing.

Dates for services. The specific dates for when services begin and end, and dates to conduct evaluations, are listed in this section of the IFSP. As LaCour (1982) indicates, clear delineation of services—especially by agency—greatly facilitates interagency communication, thereby increasing the chances for successful interventions.

Name of Case Manager

The case manager is supposed to be from the profession most immediately relevant to the needs of the child and family. The case manager coordinates services, puts the service plan together, and makes sure all necessary people are involved. In addition, this person monitors the appropriateness and effectiveness of services.

Plan for Transition to Preschool Program

When appropriate, steps are listed for supporting the passage of the child and family from one service option to another. The loss of secure relationships with particular professionals can lead to an emotional crisis for the family, especially in the transition from toddler to preschool program. An established system for smooth transitions, involving all parties, is critical for family well-being.

Coordination of Services

Under Part H of P.L. 99–457, the state's lead agency is responsible for entering into formal agreements with other agencies within a state. Every service listed in the IFSP has costs attached, so agreements are critical. The family's time, schedule, and transportation needs are important considerations in efforts to coordinate service plans. Maintaining a sense of intimacy and support while administrating services can be very difficult, however.

INTERAGENCY COORDINATION

Lead Agencies

For preschool-aged children, the state education agency assumes the responsibility of lead agency. However, according to Part H of P.L. 99–457, states may select the lead agency for children younger than 3 years. The designated lead agency has many responsibilities and duties, including

- □ general administration of programs and activities
- □ identification and coordination of all available resources at federal, state, local and private levels and the assignment of financial responsibility to appropriate state agencies
- □ resolution of state interagency disputes and procedures for ensuring services pending the resolution of disputes

□ organizing formal interagency agreements that define the financial responsibility of each state agency for early intervention services and include procedures for resolving disputes (Smith, 1988b)

Interagency Coordinating Councils

Interagency Coordinating Councils are established to advise and assist lead agencies in their responsibilities, and to promote interagency agreements. The Councils are composed of 15 members, including at least 3 parents of children younger than 6 with disabilities, 3 providers of early intervention services, 1 legislator, and 1 person involved in personnel preparation. One of the tasks of Interagency Coordinating Councils is to resolve interagency disputes. One mechanism to ease interagency costs is the possibility of using Medicaid and other third-party payments to support early intervention services (Smith, 1988a).

No matter how well program procedures and outcomes are written, interagency agreements will affect the quality of services offered families. In 1979 California's failure to provide occupational therapy and physical therapy to handicapped children caused the U.S. Bureau of Education for the Handicapped to cut off millions of dollars in funding (LaCour, 1982). At the same time, the U.S. Department of Health, Education and Welfare published documents explaining the process of developing interagency agreements to assure services for children. Clearly, having a well-written and signed document does not necessarily assure services.

Writing interagency agreements.   Interagency agreements are designed to promote discussion of goals and functions, promote cooperation rather than competition, and encourage rational problem solving to reduce conflicts (LaCour, 1982). Families have diverse needs and resources, so it is highly unlikely that one program can provide all the services a family may need. Three main types of interagency agreements have been identified by Smith (1988a)

□ agreements between state government agencies responsible for administration of the program
□ agreements between the lead agency and the service providers
□ agreements between health service providers and local education agencies, or agreements between health service providers in the community

Elder (1980) identifies a number of elements necessary in formal interagency agreements

□ purpose of the agreement
□ definition of terms
□ program delineation (specific services provided by all agencies)
□ first dollar responsibility (which agency covers which costs)
□ roles and responsibilities of each agency
□ designation of responsible positions (who is responsible in each agency for monitoring or modifying the agreement)
□ administrative procedures (procedures for administering the agreement)

SAMPLE IFSP CASE

THE WEBSTER FAMILY

An update of an IFSP written for the Webster family was presented in Figure 13–2. Michael (28) and Jenny (38) Webster live in an urban city with Jenny's 16-year-old son from a previous marriage, Walton, and the Webster's 18-month-old son, Jesse. They have been married 2 years. Jesse, born with Down Syndrome after a normal pregnancy and delivery, weighed 6 pounds 9 ounces. The day after Jesse's birth, the mother's doctor told the Websters she suspected Down Syndrome. While still in the hospital and waiting for a final diagnosis, the floor nurse, with the family's permission, called a local infant intervention program. The infant program director asked the Smiths, a family with a 10-month-old daughter with Down Syndrome and who shared the same ethnic background as the Websters, to visit the Websters. The Websters agreed to meet the Smiths.

When the Smiths arrived, Jenny said she had changed her mind and did not meet them. Michael, however, talked with the family for nearly an hour. He later told Jenny he felt more optimistic after meeting the Smith's daughter.

Shortly after Jesse's birth, Michael began working overtime at his insurance job so Jenny could change to part-time work to have more time with Jesse. When Jesse was 2 months old, the family followed up on the hospital's referral and enrolled Jesse in the infant program. Since enrollment in the program, the family has received once-a-week home visits from their interventionist, Bella. Bella is trained as a speech therapist and implements an IFSP developed by the transdisciplinary team and the family. The infant program's physical therapist released certain motor planning and strengthening skills for Bella to share with the family. The physical therapist and Bella meet weekly at the infant program to re-train and follow up on the released skills. The Webster's case manager is a social worker from their area's lead agency.

From the beginning, the Websters have been active members of the infant program's family support group and the regional Down Syndrome group. Jesse's older brother, Walton, has also been involved in intervention activities and is very protective of his little brother. Other than two ear infections and one upper respiratory infection, Jesse has been healthy. The IFSP shown in Figure 13–2 is an update IFSP requested by the family and their case manager. During an interview with their case manager, Jenny communicated that she was not happy with her adjustment. She stated that she believed her age was a factor in Jesse's condition and she felt responsible. Neither parent has other handicapping conditions in their families, so Mrs. Webster indicated the need for more information about what to expect for Jesse's future.

☐ evaluation design (procedures to monitor and evaluate outcomes and success of agreement).

Shelton and Sorter (1980) suggest that communication and leadership have a profound influence on effective interagency teamwork. Highlighting mutual benefits often encourages future interagency agreements. Smooth transitions between agencies for families are closely linked to the support networks agencies have established. Support networks are often built upon the communication skills of the professionals involved.

SUMMARY OF PROCEDURES

Infant interventionists must be empathetic listeners, teacher-therapists, consultants, resources, enablers, mobilizers, mediators, and advocates. These roles are reflected in how IFSPs are now written and implemented. A list of some of the key concepts in this chapter follows:

1. In the IFSP process, assess the family's needs and resources as well as the needs and resources of the child.
2. Write and implement intervention programs for the family that are as clearly defined and systematically implemented as the intervention plans for the child.
3. *Actively* seek the family's input on all aspects of the IFSP process by asking their evaluation of the child's strengths and weaknesses, asking them to prioritize their goals for their child and themselves, carefully listening to their responses, giving them time to respond, and genuinely attending to their concerns. To maximize family input, invite families to speak first in team meetings before professionals give their observations.
4. Translate any medical or technical jargon each time it is used so all members of the team are comfortable and understand.
5. Make whatever special efforts are required so that case management practices do not cause an additional burden or strain on the family.
6. When appropriate, seek specialized training in case management skills so interactions with the family and other professionals from different disciplines and agencies are facilitated.
7. Make assessment an evolving and continuous process, rather than a discrete activity with a prescribed beginning and end, so program evaluation data is available for program modifications at any time desired.
8. Accept the fact that it was not the goal of P.L. 99–457, Part H, to meet all the family's needs. Emphasize only family goals that can be changed so that the child's functioning is maximized. Addressing *all* the family's needs is beyond the scope of infant intervention.
9. Use both the family's and professionals' perceptions as valid means of assessing family strengths and needs.
10. Offer supports to the family that are integrated, coordinated, and continuing.

SUMMARY

The quality of collaboration may be the best yardstick for measuring the many small steps involved in the implementation of personalized Individualized Family Service Plans. Collaboration is between disciplines, agencies, professionals, and families. This type of collaboration is time consuming and may be less orderly than the way early intervention has been handled in the past. Nonetheless, most professionals contend that the outcomes of true professional-family collaboration make the challenges of reaching such a lofty objective a worthwhile endeavor.

The family-focused IFSP process not only forces professionals to re-examine their roles but to redefine and re-examine their demands on families, and how those demands are played out within the family system. Turnbull and Summers (1985) stated this well when they reacted to the demands some interventionists have placed on families' time at home: "Anything is possible to those with no responsibility for implementation" (p. 10). Interventionists are advocates for families. Consequently, professionals must encourage families to invest their energies in a reasonable way to avoid burn out. Ideally, the IFSP process should begin a pattern of balanced involvement for families of children who have disabilities.

DISCUSSION QUESTIONS

1. What major procedural and philosophical changes have IFSPs introduced to infant intervention services?
2. What are some of the potential difficulties of the IFSP process?
3. What are the benefits of interagency agreements?

APPLIED ACTIVITIES/PROJECTS

1. You are a case manager for a family with a foster child with cerebral palsy and other developmental delays. Using your local system of infant services, design an IFSP, improvising child and family resources, strengths, and needs.
2. Role play a family-focused intake team meeting. Be sensitive to the nature of your questions and parents' reactions to them.
3. Go on a home visit with an infant interventionist to observe the administration of a verbal, self-report family resource/needs assessment. Observe a transdisciplinary team, with the parents' participation, involved in the process of generating family goals and outcomes from the information gathered.

SUGGESTED READINGS

Bailey, D., & Simeonsson, R. (1988). *Family assessment and early intervention*. Columbus, OH: Merrill.

Garwood, S., & Sheehan, R. (1989). *Designing a comprehensive early intervention system: The challenge of Public Law 99–457*. Austin, TX: PRO-ED.

Johnson, B., McGonigel, M., & Kaufmann, R. (Eds.), (1989). *Guidelines and recommended practices for the Individualized Family Service Plan*. Order from: American Association for the Care of Children's Health, 3615 Wisconsin Ave., N.W., Washington, DC 20016.

Strickland, B. B., & Turnbull, A. (1990). *Developing and implementing Individualized Education Programs*. Columbus, OH: Merrill.

Weiss, H., & Jacobs, F. (Eds.). (1988). *Evaluating family programs*. Hawthorne, NY: Aldine De Gruyter.

Yogman, M., & Brazelton, T. (1986). *In support of families*. Cambridge, MA: Harvard University Press.

REFERENCES

Bailey, D., & Simeonsson, R. (1985). *Family Needs Survey*. Chapel Hill: University of North Carolina, FAMILIES Project, Frank Porter Graham Child Development Center.

Bailey, D., & Simeonsson, R. (1988). *Family assessment in early intervention*. Columbus, OH: Merrill.

Bailey, D., Simeonsson, R., Winton, P., Huntington, G., Comfort, M., Isbell, P., O'Donnell, K., & Helm, J. (1986). Family-focused intervention: A functional model for planning, implementing, and evaluating individualized family services in early education. *Journal of the Division for Early Childhood, 10,* 156–171.

Bernheimer, L., Young, M., & Winton, P. (1983). Stress over time: Parents with young handicapped children. *Journal of Developmental and Behavioral Pediatrics, 4,* 177–181.

Calhoun, M., Rose, T., & Armstrong, C. (1989). Getting an early start on community participation. *Teaching Exceptional Children, 21,* 51–53.

Cooper, M., & Ward, M. (1974). Effects of member participation and commitment in group decision making on influence, satisfaction, and decision riskiness. *Journal of Applied Psychology, 59,* 123–134.

Deal, A., Dunst, C., & Trivette, C. (in press). A flexible and functional approach to developing Individualized Family Support Plans. *Infants and Young Children.*

Dunst, C., Trivette, C., & Deal, A. (1988). *Enabling and empowering families.* Cambridge, MA: Brookline Books.

Elder, J. O. (1980). Writing interagency agreements. In J. O. Elder & P. Magrab (Eds.), *Coordinating services to handicapped children: A handbook for interagency collaboration* (pp. 244–271). Baltimore: Paul H. Brookes.

Fewell, R., & Sandall, S. (1986). Developmental testing of handicapped infants: A measurement dilemma. *Topics in Early Childhood Special Education, 6,* 86–99.

Garland, C., Woodruff, G., & Buck, D. (1988). Case management (Division for Early Childhood Special Education White Paper). Reston, VA: The Council for Exceptional Children.

Garwood, S. G., & Sheehan, R. (1989). *Designing a comprehensive early intervention system: The challenge of Public Law 99–457.* Austin, TX: PRO-ED.

Hanline, M. (1988). Making the transition to preschool: Identification of parent needs. *Journal of the Division for Early Childhood, 12,* 98–107.

Hochman, J., McGonigel, M., Toole, A., Paden, L., Foley, G., Metakes, M., Zeitlin, S., & Quigley, A. (1987). *Planning programs for infants, II.* East Brunswick, NJ: INTERACT.

Itagliata, J. (1982). Improving the quality of community care for the chronically mentally disabled: The role of case management. *Schizophrenia Bulletin, 8,* 655–673.

Johnson, B., McGonigel, M., & Kaufmann, R. (1989). *Guidelines and recommended practices for the Individualized Family Service Plan.* Washington, DC: American Association for the Care of Children's Health.

Kaiser, A., & Hemmeter, M. (1989). Value-based approaches to family intervention. *Topics in Early Childhood Special Education, 8,* 72–86.

Karnes, M., & Stayton, V. (1988). Linking screening, identification, and assessment with curriculum. In J. B. Jordan, J. J. Gallagher, P. L. Hutinger, & M. B. Karnes (Eds.), *Early childhood special education: Birth to three* (pp. 29–66). Reston, VA: The Council for Exceptional Children.

LaCour, J. A. (1982). Interagency agreement: A rational response to an irrational system. *Exceptional Children, 49,* 265–267.

McCollum, J., & Hughes, M. (1988). Staffing patterns and team models in infancy programs. In J. B. Jordan, J. J. Gallagher, P. L. Hutinger, & M. B. Karnes (Eds.), *Early childhood special education: Birth to three* (pp. 129–146). Reston, VA: The Council for Exceptional Children.

McGonigel, M., & Garland, C. (1988). The Individualized Family Service Plan and the early intervention team: Team and family issues and recommended practice. *Infants and Young Children, 1*(1), 10–21.

Odom, S. L., & Schuster, S. K. (1986). Naturalistic inquiry and the assessment of young handicapped children and their families. *Topics in Early Childhood Special Education, 6*(2), 68–82.

Olson, D., McCubbin, H., Barnes, H., Larsen, A., Muxen, M., & Wilson, M. (1982). *Family inventories*. St. Paul: University of Minnesota.

Rosenberg, S., Robinson, C., & Beckman, P. (1986). Measures of parent-infant interaction: An overview. *Topics in Early Childhood Special Education, 6*(2), 32–43.

Rosenberg, S., Robinson, C., Finkler, D., & Rose, J. (1987). An empirical comparison of formulas evaluating early intervention program impact on development. *Exceptional Children, 54*(3), 213–219.

Sheehan, R. (1989). Implications of P.L. 99–457 for assessment. *Topics in Early Childhood Special Education, 8,* 103–115.

Shelton, H., & Sorter, B. (1980). Improving interagency teamwork. *Journal of Extension, 12* (Nov./Dec.) 18–23.

Shelton, T., Jeppson, E., & Johnson, B. (1987). *Family-centered care for children with special health care needs*. Washington, DC: American Association for the Care of Children's Health.

Smith, B. J. (Ed.). (1988a). *Mapping the future for children with special needs: P.L. 99–457*. Iowa City: The University of Iowa.

Smith, B. J. (1988b). Early intervention public policy: Past, present, and future. In J. B. Jordan, J. J. Gallagher, P. L. Hutinger, & M. B. Karnes (Eds.), *Early childhood special education: Birth to three* (pp. 213–228). Reston, VA: The Council for Exceptional Children.

Thomas, A., & Chess, S. (1977). *Temperament and development*. New York: Brunner/Mazel.

Turnbull, A., & Summers, J. (1985, April). From family involvement to family support: Evolution to revolution. Presented at the Down Syndrome State-of-the-Art Conference, Boston, MA.

Winton, P., & Bailey, D. (1988). The family-focused interview: A collaborative mechanism for family assessment and goal-setting. *Journal of the Division for Early Childhood, 12,* 195–207.

Witt, J., Miller, C., McIntyre, R., & Smith, D. (1984). Effects of variables on parental perceptions of staffings. *Exceptional Children, 51,* 27–32.

Woodruff, G., & McGonigel, M. (1988). Early intervention team approaches: The transdisciplinary model. In J. B. Jordan, J. J. Gallagher, P. L. Hutinger, & M. B. Karnes (Eds.), *Early childhood special education: Birth to three* (pp. 163–182). Reston, VA: The Council for Exceptional Children.

APPENDICES

Critical Skills List

	COGNITIVE	
Age	**Skill Category**	**IEP Long-Term Goals Sample Activity**
Birth–12 months	causality	acts on objects to produce effect
		uses locomotion as means to end
		pulls to support to obtain objects
	imitation	imitates new, visible movements
	object permanence	searches for object after it disappears
	imitation	imitates new, invisible movements
12–24 months	object differentiation	uses at least 10 objects functionally
	means ends	obtains objects through use of tools
	imitation	defers motor imitation
	object permanence	systematically searches for objects
24–36 months	object differentiation	matches and sorts objects
		matches pictures
		classifies objects and/or pictures by function
		concept of 1 vs. many

Source: Bruder, M. B. (1990). Working document. Reprinted with permission.

RECEPTIVE LANGUAGE

Age	Bricker Language Skill Category	IEP Long-Term Goals Sample Activity
Birth–12 months	pre-instructional attention	turns to sounds outside visual range
	synchrony of actions	plays social ritual games (i.e., Peek-A-Boo)
	functional use of objects	demonstrates action schemes on objects
	multiword comprehension	demonstrates understanding of more than 3 words out of context (i.e., turns to name when called, points to or looks at objects named)
		responds to simple commands
12–24 months	functional use of objects	functionally uses 10 objects
	multiword comprehension	demonstrates 50-word receptive vocabulary (nouns, verbs, adjectives): a. in context b. out of context
		responds appropriately to simple questions/commands of at least 2 words
24–36 months	multiword comprehension	demonstrates 250-word receptive vocabulary (nouns, verbs, prepositions, and adjectives)
		responds correctly to multiword phrases and sentences (i.e., Put the spoon on the table. Are you hungry?)

EXPRESSIVE LANGUAGE

Age	Bricker Language Skill Category	IEP Long-Term Goals Sample Activities
Birth–12 months	speech sound production	vocalizes vowel sounds
		babbles speech sounds
		imitates familiar sounds
	establish prelinguistic signals	uses vocal/gestures to indicate needs (i.e., bounces and cries to be removed from high chair)
12–24 months	speech sound production	imitates vowel sounds
	increase frequency and diversity of signals	uses at least 5 different vocal/gestural combinations for communication purposes (i.e., points and says "da" for desired object)
	conventional word production	labels objects, persons, and events
	multiword production	strings two words together
	speech sound production	uses understandable articulation for easy-to-produce sounds
24–36 months	conventional word production	uses a variety of pragmatic functions such as requesting, calling, repeating, labeling, attending
	speech sound production	uses understandable articulation for the majority of consonants
	multiword production	produces multiword phrases (e.g., "boy sit chair"; "girl sleep") representing semantic categories

GROSS MOTOR

Age	Skill Category	IEP Long-Term Goals Sample Activity
Birth–12 months	head control	holds head upright and steady when in sitting position
	mobility	rolls in both directions
	trunk stability	sits independently
	mobility	crawls
		creeps using alternative hand-knee movement
	mobility, trunk stability	transitions from various positions: stand, sit, crawl
	mobility	steps sideways with support
12–24 months	trunk stability	stands independently
		stoops and returns to upright position
	mobility on stability	walks as means of locomotion, minimum of 5 steps
	mobility	gets on and out of chair (child size)
	ball skills	rolls ball to person
	balance	kicks stationary ball
24–36 months	mobility on stability	runs—avoids obstacles
	ball skills	throws ball—2 hands overhand
	balance	jumps on 2 feet (down or in place)
	dynamic skills	walks up and down stairs
	ball skills	catches large ball in arms from 3 feet

FINE MOTOR

Age	Skill Category	IEP Long-Term Goals Sample Activity
Birth–12 months	eye tracking	tracks 90° all directions
	midline orientation	manipulates objects with both hands at midline
	visually directed grasp	reaches and grasps objects
	object transfer	uses both hands to transfer objects
	voluntary release	releases objects into cup
12–24 months	pincer grasp	picks up item with pincer
	wrist rotation	turns lid on jar; opens door
	refined pincer grasp	turns one page at a time in book; scribbles with crayon
	controlled release	builds tower of 2–3 blocks
	eye-hand coordination/ controlled release	places shapes in a puzzle
24–36 months	eye-hand coordination and pincer grasp	places 2 small pegs in pegboard
		imitates directional movements for writing tasks: vertical, horizontal, and circular strokes
	visual motor	uses scissors to snip paper
		completes 3–piece interlocking puzzle

SELF-HELP—EATING

Age	IEP Long-Term Goals Sample Activity
Birth–12 months	sucks swallows uses tongue to move food finger feeds drinks from cup
12–24 months	rotary chews solid foods uses spoon with solid food independently drinks with cup
24–36 months	scoops with spoon to feed independently gets drink independently uses fork

SELF-HELP—DRESSING

Age	IEP Long-Term Goals Sample Activity
Birth–12 months	cooperates while being dressed (helps put arms into sleeves)
12–24 months	takes off shoes, socks, hat puts on hat obtains article of own clothing (i.e., coat, boots)
24–36 months	unzips pulls pants down pulls pants up from ankles removes coat hangs up coat puts on socks

SELF-HELP—TOILETING

Age	IEP Long-Term Goals Sample Activity
12–24 months	sits on potty indicates wet pants
24–48 months	daytime control when adult regulates toilet trip anticipates need to urinate

SOCIAL-EMOTIONAL

Age	IEP Long-Term Goals Sample Activity
Birth–12 months	spontaneously shows pleasure (i.e., social smile, vocalizes) when talked to
	manipulates simple toys (sensorimotor actions such as mouthing, banging, shaking)
	takes turns in games (i.e., Patty-Cake, Peek-A-Boo)
12–24 months	pulls adult to "show" or help
	uses toys functionally (i.e., pushes a car, bangs a xylophone)
	uses two toys together (puts balls in bucket, pushes car over blocks)
	initiates play activities
24–36 months	plays in parallel with two other children
	defends possessions
	uses objects for representational play (i.e., puts doll to bed; tea party)
	plays simple games

B

Resources for Families

General

Directory of National Information Sources on Handicapping Conditions and Related Services (2nd ed., 1980)
Clearinghouse on the Handicapped
Office of Human Development Services
U.S. Government Printing Office
Washington, DC 20401

A Training Resource Directory for Teachers Serving Handicapped Students, K–12 (1977)
Office of Civil Rights
Department of Health and Human Services
Room 5146
330 Independence Ave., S.W.
Washington, DC 20201

Special Education Programs for Severely Handicapped Students: A Directory of State Education Agency Services
National Association of State Departments of Education
1202 16th St., N.W.
Washington, DC 20036

Directory of Services and Facilities for Handicapped Children
Council for Exceptional Children
1920 Association Dr.
Reston, VA 22091

Other information can be obtained from:

The American Humane Association
Children's Division
P.O. Box 1266
Denver, CO 80201

American Association for the Care of Children's Health
3615 Wisconsin Ave.
Washington, D.C. 20016

Association for Childhood Education International
11141 Georgia Ave., Suite 200
Wheaton, MD 20902

Association for Persons with Severe Handicaps
7010 Roosevelt Way N.E.
Seattle, WA 98115

Child Welfare League of America
67 Irving Pl.
New York, NY 10003

Children's Defense Fund
122 C St. N.W.
Washington, DC 20001

Council for Exceptional Children
1920 Association Dr.
Reston, VA 22091

National Association for the Education of
Young Children
1834 Connecticut Ave., N.W.
Washington, DC 20009–5786

National Information Center for Handicapped
Children and Youth (NICHCY)
P.O. Box 1492
Washington, DC 20013

National Rehabilitation Association
1522 K St., N.W., Suite 1120
Washington, DC 20005

Special Olympics, Inc.
1701 K St. N.W., Suite 203
Washington, DC 20006

Toll-free numbers:

ERIC Clearinghouse on Adult Career and
Vocational Education
800–848–4815

Higher Education and Adult Training for
People with Handicaps
800–54–HEATH

National Health Information Clearinghouse
800–336–4797

National Organization on Disability
800–248–ABLE

National Rehabilitation Information Center
800–34–NARIC

National Speech Needs Center
800–233–1222
800–833–3232 (TDD)

For teachers and parents of the vision impaired:

American Council for the Blind
1211 Connecticut Ave., N.W., Suite 506
Washington, DC 20036

American Foundation for the Blind
15 West 16th St.
New York, NY 10011

American Printing House for the Blind
1839 Frankfort Ave.
Louisville, KY 40206

Association for Education of the Visually
Handicapped
919 Walnut St.
San Francisco, CA 94121

Blind Children's Center, Inc.
4120 Marathon St.
Los Angeles, CA 90029

Hadley School for the Blind
700 Elm St., P.O. Box 299
Winnetka, IL 60093

National Association for the Deaf-Blind
2703 Forest Oak Circle
Norman, OK 73071

National Association for the Visually Handicapped
3201 Balboa St.
San Francisco, CA 94121

National Society for the Prevention of Blindness, Inc.
79 Madison Ave.
New York, NY 10016

Canadian National Institute for the Blind
1929 Bayview Ave.
Toronto, 350, Ontario, CANADA

World Council for the Welfare of the Blind
56 Avenue Bosquet
75007 Paris, FRANCE

Materials of particular interest:

*Reach Out and Teach: Meeting the Training Needs
of Parents of Visually and Multiply Handicapped
Young Children* (Ferrell, 1985). Available from the
American Foundation for the Blind. A highly useful
and readable set of materials including a Parent
Handbook and Reachbook, in which parents apply
specific activities and record their progress. Other
related resources include an introductory slide
presentation and a Teacher's Manual that enable
teachers to use all the *Reach Out* materials in early
education programs.

Move It and *Get a Wiggle On* (Drouillard and
Raynor); *Learning to Play* (Recchia); and *Take
Charge* (Nousanen and Robinson). These and other
pamphlets are available from Hadley School for the
Blind.

*Talk to Me: A Language Guide for Parents of Blind
Children; Talk to Me II;* and *Move With Me*. These
brief booklets are available from the Blind
Children's Center.

For parents and teachers of hearing-impaired children:

Alexander Graham Bell Association for the Deaf
3417 Volta Pl., N.W.
Washington, DC 20007

American Speech-Language-Hearing Association
9030 Old Georgetown Rd.
Washington, DC 20014

National Association of the Deaf
814 Thayer Ave.
Silver Spring, MD 20910

National Association for the Deaf-Blind
2703 Forest Oak Circle
Norman, OK 73071

For teachers and parents of motor- and physically impaired children:

American Physical Therapy Association
1156 15th St., N.W., Suite 500
Washington, DC 20005

Epilepsy Foundation of America
4351 Garden City Dr.
Landover, MD 20785

March of Dimes Birth Defects Foundation
1275 Mamaroneck Ave.
White Plains, NY 10605

Muscular Dystrophy Association
810 7th Ave.
New York, NY 10019

National Easter Seal Society for Crippled Children and Adults
2023 West Ogden Ave.
Chicago, IL 60612

Spina Bifida Association of America
343 S. Dearborn St., Suite 319
Chicago, IL 60604

United Cerebral Palsy Association
666 East 34th St.
New York, NY 10016

Resource materials of particular interest:

Anderson, R. D., Bale, J. F., Blackman, J. A., & Murphy, J. R. (1986). *Infections in Children: A Sourcebook for Educators and Child Care Providers*. Rockville, MD: Aspen.

Batshaw, M. L., & Perret, Y. M. (1986). *Children with Handicaps: A Medical Primer*. Baltimore: Paul H. Brookes.

Blackman, J. A. (Ed.) (1984). *Medical Aspects of Developmental Disabilities in Children Birth to Three*. Rockville, MD: Aspen.

Bleck, E. E., & Nagel, D. A. (Eds.) (1982). *Physically Handicapped Children: A Medical Atlas for Teachers*. New York: Grune & Stratton.

Finnie, N. (1975). *Handling the Young Cerebral Palsied Child at Home*. New York: E. P. Dutton.

Williamson, G. G. (1987). *Children with Spina Bifida: Early Intervention and Preschool Programming*. Baltimore: Paul H. Brookes.

For teachers and parents of developmentally-delayed or behaviorially-impaired children:

American Association on Mental Deficiency
5101 Wisconsin Ave., N.W.
Washington, DC 20007

American Association of Psychiatric Services for Children
1701 18th St. N.W.
Washington, DC 20009

American Psychological Association
9030 Old Georgetown Rd.
Washington, DC 20014

Association for Children and Adults with Learning Disabilities
4156 Library Rd.
Pittsburgh, PA 15234

International Directory of Mental Retardation Sources (ed. R. F. Dybwad).
President's Committee on Mental Retardation
U.S. Dept. of Health and Human Services
Office of Human Services
Washington, DC 20006

National Association for Retarded Citizens
P.O. Box 6109
2501 Avenue J
Arlington, TX 76011

National Association of School Psychologists
1511 K St. N.W.
Washington, DC 20005

National Society for Children and Adults with Autism
1234 Massachusetts Ave. N.W., Suite 1017
Washington, DC 20005

Selected resources for teachers
in integrated classrooms:

"My Friends and Me"
Duane E. Davis: American Guidance Service, Inc.
P.O. Box 99
Circle Pines, MN 55014–1796
   Kit including 190 activities and lesson plans
(activity manuals, dolls, magnetic shapes, recorded
songs, etc.) intended to help children develop
positive, confident, and realistic personal identity
and essential social skills and understandings.

"Hal's Pals"
Mattel: Therapy Skill Builders
3830 E. Bellevue, P.O. Box 42050–A
Tucson, AZ 85733
   Five sets of materials dealing with amputation,
hearing impairment, leg braces, blindness, and
wheelchairs.

Some specific books of potential value to teachers
of young children include the following:

Baslin, B., & Harris, K. (1984). *More Notes From A
Different Drummer: A Guide to Juvenile Fiction
Portraying the Disabled*. Ann Arbor, MI: Bowker.

Buchbinder, D. (1984). *Special Kids Make Special
Friends*. Association for Children with Down's
Syndrome. 2616 Martin Ave., Bellmore, NY 11710.

Feshbach, N., Feshbach, S., Fauvre, M., & Ballard-
Campbell, M., (1984). *Learning to Care*. Glenview,
IL: Goodyear Books.

Field, T., Roopnarine, J., & Segal, M. (1984).
Friendships in Normal and Handicapped Children.
Norwood, NJ: Ablex.

Krause, Bob (Ed.). (1977). *An Exceptional View of
Life: The Easter Seal Story*. Norfolk Island, Australia:
Island Heritage Limited.

McElmurry, M. (1983). *Belonging*. Good Apple, Inc.
Box 299, Carthage, IL 62321–0299.

Schuncke, G., & Krough, S. (1983). *Helping Children
Choose*. Glenview, IL: Goodyear Books.

C

National Professional Associations and Voluntary Organizations

Affiliated Leadership League of and for the Blind of America (ALL)
2025 I St., N.W.
Suite 405
Washington, DC 20006
202–775–8262

Alexander Graham Bell Association for the Deaf
3417 Volta Pl., N.W.
Washington, DC 20007
202–337–5520

Alliance of Genetic Support Groups
38th and R Sts., N.W.
Washington, DC 20057
202–625–7853

American Academy for Cerebral Palsy and Developmental Medicine
2405 Westwood Ave., Suite 205
P.O. Box 11083
Richmond, VA 23230
804–355–0147

American Academy of Pediatrics
141 Point Blvd., N.W.
P.O. Box 927
Elk Grove Village, IL 60009
312–288–5005

American Amputee Foundation, Inc. (AAF)
Box 55218
Little Rock, AR 72225
501–666–2523

American Brittle Bone Society (ABBS)
1256 Merrill Dr.
Marshallton
West Chester, PA 19380
215–692–6248

American Cancer Society (ACS)
90 Park Ave.
New York, NY 10016
212–599–8200

American Cleft Palate Educational Foundation (ACPEF)
331 Salk Hall
University of Pittsburgh
Pittsburgh, PA 15261
412–681–9620

American Coalition of Citizens with Disabilities (ACCD)
1012 14th St., N.W.
Suite 901
Washington, DC 20005
202–628–3470

American Council for the Blind (ACB)
1010 Vermont Ave., N.W.
Suite 1100
Washington, DC 20005
202–393–3666
800–424–8666

American Council on Rural Special Education
(ACRES)
Western Washington University
Bellingham, WA 98225
206–676–3576

American Diabetes Association, Inc. (ADA)
National Service Center
P.O. Box 25757
Alexandria, VA 22313
202–331–8303
800–232–3472

American Foundation for Maternal and Child Health
439 E. 51st St.
New York, NY 10022
212–759–5510

American Foundation for the Blind (AFB)
15 West 16th St.
New York, NY 10011
212–620–2000

American Home Economics Association (AHEA)
2010 Massachusetts Ave., N.W.
Washington, DC 20036
202–862–8330

American Nurses' Association
2420 Pershing Rd.
Kansas City, MO 64108
816–474–5720

American Occupational Therapy Association
1383 Piccard Dr.
P.O. Box 1726
Rockville, MD 20850–4375
301–948–9626

American Orthopsychiatric Association (AOA)
19 W. 44th St., #1616
New York, NY 10036
212–354–5770

American Physical Therapy Association
1111 N. Fairfax St.
Alexandria, VA 22314
703–684–2782

American Printing House for the Blind (APHB)
1839 Frankfort Ave.
P.O. Box 6085
Louisville, KY 40206–0085
502–895–2405

American Psychological Association
1200 17th St., N.W.
Washington, DC 20036
202–955–7600

American Society for Deaf Children (ASDC)
814 Thayer Ave.
Silver Spring, MD 20910
301–585–5400

American Speech-Language-Hearing Association
10801 Rockville Pike
Rockville, MD 20852–3279
800–638–8255

Arthritis Foundation
1314 Spring St., N.W.
Atlanta, GA 30309
404–872–7100

Association for Persons with Severe Handicaps
7010 Roosevelt Way, N.W.
Seattle, WA 98115
206–523–8446

American Association for the Care of Children's
Health (ACCH)
3615 Wisconsin Ave., N.W.
Washington, DC 20016
202–244–1801

Association for Childhood Education Internationa
(ACEI)
11141 Georgia Ave., #200
Wheaton, MD 20902
301–942–2443

Association of Birth Defect Children (ABDC)
3526 Emerywood Lane
Orlando, FL 32806
305–859–2821

The Candlelighters Childhood Cancer Foundation
2025 I St., N.W.
Washington, DC 20006
202–659–5136

Center for Birth Defects Information Services
Dover, MA 02030
617–785–2525

Center for Parent Education
55 Chapel St.
Newton, MA 02160

Child Welfare League of America (CWLA)
67 Irving Place
New York, NY 10003
212–254–7410

Clearinghouse on the Handicapped
Office of Special Education and Rehabilitative
Services
Department of Education
Switzer Building, Room 3119–S
Washington, DC 20202
202–245–0080

Closer Look Information Center
Parents Campaign for Handicapped Children
and Youth
1201 16th St., N.W.
Washington, DC 20036
202–822–7900

Compassionate Friends, Inc.
P.O. Box 1347
Oak Brook, IL 60521
312–323–5010

Consumers Organization for the
Hearing Impaired, Inc.
c/o National Association for Hearing
and Speech Action
10801 Rockville Pike
Rockville, MD 20852
800–638–8255
301–897–8682

Cornelia deLange Syndrome Foundation
60 Dyer Ave.
Collingsville, CT 06022
203–693–0159

The Council for Exceptional Children
1920 Association Dr.
Reston, VA 22091
703–620–3660

Deaf Communications Institute
P.O. Box 247
Fayville, MA 01745
617–872–9406

Disability Rights Center
1346 Connecticut Ave., N.W.
Suite 1124
Washington, DC 20036
202–223–3304

Epilepsy Foundation of America
4351 Garden City Dr.
Suite 406
Landover, MD 20785
301–459–3700

Family Resource Coalition
230 N. Michigan Ave.
Suite 1625
Chicago, IL 60601
312–726–4750

The Family Survival Project
1736 Divisadero St.
San Francisco, CA 94115
415–921–5400

Foundation for Children with Learning Disabilities
Grand Central Station
P.O. Box 2929
New York, NY 10163
212–687–7211

International Association for Infant Mental Health
Department of Psychology
Psychology Research Building
Michigan State University
East Lansing, MI 48824–1117

Joseph P. Kennedy, Jr. Foundation
1350 New York Ave., N.W.
Suite 500
Washington, DC 20005
202–393–1250

Junior National Association for the Deaf
445 N. Pennsylvania
Suite 804
Indianapolis, IN 46204
317–638–1715

Juvenile Diabetes Foundation International
60 Madison Ave.
New York, NY 10010

Leukemia Society of America
733 Third Ave.
New York, NY 10017
212–573–8484

Little People of America
Box 633
San Bruno, CA 94066
415–589–0695

Mainstream, Inc.
1200 15th St., N.W.
Washington, DC 20005
202–833–1136

March of Dimes Birth Defects Foundation
1275 Mamoroneck Ave.
White Plains, NY 10603
914–428–7100

Muscular Dystrophy Association
810 Seventh Ave.
New York, NY 10019
212–586–0808

National Amputation Foundation
12045 150th St.
Whitestone, NY 11357
718–767–8400

National Association for Retarded Citizens
2501 Ave. J
Arlington, TX 76006
817–640–0204

National Association for Sickle Cell Disease, Inc.
4221 Wilshire Blvd.
Suite 360
Los Angeles, Ca 90010
213–936–7205
800–421–8453

National Association for the Deaf
814 Thayer Ave.
Silver Spring, MD 20910
301–587–1788

National Association for the Education of Young
Children (NAEYC)
1834 Connecticut Ave., N.W.
Washington, DC 20009–5786
202–232–8777
800–424–2460

National Association for the Visually Handicapped
22 West 21st St., 6th Floor
New York, NY 10010
212–889–3141

National Association of Developmental Disabilities
Council
1234 Massachusetts Ave., N.W.
Suite 203
Washington, DC 20005
202–347–1234

National Association of Social Workers
7981 Eastern Ave.
Silver Spring, MD 20910
301–565–0333

National Ataxia Foundation
600 Twelve Oaks Center
15500 Wayzata Blvd.
Wayzata, MN 55391
612–473–7666

National Center for Clinical Infant Programs
2000 14th St., N., Suite 380
Arlington, Va 22201–2500
703–528–4300

National Center for Education in Maternal and Child
Health
38th and R Sts., N.W.
Washington, DC 20057
202–625–8400

National Council on Stuttering
P.O. Box 8171
Grand Rapids, MI 49508
616–241–2372

National Down Syndrome Congress
1800 Dempster St.
Park Ridge, IL 60068–1146
800–232–NDSC

National Down Syndrome Society
141 Fifth Ave.
New York, NY 10010
212–460–9330
800–221–4602

National Easter Seal Society
2023 West Ogden Ave.
Chicago, IL 60612
312–243–8400

National Education Association
1201 16th St., N.W.
Washington, DC 20036
202–833–4000

National Federation of the Blind
1800 Johnson St.
Baltimore, MD 21230
301–659–9314

National Head Injury Foundation
P.O. Box 567
Framingham, MA 01701
617–679–7473

The National Hemophilia Foundation
The Soho Building
110 Greene St., Room 406
New York, NY 10012
212–219–8180

National Information Center for Handicapped
Children and Youth
P.O. Box 1492
Washington, DC 20013
703–522–0870

National Institute of Child Health and
Human Development
9000 Rockville Pike
Building 31, Room 2A32
Bethesda, MD 20205
301–496–4143

National Mental Health Association
1021 Prince St.
Alexandria, VA 22314–2971
703–684–7722

National Network to Prevent Birth Defects
Box 15309
Southeast Station
Washington, DC 20003

National Neurofibromatosis Foundation
141 Fifth Ave.
Suite 7–S
New York, NY 10010
212–460–8980

National Organization for Rare Disorders
P.O. Box 8923
New Fairfield, CT 06812
203–746–6518

National Organization on Disability
2100 Pennsylvania Ave., N.W.
Suite 234
Washington, DC 20037
202–293–5968

National Perinatal Association
101–1/2 South Union St.
Alexandria, VA 22314–3323
703–549–5523

National Retinitis Pigmentosa Foundation
(RP Foundation Fighting Blindness)
1401 Mt. Royal Ave.
Fourth Floor
Baltimore, MD 21217
800–638–2300

The National Society for Children and
Adults with Autism
1234 Massachusetts Ave., N.W.
Suite 1017
Washington, DC 20005–4599
202–783–0125

National Society to Prevent Blindness
79 Madison Ave.
New York, NY 10016
212–684–3505

National Tay-Sachs and Allied Diseases Association,
Inc.
92 Washington Ave.
Cedarhurst, NY 11516
516–569–4300

National Tuberous Sclerosis Association, Inc.
National Headquarters
P.O. Box 612
Winfield, IL 60190
312–668–0787

Osteogenesis Imperfecta Foundation, Inc.
P.O. Box 838
Manchester, NH 03105
516–325–8992 (Administrative Office)

Parent Advocacy Coalition for Education Rights
4826 Chicago Ave.
Minneapolis, MN 55417

Parent Care
University of Utah Medical Center
Suite 2A210
Salt Lake City, UT 84132
801–581–5323

Parentele
1301 E. 38th St.
Indianapolis, IN 46205
317–926–4142

Parents Helping Parents
47 Maro Dr.
San Jose, CA 95127
408–272–4774

Parents of Premature and High Risk Infants
International, Inc.
33 West 42nd St.
New York, NY 10036
606–277–0008

Parent to Parent
301 W. Franklin St., Room 1608
Virginia Commonwealth University
Box 3020
Richmond, VA 23284–3020
804–225–3875

Prader-Willi Syndrome Association
5515 Malibu Dr.
Edina, MN 55436
612–933–0113

Rural Network
c/o Child Development Resources
P.O. Box 306
Lightfoot, VA 23090
804–565–0303

Sensory Aids Foundation
399 Sherman Ave.
Suite 12
Palo Alto, CA 94306
415–329–0430

Sick Kids (Need) Involved People, Inc.
216 Newport Dr.
Severna Park, MD 21146
301–647–0164

Spina Bifida Association of America
343 South Dearborn St.
Room 310
Chicago, IL 60604
312–663–1562
800–621–3141

Spinal Cord Society
2410 Lakeview Dr.
Fergus Falls, MN 56537
218–738–5252

Tourette Syndrome Association
41–02 Bell Blvd.
Bayside, NY 11361
718–224–2999

United Cerebral Palsy Associations
66 East 34th St.
New York, NY 10016
212–481–6300

United Ostomy Association
2001 W. Beverly Blvd.
Los Angeles, CA 90057
213–413–5510

Very Special Arts
1825 Connecticut Ave., N.W.
Suite 417
Washington, DC 20009
202–332–6960

Vision Foundation, Inc.
818 Mt. Auburn St.
Watertown, MA 02172
617–926–4232
800–852–3029 (Toll free in Massachusetts)

D

Analysis of Individualized Family Service Plans

Instructions. The purpose of this instrument is to review the content of *each* infant's or toddler's Individualized Family Service Plan. Children's names may, at the discretion of the early intervention program staff, be included in this analysis. In the event that a child's name is included in the analysis, program staff *must* still assign a unique identifier number to each child being served by the demonstration program. If any early intervention program chooses to only record identification numbers in the analysis, the program staff assume responsibility for maintaining a master record of children's identities and their respective identification numbers.

Program title: _____

Program address: _____

Person completing this analysis: _____

  Telephone during day: (_____) _____
                  Area   Number

Date of analysis: _____ / _____ / _____

Child's name: _____ Child's ID: _____ Birth date: ____ / ____ / ____

Child has an IFSP   _____ Yes   _____ No   If yes, go on.

IFSP Component	Yes	No
1. Child's name is on the form.	____	____
2. Parents' names are on the form.	____	____
3. Contains report of multidisciplinary assessment of child.	____	____
4. Parents participated in the IFSP development (documented on the IFSP).	____	____
5. IFSP reviewed with the parents in the past 6 months.	____	____
6. Multidisciplinary assessment occurred in a reasonable time after the initial referral (e.g., 4 weeks).	____	____
7. Contains present level of infant's:	____	____
a. physical development	____	____
b. cognitive development	____	____
c. language/communication development	____	____
d. psychosocial development	____	____
e. self-help skill acquisition	____	____
8. Statement of families' strengths and needs is contained in the IFSP.	____	____
9. Statement of major outcomes to be achieved by the parents, with criteria and time lines, is contained in the IFSP.	____	____
10. Statement of the nature and intensity of the service provided to infants and parents is contained in the IFSP.	____	____
11. Projected or actual dates of initiation of services are contained.	____	____
12. Case manager is named.	____	____
Please state that person's title: _____		
13. Statement for supporting transition to other agencies if needed is contained.	____	____

Source: From *Designing a Comprehensive Early Intervention System: The Challenge of Public Law 99-457* (pp. 104–105) by S. G. Garwood and R. Sheehan, 1989, Austin, TX: PRO-ED. Copyright © 1989 by PRO-ED. Reprinted by permission.

E

Early Intervention Program Description

Instructions. The purpose of this instrument is to describe in a quick fashion the services provided by early intervention programs operating in the state. These programs serve infants and toddlers and their families. Please check below the activities (as they apply to infants and toddlers and families) in which your program is engaged.

Program title: _____   Date of submission: _____ / _____ / _____

Program address: _____   Check if submission is an update: _____

Person completing this description: _____   Geographic area served by program: _____

Telephone during day: (_____) _____
                          Area   Number

Please check below the activities conducted by your early intervention program. If you have specific information to share about any of those activities, please do so in the comments column below.

Child Find/Screening	**Comments**
1. ____ Advertisement	_____
2. ____ Screening clinics	_____
3. ____ Home visit by public health nurse	_____
4. ____ Well-baby clinic	_____
5. ____ Other: _____	_____
6. ____ Other: _____	_____
7. ____ Other: _____	_____

Screening and Diagnostic Services

Comments

1. ____ Screening of risk factors

2. ____ Screening of infant and toddler performances

3. ____ Multidisciplinary diagnostic assessment of developmental delay

4. ____ Other: _____

5. ____ Other: _____

6. ____ Other: _____

Referral Services

1. ____ Infants and families are referred to another agency.

2. ____ Infant and family participation in another agency is tracked through organized referral system.

3. ____ Infants and families are accepted on a referral basis from other agencies.

4. ____ A procedure is employed to determine how long after referral *to* another agency services are provided.

5. ____ A procedure is employed to determine how long after referral *from* another agency services are provided.

6. ____ Other: _____

7. ____ Other: _____

8. ____ Other: _____

Programmatic Assessment as a Part of Intervention   **Comments**

1. ____ Ongoing developmental monitoring of   _____
children not in program but being
monitored

2. ____ Ongoing developmental monitoring of   _____
children in program

3. ____ Other: _____   _____

4. ____ Other: _____   _____

5. ____ Other: _____   _____

Service Delivery Programs

1. ____ Home visits   _____

2. ____ Center-based services/child alone   _____

3. ____ Center-based services/child and family   _____
alone

4. ____ Center-based services/individual parents   _____
(alone)

5. ____ Visits to other child care programs   _____

6. ____ Specialized services to particular groups   _____
of parents (e.g., MR parents)

7. ____ Center-based services to all parents in   _____
groups

8. ____ Transitional programming for children   _____
moving to preschool programs

9. ____ Other: _____   _____

10. ____ Other: _____   _____

11. ____ Other: _____   _____

Case Management	**Comments**

1. _____ Professional case manager (i.e., person whose primary responsibilities are case management)   _____

2. _____ One member of interdisciplinary team serves as case manager   _____

3. _____ Entire team acts as case managers   _____

4. _____ Parents are own case managers   _____

5. _____ Other: _____   _____

Training

1. _____ Train staff at day care centers for normally developing children in which developmentally delayed or at-risk children are enrolled.   _____

2. _____ Train pediatricians.   _____

3. _____ Train staff in other programs serving developmentally delayed, handicapped, or at-risk children but not receiving 99–457 funds.   _____

4. _____ Other: _____   _____

5. _____ Other: _____   _____

6. _____ Other: _____   _____

Source: From *Designing a Comprehensive Early Intervention System: The Challenge of Public Law 99–457* (pp. 118–122) by S. G. Garwood and R. Sheehan, 1989, Austin, TX: PRO-ED. Copyright © 1989 by PRO-ED. Reprinted by permission.

F

Individualized Family Service Plan Form

Instructions. This form must be completed at onset of early intervention (or as soon as possible thereafter) for every infant and toddler in the program. The form is to be completed with the full participation of children's parents and staff, and parents are expected to sign and date the form when it is complete. The form is to be reviewed after 6 months (again, signatures are necessary) and revised, as needed, after 12 months.

Child's name _____ Child's ID: _____ Birth date: _____ / _____ / _____

Date IFSP completed: _____ / _____ / _____

Early intervention program staff completing IFSP:

_____   _____
              Signature   Discipline

_____   _____
              Signature   Discipline

_____   _____
              Signature   Discipline

_____   _____
              Signature   Discipline

Parent(s): I (We) have reviewed the Individualized Family Service Plan and approve of this plan.

_____ _____ / _____ / _____   _____ _____ / _____ / _____
     Signature   Date   Signature   Date

Part I: Child Assessment

**Instruments/
Procedures**

Present level of functioning

1. Physical development: _____   _____

2. Cognitive development: _____   _____

3. Speech/language development: _____   _____

4. Psychosocial development: _____   _____

5. Self-help skills: _____   _____

Part II: Family Assessment—Family members: _____

A. **Family strengths**   **Method Used to Assess**

1. _____   _____

2. _____   _____

3. _____   _____

B. **Family needs, as expressed by family**

1. _____

2. _____

3. _____

Part III: Team Recommendations for Services to Child/Family

1. _____

2. _____

3. _____

Part IV: Major Expected Child Outcomes

1. Outcome: _____

   a. Intervention procedures/services: _____

   b. Assessment criteria, procedures: _____

   c. Timelines: _____

Part IV: Major Expected Child Outcomes (continued)

2. Outcome: _____

   a. Intervention procedures/services: _____

   b. Assessment criteria, procedures: _____

   c. Timelines: _____

3. Outcome: _____

   a. Intervention procedures/services: _____

   b. Assessment criteria, procedures: _____

   c. Timelines: _____

Part V: Major Expected Family Outcomes

1. Outcome: _____

   a. Intervention procedures/services: _____

   b. Assessment criteria, procedures: _____

   c. Timelines: _____

2. Outcome: _____

   a. Intervention procedures/services: _____

   b. Assessment criteria, procedures: _____

   c. Timelines: _____

Part VI: Role of Parents in Developing the IFSP (Optional)

Please provide a short, descriptive statement of the parents' role in developing this IFSP.

_____

_____

_____

Part VII: Case Manager Information

1. Name of Case Manager: _____

2. Title of Case Manager: _____

Part VIII: Review and Annual Re-evaluation and Revision Timelines

1. Date of next review: _____ / _____ / _____

2. Date of next revaluation: _____ / _____ / _____

3. Date of next revision of IFSP: _____ / _____ / _____

Part IX: Statement of Anticipated Transition Services

_____

_____

_____

_____

_____

_____

_____

_____

_____

_____

_____

_____

_____

_____

Source: From *Designing a Comprehensive Early Intervention System: The Challenge of Public Law 99–457* (pp. 108–112) by S. G. Garwood and R. Sheehan, 1989, Austin, TX: PRO-ED. Copyright © 1989 by PRO-ED. Reprinted by permission.

Glossary

Acquired Immune Deficiency Syndrome (AIDS): A communicable illness that reduces the body's ability to fight some types of infection and cancers.

Activity-based Instruction: The process of teaching skills, from a number of developmental domains, within the same age-appropriate activity.

Adaptive Equipment: Any device or material that is modified to enhance the independence of a child by controlling for abnormal postural responses.

Amblyopia: Reduction of visual acuity in the absence of any organic lesion.

American Sign Language (ASL or Ameslan): A communication system in which everything that a speaker says is not included and gestures are used.

Anomaly: A malformation or deviation from the normal.

Anoxia: The lack of oxygen.

Anticipatory Guidance: The process of predicting upcoming issues and problems for families and taking steps to prevent or minimize these difficulties.

Aorta: The major vessel carrying oxygenated blood from the heart to the rest of the body.

Apgar Scores: A measure that evaluates the effect of loss of oxygen and damage to the circulation of newborns.

Apnea: The cessation of breathing.

Arena Assessment: The process of one professional conducting an evaluation while other team members, including the family, observe and contribute.

Asphyxia: Suffocation; a condition in which there may be lack of oxygen with a build-up of carbon dioxide that may occur at any time during life, including before labor and birth into adulthood.

Aspiration: The act of inhaling or drawing in air. (If there is a foreign substance in the area above the windpipe [trachea], it too will be aspirated as air is drawn into the lungs.)

Asthma: A disease characterized by airways that react allergically or react to the environment by constricting, causing wheezing and difficulty catching a breath.

Asymmetric Tonic Neck Response: A primitive reflex seen in the newborn period.

Asymptomatic HIV Infection: The presence of HIV antibodies without subjective or objective signs of illness.

Ataxia: Failure or irregularity of muscle coordination and muscle action.

Athetosis: Ceaseless, slow, writhing movements.

Atonic: Without tone.

Atrophy: Wasting away or diminution in size of an organ.

Attachment: An intense relationship that persists over time.

Auditory Brainstem Response (ABR) Testing: A screening tool used with infants and older children when a voluntary response to sound is not evident.

Auditory Evoked Response: The electrical response of the brain to a standard sound.

Auditory Habilitation: Learning to use one's hearing as efficiently as possible.

Behavioral Intervention Specialist: Infant interventionist who works in the NICU and assists the staff in identifying environmental manipulations and handling strategies that better support the developing infant.

Bilateral: Both sides.

Bilirubin: A chemical breakdown product of hemoglobin (red blood cells) that is evidenced by yellow pigment.

Bilirubin Encephalopathy: A change in brain activity due to poisoning from bilirubin.

Biological Risk: Insult to the nervous system during prenatal, perinatal, neonatal, or early infancy period that makes normal development problematic.

Bradycardia: Slowing of the heart rate.

Bronchiolitis: Inflammation of the small airways associated with wheezing.

Bronchopulmonary Dysplasia (BPD): A chronic lung condition primarily involving the airways of premature infants who have required mechanical ventilation and oxygen therapy.

Bulbar: Pertaining to the region of the brain known as the medulla oblongata and its nerve centers, in particular, the centers for the nerves supplying the areas of the throat and vocal cords.

Bulbar Nerve Damage: Damage to the medulla oblongata area of the brain (between the pons and the spinal cord) that contains nerve cells that deal with vital functions such as breathing, circulation, and certain senses.

Cardiac: Pertaining to the heart.

Cardiac Catheterization: Procedure in which a long, small tube is passed through a vessel into the heart and the vessels near it and contrast material is injected, allowing visualization of the heart anatomy on radiograph.

Cardiopulmonary Resuscitation (CPR): Artificial breathing and heart pumping, sometimes administered along with medications, in an attempt to restore normal function of the heart and lungs.

Case Manager: An early intervention professional who assumes primary responsibility for coordinating infant and toddler services for a family, and ensuring the IFSP is written and all aspects are met.

Child Find: A system of locating children who are eligible, or potentially eligible, for services.

Cerebral Palsy: Disorder of movement and posture due to a nonprogressive defect of the immature brain.

Clonus: Spasm in which there is rigidity alternating with relaxation.

Coacting Teams: A process in which all communication flows through a central person.

Coactive Movements: Occur when an adult moves a child through a movement.

Cognitive Development: Progressive change in internal mental processes such as thinking, reasoning, remembering, and the ability to function adaptively.

Cohesiveness: A sense of "oneness" team members experience that results in their willingness to work harder toward the group's goals and their desire to remain part of the group.

Communicable or Contagious Disease: Illness caused by a specific infectious agent (i.e., a virus, bacteria, fungus) that is transmitted, directly or indirectly, from an infected person to another person.

Communication: A process by which information and feelings are received and sent between individuals.

Communication Hydrocephalus: A buildup of fluid within the brain caused when the normal absorption process is interrupted. In this condition there is no blockage of flow of the cerebral spinal fluid, but the fluid does not circulate. This commonly develops after meningitis.

Conductive Hearing Loss: Characterized by a decreased sensitivity to sound but does not generally affect word recognition abilities.

Conflict Resolution Strategies: The process of stating the conflict as explicitly as possible, generating several means of resolving the conflict, and then conscientiously following the agreed solution.

Congenital: Existing at birth, but not necessarily hereditary or evident at birth.

Congenital or Prenatal Transmission: Transmission of infection occurring prior to birth, causing an infant to be born with the infection.

Congenitally Blind: Blind from birth.

Congestive Heart Failure: Inability of the heart to perform its normal pumping activity, causing a backing up of blood in the circulation.

Contingency Experiences: Experiences that occur because of the infant's actions or behavior.

Contingent Responsivity: Parental behavior that is temporally and functionally related to an infant's signals.

Contraindication: Any condition, especially any condition of disease, which renders some particular line of treatment improper or undesirable.

Cooperative Scribbling: When an adult and child scribble on the same piece of paper and may take turns scribbling in the same area.

Corrected Age (of Infants):   Calculated by subtracting the number of weeks of prematurity from the infant's chronological age.

Cortical Blindness: A disturbance of the visual cortex in the absence of any other known pathology.

Cortical Sensory Deficits: Loss of function of the senses because of loss within the brain, as opposed to loss of function within the sensory organ itself.

Critical Skills: Broad, activity-based competencies.

Cross-modal Transfer: The ability to take information obtained through one sensory modality and apply it to another.

Croup: A disorder occurring in infants and young children that has a characteristic barking cough because of narrowing of the larynx (voice box) due to allergy or infection.

Cyst: A sac containing fluid or semisolid material. It may develop within normal tissue as a result of breakdown of the area from infection or loss of blood flow.

Cytomegalovirus (CMV):   One of a group of viruses that causes specific changes in cells, enlarging them.

Deferred Imitation: Occurs when a child reproduces an action or sound some time after observing it performed.

Developmental Delay: Children with or without an established diagnosis who have fallen significantly behind developmental norms.

Developmental Therapist: Term used to describe the overlapping roles of occupational and physical therapists in their work with very young children with special needs.

Diaphragmatic Hernia: A congenital absence of all or part of the diaphragm that allows the abdominal contents to get into the chest cavity and compress the lungs.

Disassociation: The ability to move one segment of the body while holding another segment still or moving it in the opposite direction.

Domains: Different components of a child's development.

Dysplasia: An abnormal growth pattern.

Early Facilitation: Infant interventionists' style of supporting the development of infants and their families.

Early Intervention: Services for children from birth to school age.

Effective Questioning: The ability to ask questions in a manner in which information is shared.

Efficacy: Positive effects or impact of a program, strategy, approach, or procedure.

Empowerment: The process of assisting families in recognizing and developing their own competence.

Enablement: Creating opportunities for family members to become more competent and self-sustaining to get their needs met and attain desired goals.

Encephalitis: An inflammation of the brain tissue, usually caused by viruses.

Encephalopathy: A degenerative disease of the brain.

Endocardial Cushion: The embryologic area of the heart from which the valves and the walls between the heart tissues form.

Endotracheal Tubes: Tubes through the mouth into the trachea or windpipe that assist in artificial ventilation.

Environmental Risk Conditions: The presence of factors in the family, community, social, or economic system that predict early life experiences that may result in developmental delay.

Epilepsy: Recurrent convulsions or seizures.

Established Risk Conditions: The presence of a diagnosed physical or medical condition that is likely to lead to developmental delay.

Etiology: Cause.

Exosystem: Settings that do not involve the developing person as an active participant, but in which events occur that affect, or are affected by, what happened in the setting containing the developing person.

Expressive Language: Child's ability to produce language.

Extended Family: Family members outside the immediate family.

Extension: To straighten out.

Extensor Posturing: Maintenance of a straight position.

Extrafamilial: Extended family members.

Extrapulmonary: Outside the lungs or airways.

Extrapyramidal: Outside the pyramidal tracts, which carry the motor fibers from the cerebral cortex to the spinal cord.

Extrauterine: Outside the uterus; therefore, when describing infants, means after birth.

Extubation: Removal of a tube.

Family's Agenda: The family's priorities for how early intervention will be involved in their life.

Family-focused Approach: Involves concentrating intervention equally on the child and the child's family.

Family Functions: The tasks necessary for a family to maintain itself.

Family Interaction: The relationships between individual family members.

Family Life Cycle: Sequence of changes that occur in families at different times.

Family Needs: The process of identifying and satisfying the needs of family members so that they may more fully participate in the intervention activities of their child.

Family Resources: Characteristics of the family, child's exceptionality, personal characteristics of family members, and how the family addresses the needs of its family members.

Family Strengths: The characteristics of a family that assist them in functioning and meeting each other's needs, especially those of the handicapped family member.

Family Subsystems: Subgroups found in every family (e.g., parental, sibling).

Family Systems Approach: Considers the roles of different family members, the role of the family on larger social networks, and the impact of family and social networks on intervention efforts.

Fetal Alcohol Syndrome: Characterized by infants who are small for gestational age, have mild to moderate mental retardation, congenital heart defects, droopy eyelids, microcephaly, and joint abnormalities.

Fingerspelling: Hand and finger shapes used to represent each of the 26 letters of the alphabet to form words, phrases, and sentences.

Flexion: Bending of a part of the body at a joint.

FM System: An assistive listening device that transmits the speaker's voice directly to the child's hearing aid, thereby minimizing the common problems associated with reverberation, distance, and background noise.

Functional Skills: Abilities that will be immediately useful to the infant and that will be relatively frequently used in the infant's typical environment.

Functional Vision Inventory: An assessment that provides information on how much vision a person has and how well the person uses that vision.

Functionally Blind: Individual with limited vision who under some circumstances must rely on senses other than vision.

Gastroenteric: Pertaining to the stomach and intestines.

Gastrostomy Feedings: Rubber tube going through a gastrostomy that has one end within the stomach and the other outside the abdominal wall, permitting feeding directly into the stomach.

Gavage: Forced feeding through a tube into the stomach so that feeding is pushed or allowed to drip through a tube as opposed to feeding by sucking.

Growth Failure: When growth does not follow the rate expected for age.

HIV Positive: When test results from an individual indicate the presence of HIV infection.

Human Immunodeficiency Virus (HIV):   The specific AIDS virus that has been identified as destroying the body's immune system, making a person susceptible to life-threatening opportunistic infections or rare cancers.

Hyaline Membrane Disease (HMD):   Lung disease of biochemical immaturity where the lungs have a tendency to deflate abnormally. HMD is used interchangeably with Respiratory Distress Syndrome (RDS).

Hydrocephalus: Abnormal accumulation of fluid within the vault containing the brain.

Hyperextension: Straightening out a part of the body beyond the range considered typical.

Hypertonia: High resting activity or tension of muscle; spasticity.

Hypertonic Profile: A child who is irritable, tolerates minimal handling, shows disorganized movements, extensor posturing, and may have decreased mobility of oral musculature.

Hypoglycemia: Low blood sugar.

Hypotonia: Low resting activity or tension of muscle.

Hypotonic Profile: A child who is difficult to arouse, molds easily, fixates at the shoulders and hips (stiffens the muscles around the joints), and may have a weak suck or poorly coordinated suck-swallow mechanism.

Hypoxemia: Low level of oxygen in the blood.

Imitation/Modeling: Performing an action and expecting the child to repeat it.

Immature Infants: Infants born at less than 28 weeks gestational age.

Immediate Imitation: Repeating an action or word as soon as it is produced.

Immittance (Impedance) Testing: An assessment that allows audiologists or physicians to determine whether there are physical problems in an infant's middle ear.

Immune System: The natural system of defense mechanisms in which specialized cells and proteins in the blood and other body fluids work together to eliminate disease-producing micro-organisms and other foreign substances.

Incidental Language Teaching: Involves achieving communication goals by arranging activities or focusing on spontaneous activities.

Incidental Teaching: Involves the arrangement of the environment so that chances of child-initiated, spontaneous interactions are increased.

Individualized Family Service Plan: A list of formal and informal goals, resources, and services (prepared jointly by the family and professionals) for the family and their handicapped or at-risk child.

Infant Intervention: Any service, or cluster of services, made available to at-risk and disabled children and their families at any time from the child's birth to the time of the child's third birthday.

Infection: Conditions that are caused by organisms that may be viral, parasitic, bacterial, or fungal.

Infectious Disease: An illness that results from the entry, development, or multiplication of a communicable disease-causing organism.

Insult: An injury, irritation, or trauma.

Intake: Initial introduction to infant/toddler services.

Interacting Team: Team that is characterized by relaxed, direct communication.

Interdisciplinary Approach: A process in which professionals from different, but related, disciplines work together to assess and manage problems by actively participating in mutual decision making.

Intervention Coaching: Assisting parents and family members in identifying and promoting interactions that appear to facilitate learning in at-risk or special needs children.

Intervention Matrix: A strategy for combining intervention targets/goals with children's daily routines so learning occurs throughout the day.

Intervention Teaming: Professionals, often from different disciplines, working collaboratively to identify and implement services for children and families.

Intracranial Hemorrhage: Bleeding in the head.

Intrafamilial: Immediate relatives.

Intrapulmonary: Inside the lungs or airways.

Intraventricular Hemorrhage (IVH):   Bleeding occurring in or around the ventricles of the brain.

Intubation: Placing a tube within the body; usually applies to inserting a tube through the mouth into the trachea (endotracheal intubation).

Itinerant Teachers: Educators trained in the specific needs of children and adults with specialized needs, such as visual impairments, who travel between schools/programs to serve children.

Jejunal: Tube ending in small intestine; may be nasal or oral.

Labyrinthine Reflex: A primitive reflex that usually is lost by 3 months of age in nondisabled children.

Language Expansion: Technique that involves retaining the words given by a child and adding to them to make better formed responses that match the circumstances.

Lead Agency: A State agency that assumes the general administration of infant/toddler program services and coordinates services.

Learned Helplessness: Belief that an individual lacks control over life's events.

Least Restrictive Environment: The most integrated placement in which a child may function successfully.

Leukomalacia: Softening of the white matter of the brain, usually because of loss of viability and function of the tissue.

Ligation: Closing off a vessel, fistula, etc., by placing a tie around it.

Limit Setting: The process by which team members establish a procedure for identifying individual responsibility.

Low Birthweight (lbw) Infants: Those who weigh between 1,500 and 2,500 g or $3\frac{1}{2}$ to $5\frac{1}{2}$ pounds.

Low Vision Infant: Child whose sight is severely limited, but who is able to use vision to some extent in conjunction with other senses.

Macrocephaly: A large head, not necessarily equivalent to hydrocephalus.

Macrosystem: The form and content of one's subculture or the culture as a whole, and one's belief systems or ideology.

Mainstreamed: Placement of handicapped and nonhandicapped children together.

Mechanical Adaptation: Making changes to a toy to allow a child to control the toy independently.

Meninges: Membrane covering the brain and spinal cord.

Meningitis: An inflammation of the lining of the brain; may be bacterial or viral.

Meningocele: A type of spina bifida in which only the coverings of the spinal cord protrude at birth.

Mesosystem: The interrelations among two or more settings in which the developing person actively participates.

Microcephaly: Head and, therefore, brain size far below average.

Microsystem: The pattern of activities, roles, and interpersonal relations experienced by the developing person in a given setting.

Midline: The middle segment of the body.

Minimal Encouragers: Brief responses by a listener that invite family members to continue talking.

Mixed Hearing Loss: Loss of hearing that is due to motor, sensorineural, and conductive origins.

Morbidity: Rate of disease.

Mortality: Rate of death.

Multidisciplinary Approach: Team evaluation and management process in which individual consultations from different disciplines are obtained, but in which evaluations are carried out independently with little opportunity for professional interaction or integrated planning.

Muscle Balance: Occurs when there is neither too much nor too little tension in a muscle.

Muscular Dystrophy: Condition that produces progressive muscle weakness, respiratory difficulty, heart failure, and often mental retardation.

Myelination: Maturation of nerve fibers involving formation of an outer sheath.

Myelomeningocele: A type of spina bifida that involves a protrusion of the spinal cord.

Nasogastric: Tube through nose into stomach.

Naturalistic Time-delay: Caregivers withhold assistance from the child in an effort to encourage spontaneous behavior.

Necrosis: Tissue death.

Necrotizing Enterocolitis (NEC):   A disease process in the bowel characterized by bloody stool, distention, and tissue death.

Neonate: Infant from birth to 28 days of age.

Neural Tube Defects: Abnormal fetal development that results in a lack of bony closure around the spinal cord.

Neurodevelopmental Treatment Approach (NDT):   A process to facilitate muscle tone and automatic postural responses, and prevent secondary deformities.

Noncategorical: Children with a wide array of disabilities are served as a group.

Noncontingent Help: Assisting a child without the child indicating or requesting assistance.

Nonprogressive: A condition that does not worsen over time.

Nonverbal Communication: The use of body language including gestures, facial expressions, posture, and body movements to convey information.

Norm-referenced Scales: Measures that statistically compare a child's performance to other children of the same chronological age.

Nystagmus: Involuntary, rapid movements of the eyes.

Object permanence: The knowledge that items or persons exist when they are not in sensory contact with the individual.

Occlusion: Blockage.

Optic Atrophy: Wasting away of the optic nerve.

Oral Gastric Gavage Feeding: Forced feeding through a tube into the stomach in which formula is either dripped or pushed so sucking is not required.

Orientation and Mobility Specialist: A professional trained to teach visually impaired children and adults independent travel.

Orogastric: Tube through mouth into stomach.

Orthotics: Orthopedic appliances used to support, align, prevent, or correct deformities or to improve the functioning of movable parts of the body.

Osteogenesis Imperfecta: A syndrome that creates an increased susceptibility to fractures that result in bone deformities; often children are deaf.

Ostomy: Surgical procedure for treatment of NEC in which healthy intestine is temporarily attached to the surface of the abdominal wall where a sac catches stool until the diseased intestine is removed.

Otitis: Inflammation of the ear.

Otitis Media: Inflammation of the middle ear; a common infection.

Otologic History: A medical examination by an otologist that indicates information related to ear abnormalities, middle ear infections, and other physical problems related to the ear.

Palmar Grasp: A primitive reflex in which an infant curls the fingers around whatever strokes the palm.

Paralanguage: The manner of speech or optional vocal effects, such as voice tone, volume, or intonation, that accompany or modify an utterance and communicate meaning.

Paraphrasing: Sending an abbreviated version of the message back to the speaker in an attempt to continue the verbal interaction.

Parenteral: Not through the gastrointestinal tract, but rather by injection through skin, muscle, or vessel (intravenous).

Patent Ductus Arteriosus (PDA):   The ductus arteriosus is a fetal vessel connecting the pulmonary artery to the aorta. If it remains open, it is patent. After birth, a PDA allows blood to flow in inappropriate directions.

Pediatric AIDS: Clinical AIDS in children younger than 13.

Perinatal: Around the time of birth.

Perinatal Asphyxia: Suffocation occurring around the time of birth.

Personal Resources: Characteristics that give meaning to life and allow individuals to address problems constructively.

Physical Accessibility: Changing the position of the toy or material, or the position of the child, to allow the child better access to the material.

Placenta Abruptio: A detaching of the placenta before birth.

Placenta Previa: A placenta that is low within the uterus, overlying the cervix. It can lead to bleeding and prevents a normal delivery.

Pneumonia: An infection in the lungs.

Positioning: Placing the child in certain postures in an attempt to promote symmetrical body alignment, normalize muscle tone, and promote functional skills.

Postlingually: After one has developed communication skills.

Postnatal: Following birth.

Pragmatics: The use of language in social contexts that includes the rules for how language is used for communication.

Precipitous: Rapid and usually uncontrolled.

Prelinguistic Development: Communication abilities that precede verbal communication.

Prenatal: Before birth.

Preschool Intervention: A term used to describe services provided for at-risk and handicapped children between 3 and 5 years of age.

Preterm Infants: Gestational age of 37 weeks (or less). When less than 28 weeks, the term immature may be used.

Primary Care Physician: A family's pediatrician and/or family practitioner who communicates regularly with medical specialists attending to medically complex infants.

Primary Nurse: The hospital nurse that is assigned primary care for a given child.

Primary Prevention: Efforts to keep a risk condition from occurring.

Primary Service Provider: A team member authorized by the team to work directly with the family.

Process-oriented Assessment: Method to evaluate child's ability to perform tasks and how the child achieves tasks in natural settings.

Program Evaluation: An objective systematic process for gathering information about a service or set of activities.

Prone: Lying on the stomach.

Proprioceptive: Term used to describe the sensory receptors found in joints that sense where the body is in space.

Proprioceptive Neuromuscular Facilitation Approach (PNF): Techniques that involve motor learning and incorporate both volitional control and automatic reactions to specific stimulation.

Protracted: Prolonged or drawn out.

Pulmonary Air Leaks: Leakage of air outside the normal air spaces within the lungs.

Pulmonary Hypertension: Increase in the pressure of the vessels in the lungs. When the pressure is too high, blood flow to pick up oxygen is inhibited.

Pulmonary Hypoplasia: Lack of growth and development of the lungs, making extrauterine survival difficult or impossible.

Pulmonary Immaturity: Biochemical and physical inability of the lungs to perform normally after birth.

Questioning (in Naturalistic Teaching): Asking the child to respond about an activity in which the child is currently engaged.

Receptive Language: Child's ability to understand spoken words.

Reflecting: A method of checking with the speaker to determine if the listener understood what was said.

Representative Language Sample: A collection of the child's spoken words that reflects the child's optimal performance, portrays the child's usual performance, and includes the child's usual productive speaking ability, including performance that may be somewhat below or above usual abilities.

Residual Vision: Any sight or light perception.

Respiratory Distress Syndrome (RDS): A combination of symptoms due to immaturity of the lungs, making breathing after birth difficult.

Respiratory Syntitial Virus: A virus causing respiratory infections, notably bronchiolitis in infants.

Respite Care: Child care arrangements that permit parents and/or families to have time away from a handicapped family member.

Response-contingent Learning Episodes: Experiences that offer interesting consequences as a result of the child's actions on the environment.

Responsivity: A tendency for a parent to quickly follow infant signaling behaviors with a behavior by the parent.

Retina: The lining of the inside of the eye glove where special cells convert visible light into nerve impulses.

Retinopathy of Prematurity (ROP): Abnormality of maturation of the retinal vessels.

Rickets: A weakening of bones due to inadequate calcium/phosphorus/vitamin D.

Role Release (Sharing): The systematic training and monitoring of other professionals in one's discipline-specific skills.

Rubella: German measles; when occurring during pregnancy, the fetus may develop abnormally and have deafness, cataracts, and retardation.

Schemas: Patterns.

Scoliosis: Lateral deviation of the spine.

Secondary Prevention: Efforts that improve the prognosis for infants who have been identified through prenatal, perinatal, neonatal, or early infant screening as having a high risk of disability.

Sensorimotor Stage: Piaget's first period of intellectual development, birth to about 2 years of age.

Sensorineural Deafness: Loss of hearing due to loss of nerve function.

Sensorineural Hearing Loss: Caused by damage to the inner ear.

Sentence Completion: A nonthreatening way to elicit one- or two-word responses from a child in which a child finishes a statement made by an adult.

Sepsis: A combination of signs and symptoms due to the release of toxins during a severe infection.

Shunt: A bypassing or diversion from the usual path. A shunt may be naturally occurring, involving blood vessels bypassing a normal distribution, for example, or it may be surgically created.

Simultaneous Communication: A method of communication which refers to the use of both speech and signs at the same time.

Sleep Apnea Test: A recording of heart and respiratory rates taken over a 6- to 12-hour period, usually including periods of sleep.

Socio-communicative Development: Involves attachment and interaction-communication skills in the young child.

Spastic: Increased tone so that muscles are stiff and movements are awkward.

Spastic Diplegia: A classification of cerebral palsy where there is stiffness and weakness or paralysis, primarily of the lower extremities.

Spastic Hemiplegia: Stiffness and weakness or paralysis of one side.

Spastic Quadriplegia: Paralysis of all four extremities with muscle rigidity.

Speechreading: Recognizing spoken words by watching the speaker's lip and mouth movements, and facial expressions.

Spina Bifida: A developmental anomaly characterized by a defect in the bony encasement of the spinal cord.

Spina Bifida Occulta: Type of spina bifida in which there is a failure of the posterior bones of the spinal cord to form.

Staffings: Meetings in which team members admit a child for services and/or discuss a child and family's IFSP and services.

Stenosis: A narrowing.

Strabismus: Abnormal adjustment of the eye.

Subdural: Under the dura, one of the three membranes lining the brain and spinal cord.

Sudden Infant Death Syndrome (SIDS): A sudden and unexplained death occurring in a seemingly well infant.

Supine: Lying on the back.

Symbolic Representation: The substitution of a mental image, word, or object for something that is not immediately present.

Systematic Fading: The gradual removal of any support that assists a child's learning.

Tachycardia: Rapid heart rate.

Task Analysis: Breaks a skill into small steps in order to teach the skill step by step.

Team Building: The process of helping a team engage in continuous self-examination, gathering information about themselves as individuals and as a group, and using those data to make decisions.

Temperament: Individual differences in the behavioral style of child.

Teratogenic: Capable of causing physical defects in the developing embryo.

Total Communication: The choice of a combination of methods to communicate effectively in a given situation.

Toxemia: A reaction in pregnancy affecting the mother's nervous system, kidneys, blood pressure, and placental blood flow.

Toxoplasmosis: A parasite that causes disease in birds and mammals and is most commonly acquired from cat feces or ingestion of undercooked meats.

Tracheostomy: An artificial opening through the neck into the trachea that allows air to enter and leave the lungs without going through the upper airways (nose, mouth, or voice box), requiring less work for breathing.

Tracking: Following an object or person with one's eyes.

Trailing: The process of following the walls with one's hands/body as a guide; used by visually impaired children and adults.

Transdisciplinary Approach: A term used to describe a type of interdisciplinary team functioning that involves mutual sharing of assessment, planning, and intervention that crosses traditional disciplines boundaries.

Transdiscipinary Team: A team that shares assessment, planning, and intervention responsibilities and shares discipline-specific expertise among team members.

Transpyloric: Tube crossing the pyloric exit of the stomach.

Trisomy 21:   Type of Down Syndrome that results due to a nondisjunction of 2 chromosomes upon conception.

Unidisciplinary Approach: Independent evaluation and planning by a single professional without input or consultation from other child development professionals.

Ventilator: A mechanical device that supplies oxygen and air under pressure to inflate the lungs; often called respirator.

Ventricle: A small chamber: in the heart it is one of the two lower chambers; in the head, the ventricles are four fluid-filled cavities in the center.

Ventricular Septal Defect (VSD):   A hole in the wall between the two lower chambers of the heart.

Very Low Birthweight (vlbw) Infants: Those weighing less than 1,500 g or $3\frac{1}{2}$ pounds.

Visual Functioning: Term frequently used to refer to a continuum of visual ability that ranges from normal or near-normal vision to total blindness.

Visual Impairment: Used to refer to an array of eye conditions that result in less than normal sight.

Visually Handicapped: People who have a visual impairment which, even with correction, adversely affects their educational performance.

Visually Limited Infant: A child who is primarily a visual learner but who is limited visually under specific everyday conditions such as bright sunlight.

Author Index

Subject Index